Study Guide

Pharmacology

A Patient-Centered Nursing Process Approach

Study Guide

Pharmacology

A Patient-Centered Nursing Process Approach

12th Edition

Study Guide prepared by
Mary B. Winton, PhD, MSN, RN
Associate Professor
Tarleton State University
Stephenville, Texas

Textbook prepared by
Linda E. McCuistion, PhD, MSN, RN
Professor (Retired), University of Holy Cross
New Orleans, Louisiana

Kathleen Vuljoin DiMaggio, RN, MSN
Professor Emerita
University of Holy Cross
New Orleans, Louisiana

Mary B. Winton, PhD, MSN, RN
Associate Professor
Tarleton State University
Stephenville, Texas

Jennifer J. Yeager, PhD, MSN, RN
Associate Professor
Tarleton State University, School of Nursing
Stephenville, Texas

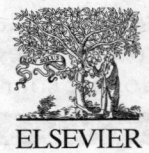

ELSEVIER

Elsevier
3251 Riverport Lane
St. Louis, Missouri 63043

STUDY GUIDE FOR PHARMACOLOGY: A PATIENT-CENTERED
NURSING PROCESS APPROACH, TWELFTH EDITION

ISBN: 978-0-443-11524-0

Previous editions copyrighted 2023, 2021, 2018, 2015, 2012, 2009, 2006, 2003, 2000, 1997, 1993

Executive Content Strategist: Lee Henderson
Senior Content Development Specialist: Elizabeth McCormac
Publishing Services Manager: Deepthi Unni
Project Manager: Nandhini Thanga Alagu
Design Direction: Gopalakrishnan Venkatraman

Printed in India

Last digit is the print number: 9   8   7   6   5   4   3   2   1

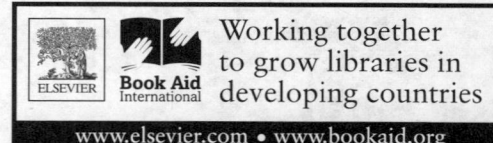

Preface

This comprehensive *Study Guide* is designed to provide the learner with clinically based situation practice problems and questions. This book accompanies the text *Pharmacology: A Patient-Centered Nursing Process Approach*, 12th Edition, and may also be used independently of the text.

Opportunities abound for the enhancement of critical thinking, clinical judgment, and decision-making abilities. Hundreds of study questions and answers are presented on nursing responsibilities in therapeutic pharmacology. Each chapter follows a format that includes NCLEX® Exam–style study questions (including multiple-choice, matching, labeling, prioritizing, select-all-that-apply, and completion exercises) and case studies. Next-Generation NCLEX® Exam–style case studies are also included.

This new edition provides more than 160 drug calculation problems and questions, many relating to actual patient care situations and enhanced with updated, authentic drug labels. The learner is also expected to recognize safe dosage parameters for the situation.

The 12th edition includes a step-by-step approach to using dimensional analysis on selected drug calculation problems, including critical care drugs. Multiple practice opportunities are provided in the areas of measurement, reading of drug labels, calculation of oral and injectable dosages (including body surface area for pediatric and critical care drugs), and flow rates of intravenous fluids.

The nursing process is used throughout the patient situation–based questions and case studies. Chapters have questions that relate to assessment data, including laboratory data and side effects, planning and implementing care, patient/family teaching, cultural and nutritional considerations, and effectiveness of the drug therapy regimen.

Because of the ever-expanding number of drugs available, pharmacology can be an overwhelming subject. To help learners grasp essential content without becoming overwhelmed, chapters have been divided into multiple smaller units. The result is a layout that is user-friendly.

Answers to all questions are presented in the Answer Key to make studying easier. The 12th edition provides rationales for every question, including the case studies.

The *Study Guide* is part of a comprehensive pharmacology package, including the textbook. Instructor and Student Resources available on the companion Evolve website, Elsevier Adaptive Quizzing, and Sherpath Vantage. This package and each of its components were designed to promote clinical judgment and learning. We are excited about this edition of the *Study Guide* because it offers the learner a variety of modalities for mastering the content.

Mary B. Winton

Contents

1 Clinical Judgment Management Model and the Nursing Process

STUDY QUESTIONS

Answer the following questions as true or false. If false, make the statement true.

1. A concept that influences patient care focuses on a disease-centered model of health care.

2. Concepts are related to patient's problems, medications, or topic of care listed within the medical diagnosis.

3. The Nursing Alliance for Quality Care (NAQC) that supports quality, patient-centered health care is partnered with the American Medical Association.

4. The NAQC believes that it is everyone's role to cultivate successful patient and family engagement.

5. The purpose of developing good clinical judgment allows nurses to recognize changes in patient's conditions and address patient's needs.

6. Cues are information the nurse provides to the patient when providing teaching on medications or treatments.

7. **Arrange the cognitive skill of the clinical judgment in the correct order.**
   a. Take action
   b. Generate solutions
   c. Evaluate outcomes
   d. Recognize cues
   e. Analyze cues and prioritize hypothesis

Match the phrases in Column I to the cognitive skill of the clinical judgment in Column II. The cognitive skills in Column II will be used more than once.

Column I

_____ 8. Decreased adherence

_____ 9. Current health history

_____ 10. Goal/outcome setting

_____ 11. Patient's environment

_____ 12. Action to accomplish goals

_____ 13. Drug allergies and reactions

_____ 14. Referral

_____ 15. Patient/significant other teaching

_____ 16. Use of teaching drug cards

_____ 17. Laboratory test results

_____ 18. Effectiveness of health teaching and drug therapy

Column II

a. Recognize cues
b. Analyze cues and prioritize hypothesis
c. Generate solutions
d. Take action
e. Evaluate outcomes

Match the clinical manifestations in Column I with the data type in Column II. The data type in Column II will be used more than once.

Column I

_____ **19.** Productive cough

_____ **20.** Pain in left ear

_____ **21.** Lab values

_____ **22.** Nausea

_____ **23.** Heart rate

_____ **24.** Patient perception of drug's effectiveness

_____ **25.** Reported allergies

Column II

a. Subjective
b. Objective

REVIEW QUESTIONS

Select the best response.

26. *Possible injury* would be included in which cognitive skill of the clinical judgment for a patient who is taking a sedative-hypnotic?
    a. Recognize cues
    b. Take action
    c. Generate solutions
    d. Analyze cues and prioritize hypothesis

27. The patient has congestive heart failure and has been prescribed a diuretic. The nurse *obtaining the patient's weight to be used for future comparison* would be included in which cognitive skill of the clinical judgment?
    a. Recognize cues
    b. Evaluate outcomes
    c. Generate solutions
    d. Analyze cues and prioritize hypothesis

28. *The patient will receive adequate nutritional support through enteral feedings* is included in which cognitive skill of the clinical judgment?
    a. Recognize cues
    b. Take action
    c. Generate solutions
    d. Analyze cues and prioritize hypothesis

29. *The patient will maintain a diastolic blood pressure between 60 and 80* is included in which cognitive skill of the clinical judgment?
    a. Recognize cues
    b. Evaluate outcomes
    c. Generate solutions
    d. Analyze cues and prioritize hypothesis

30. The patient has been diagnosed with angina and hypertension and has been started on a drug. *Instruct the patient to avoid caffeine-containing beverages* is included in which cognitive skill of the clinical judgment?
    a. Evaluate outcomes
    b. Take action
    c. Analyze cues and prioritize hypothesis
    d. Generate solutions

31. Revision of goals is included in which cognitive skill of the clinical judgment?
    a. Recognize cues
    b. Evaluate outcomes
    c. Take action
    d. Generate solutions

32. The patient has been prescribed a diuretic to treat hypertension. *Disturbed sleep* is included in which cognitive skill of the clinical judgment?
    a. Recognize cues
    b. Evaluate outcomes
    c. Take action
    d. Analyze cues and prioritize hypothesis

33. The pediatric patient has been started on antibiotics for strep throat. *Advise the child's parents to report adverse reactions such as nausea and vomiting to the health care provider* is included in which cognitive skill of the clinical judgment?
    a. Recognize cues
    b. Take action
    c. Generate solutions
    d. Analyze cues and prioritize hypothesis

34. The patient has been prescribed an opioid pain drug after hip surgery. *Psychological disturbance* is included in which cognitive skill of the clinical judgment?
a. Take action
b. Evaluate outcomes
c. Analyze cues and prioritize hypothesis
d. Generate solutions

35. *Instruct the patient not to discontinue drugs abruptly* is included in which cognitive skill of the clinical judgment for a patient with epilepsy who is taking phenytoin?
a. Recognize cues
b. Evaluate outcomes
c. Take action
d. Generate solutions

CASE STUDY: CRITICAL THINKING

Read the scenario and answer the following questions on a separate sheet of paper.

A patient has been diagnosed with diabetes and has been prescribed insulin. In speaking to the nurse, the patient says, "I don't think I can give myself shots. I can't stick myself with a needle."

1. Utilizing the cognitive skill of the clinical judgment (nursing process), how will the nurse develop a teaching plan?

2. How will the nurse determine the effectiveness of the teaching plan?

3

2 Drug Development and Ethical Considerations

Match the description in Column I with the act or amendment in Column II.

Column I

a. Determined which drugs can be sold with or without a prescription
b. Attempted to control the abuse of depressants, stimulants, and hallucinogens
c. Tightened controls on drug safety and testing
d. Mandated physicians and pharmacists to keep records of prescribed narcotics
e. Promoted the development of drugs used to treat rare illnesses
f. Attempted to remedy the escalating problem of drug abuse
g. Empowered the Food and Drug Administration (FDA) to monitor and regulate the manufacturing and marketing of drugs
h. Enhanced the FDA's ability to identify, prevent, and mitigate drug shortages

Column II

_____ 1. Kefauver-Harris Amendment

_____ 2. Federal Food, Drug, and Cosmetic Act

_____ 3. The Orphan Drug Act

_____ 4. Durham-Humphrey Amendment

_____ 5. Harrison Narcotic Act

_____ 6. Drug Abuse Control Amendments

_____ 7. Coronavirus Aid, Relief, and Economic Security Act

_____ 8. Comprehensive Drug Abuse Prevention and Control Act

Complete the following.

9. The _____ name, also known as the proprietary name, is usually a registered trademark.

10. Schedule _____ drugs are not approved for medical use.

11. The Health Insurance Portability and Accountability Act (HIPAA) allows patients more control over their _____ _____.

12. The Food and Drug Administration Safety and Innovation Act strengthens the _____ to safeguard and advance public _____ by expediting development of _____, _____, and _____ products.

13. Practicing nurses should be knowledgeable about the _____ _____ _____ in the state where they are practicing.

Answer the following questions as true or false. If false, make the statement true.

_____ 14. Substance examples of Schedule II drugs include peyote, heroin, and cannabis.

_____ 15. Examples of Schedule IV substances include the category of benzodiazepines.

_____ 16. All drugs become less effective over time.

_____ 17. A nurse advances the health care profession through research and scholarly inquiry.

_____ 18. A nurse cannot be prosecuted for omitting a drug dose.

Select the best response.

19. Which ethical principle is being observed when a nurse explains to a research participant the risks versus the benefits of participating in the research?
a. Justice
b. Beneficence
c. Autonomy
d. Respect for persons

20. Before administering controlled drugs to a patient, a nurse would perform which action?
a. Verify prescription before drug administration
b. Not document all wasted drugs
c. Keep controlled drugs accessible for patient's convenience
d. Have a witness for wastage of only Scheduled III drugs

21. Which resource provides the basis for standards in drug strength and composition throughout the world?
a. United States Pharmacopeia/National Formulary
b. American Hospital Formulary Service Drug Information
c. MedlinePlus
d. International Pharmacopeia

22. Which primary purpose of federal legislation is related to drug standards?
a. Provide consistency
b. Establish cost controls
c. Ensure safety
d. Promote competition

23. The Kefauver-Harris Amendment was passed to improve safety by requiring which information to be included in the drug's literature?
a. Recommended dose
b. Pregnancy category
c. Side effects and contraindications
d. Adverse reactions and contraindications

24. A patient presents to the emergency department with hallucinations. The patient's friend states the patient has been using lysergic acid diethylamide and mescaline. To which schedule do these drugs belong?
a. Schedule IV
b. Schedule III
c. Schedule II
d. Schedule I

25. In which schedule would the nurse find codeine, an ingredient found in many cough syrup formulations?
a. II
b. III
c. IV
d. V

26. Where must controlled substances be stored in an institution/agency?
a. In a double-wrapped and labeled container
b. In the patient's drug bin
c. Near the nurse's station
d. In a locked, secured area

27. A patient with advanced pancreatic cancer agrees to participate in a clinical research for a new chemotherapy regimen and asks the nurse which group will be assigned. The nurse would provide which correct response?
a. The patient will receive information about the study through the mail.
b. The nurse has the role in explaining the study to the patient.
c. The patient must be alert and comprehend the information being provided.
d. Information should be vague because the patient does not need to know the study protocol.

28. The nurse must be alert for counterfeit prescription drugs. Which clues help identify drugs that could be counterfeit products? **Select all that apply**.
a. Different color
b. Different dose
c. Different taste
d. Different labeling
e. Different shape

CASE STUDY: CRITICAL THINKING

Read the scenario and answer the following questions on a separate sheet of paper.

An adult patient has received a prescription for a drug to treat hypertension and is preparing for discharge from the emergency department. The patient tells the nurse, "I don't understand all of this paperwork that I have to sign. I sign this same form every time. What is HIPAA, and why should I even care?"

1. How would the nurse explain HIPAA to the patient as it pertains to the drugs prescribed?

2. What would the nurse tell the patient about the boundaries on the use and release of the health records?

3 Pharmacokinetics and Pharmacodynamics

Complete the following.

1. Pharmacokinetic phases are composed of _____, _____, _____, and _____.

2. The $t_{1/2}$ or the _____ is when 50% of the drug concentration is eliminated from the body.

3. _____ is the effect of drug action on cells (the body).

4. Drug absorption is the movement of the drug into the _____ after _____.

5. Drugs that are _____ block the drug's intended responses.

6. Cell membranes contain _____ that enhance drug actions.

Match the terms in Column I with their descriptions in Column II.

Column I

_____ **7.** Dissolution

_____ **8.** Hepatic first pass

_____ **9.** Nonselective receptors

_____ **10.** Passive absorption

_____ **11.** Protein-bound drug

_____ **12.** Unbound drug

_____ **13.** Facilitated diffusion

Column II

a. Drug absorbed by diffusion
b. Causes inactive drug action/response
c. Drugs that affect various receptors
d. Free active drug causing a pharmacologic response
e. Proceeds directly from the intestine to the liver
f. Breakdown of a drug into smaller particles
g. Drugs requiring a carrier for absorption

Match the terms in Column I with their descriptions in Column II.

Column I

_____ **14.** Duration of action

_____ **15.** Onset

_____ **16.** Peak action

_____ **17.** Therapeutic index

Column II

a. Length of time a drug has a pharmacologic effect
b. The margin of safety of a drug
c. Occurs when a drug has reached its highest plasma concentration
d. The time it takes a drug to reach a minimum effective concentration

Select the best response.

18. Which drug form is most rapidly absorbed from the gastrointestinal (GI) tract?
    a. Capsule
    b. Sublingual
    c. Liquid
    d. Tablet

19. Which organ of the body allows the disintegration of enteric-coated tablets to occur?
    a. Colon
    b. Liver
    c. Small intestine
    d. Stomach

20. Which effect does food usually have on the dissolution and absorption of oral drugs?
    a. Increases
    b. Decreases
    c. Has no effect
    d. Prevents

21. Which statement places the four processes of pharmacokinetics in the correct sequence?
    a. Absorption, metabolism, distribution, excretion
    b. Distribution, absorption, metabolism, excretion
    c. Distribution, metabolism, absorption, excretion
    d. Absorption, distribution, metabolism, excretion

22. Which type of drug passes rapidly through the gastrointestinal (GI) membrane?
    a. Lipid-soluble and ionized
    b. Lipid-soluble and nonionized
    c. Water-soluble and ionized
    d. Water-soluble and nonionized

23. Which factor most commonly affects a drug's absorption? **Select all that apply**.
    a. Body mass index
    b. Hypotension
    c. Pain
    d. Sleep
    e. Stress

24. Two days after starting diazepam for anxiety, the patient is started on ampicillin with sulbactam for an infection. Which action will happen to the diazepam in the patient's body?
    a. The diazepam remains highly protein-bound.
    b. The diazepam is deactivated.
    c. Most of the diazepam is released, and it becomes more active.
    d. The diazepam is excreted in the urine unchanged.

25. Which body organ is the primary site for drug metabolism?
    a. Kidney
    b. Liver
    c. Lung
    d. Skin

26. Which route of drug absorption has the greatest bioavailability?
    a. Intramuscular
    b. Intravenous
    c. Oral
    d. Subcutaneous

27. Which description of a drug's serum half-life is most correct?
    a. The time required for half of a drug dose to be absorbed.
    b. The time required for half of the drug to be eliminated.
    c. The time required for a drug to be totally effective.
    d. The time required for half of the drug dose to be completely distributed.

28. A patient is taking a drug that has a half-life of 24–30 hours. In preparing discharge teaching, which dosing schedule would the nurse anticipate would be prescribed for this drug?
    a. Daily
    b. Every other day
    c. Twice per day
    d. Three times per day

29. Which type of drug metabolite can be eliminated through the kidneys?
    a. Enteric-coated
    b. Lipid-soluble
    c. Protein-bound
    d. Water-soluble

30. An older adult patient with a glomerular filtration rate (GFR) of less than 30 mL/min has been prescribed trimethoprim for a urinary tract infection. If the normal dose is 200 mg per day, which dosing would the nurse anticipate?
    a. Double the dose.
    b. Decrease the dose.
    c. Keep the dose the same.
    d. Increase the dose to three times per day.

31. Which statement provides the best determinant of the biological activity of a drug?
    a. The fit of the drug at the receptor site.
    b. The misfit of the drug at the receptor site.
    c. The inability of the drug to bind to a specific receptor.
    d. The ability of the drug to be rapidly excreted.

32. Which type of drug prevents or inhibits a cellular response?
    a. Agonist
    b. Antagonist
    c. Cholinergic
    d. Nonspecific drug

33. A drug effect on receptors located in different parts of the body may initiate a variety of responses depending on the anatomic site. Which type of drug responds in this manner?
    a. Ligand-gated
    b. Nonselective
    c. Nonspecific
    d. Placebo

34. Which term is closely related to dose-response and efficacy?
    a. Therapeutic range
    b. Therapeutic index
    c. Duration of action
    d. Drug half-life

35. Which measurement checks for the highest plasma/serum concentration of the drug?
    a. Peak level
    b. Minimal effective concentration
    c. Half-life
    d. Trough level

36. Which cue would the nurse analyze before administering a drug? **Select all that apply**.
    a. Contraindications
    b. Half-life
    c. Maximum effective concentration
    d. Protein-binding effect
    e. Therapeutic range

37. Which types of physiologic effects are predictable or associated with the use of a specific drug?
    a. Severe adverse reactions
    b. Side effects
    c. Synergistic effects
    d. Toxic effects

38. Which term is illustrated when the nurse gives a large initial dose of a drug to rapidly achieve minimum effective concentration in the plasma?
    a. Therapeutic dose
    b. Toxic dose
    c. Loading dose
    d. Peak dose

39. A time-response curve evaluates parameters of a drug's action. Which parameter is part of the time-response curve? **Select all that apply**.
    a. Duration of action
    b. Onset of action
    c. Peak action
    d. Therapeutic range
    e. Minimum effective concentration

40. The nurse would *take action* on which intervention regarding drug therapy? **Select all that apply.**
    a. Assess for side effects, with a focus on undesirable side effects.
    b. Check reference books or drug inserts before administering the medication.
    c. Teach the patient to wait 1 week after the appearance of side effects to see if they disappear.
    d. Check the patient's serum therapeutic range of drugs that have a narrow therapeutic range.
    e. Evaluate peak and trough levels of drugs with a narrow therapeutic index before administering drugs.

CASE STUDY: CRITICAL THINKING

Read the scenario and answer the following questions on a separate sheet of paper.

A patient with angina has been prescribed verapamil. The nurse knows that this drug is part of the ligand-gated ion channel receptor family.

1. Explain the receptor theory and the four receptor families. Verapamil belongs to which class, and how does it work?

2. What key teaching points would the nurse provide?

4 Pharmacogenetics

Complete the following.

1. _____ is the study of how genomes affect an individual's drug response.

2. Persons with UGT1A1 gene variation may be unable to eliminate _____.

3. Patients with HLA-B*5701 allele can have fatal multi-organ hypersensitivity reactions with _____.

4. Life-threatening bleeds can occur with warfarin in patients with _____ and _____ genotypes.

Answer the following questions as true or false. If false, make it into a true statement.

5. Persons with genetic variation necessary to convert clopidogrel to the active metabolite are at risk for bleeding.

6. The CYP2D6 enzyme has little-known variants slowing down drug metabolism.

7. Everyone within an ethnic group shares the same genetic variations.

8. Insurance companies are prohibited from requiring genetic testing to obtain health insurance.

REVIEW QUESTIONS

9. Which term is the study of how a person's genetics affect drug responses?
   a. Pharmacodynamics
   b. Pharmacotherapeutics
   c. Pharmacogenetics
   d. Ethnopharmacy

10. Which patient would benefit the most from the use of pharmacogenetics?
    a. A patient with one disease process.
    b. A patient who is not on any routine drugs.
    c. A patient who is elderly.
    d. A patient on multiple drugs.

11. Patients with which gene variation may not be able to eliminate irinotecan?
    a. UGT1A1 gene
    b. CYP2D6
    c. TPMT
    d. CYP2C19 enzyme

CASE STUDY: CRITICAL THINKING

Read the scenario and answer the following questions on a separate sheet of paper.

A 54-year-old Asian who lives in a remote rural town has fibromyalgia. R.J. was prescribed tramadol 50 mg by mouth every 6 hours as needed for pain. The dose was increased to 75 mg for unrelieved pain after 14 days of treatment. After another 14 days, the dose was increased to 100 mg. The patient returns to the clinic for unrelieved pain after 2 months of treatment.

1. What is the nurse's first concern?

2. How would the nurse approach the patient in treating the unrelieved pain?

5 Complementary and Alternative Therapies

STUDY QUESTIONS

Match the description in Column I with the letter of the reference in Column II.

Column I

_____ 1. Therapeutic value of plants

_____ 2. Clarified marketing regulations for dietary supplements

_____ 3. Assures manufacturing quality controls

_____ 4. Reviews global literature on herbal studies by clinicians and researchers

_____ 5. Supports study of alternative therapies

Column II

a. Current Good Manufacturing Practices
b. Dietary Supplement Health and Education Act of 1994
c. National Center for Complementary and Integrative Health
d. Natural Standard Research Collaboration
e. Phytomedicine

Complete the following.

6. Pouring boiling water over _____ is called _____.

7. A(n) _____ is derived from soaking fresh or dried herbs in a solvent.

8. _____ of a plant added to a solvent and applied topically is called a(n) _____.

9. Tea made from boiling plants, such as bark, rhizomes, and roots, is called a(n)_____.

10. Aromatic _____ oils from plants are called _____ _____ _____.

Match the supplement in Column I with the letter of its description in Column II. Some supplements may have more than one description.

Column I

_____ 11. *Ginkgo biloba*

_____ 12. Saw palmetto

_____ 13. Dong quai

_____ 14. Garlic

_____ 15. Ginseng

_____ 16. Chamomile

_____ 17. Lavender

_____ 18. Echinacea

_____ 19. Ginger

_____ 20. St. John's wort

Column II

a. Treat diabetes
b. Nausea
c. Enhance the immune system
d. Deter intermittent claudication and Alzheimer's disease
e. Relief from stiffness and pain of osteoarthritis and rheumatoid arthritis
f. Induce sleep
g. Treat benign prostatic hypertrophy and pelvic pain
h. May interfere with anticoagulants
i. Treat mental health disorders
j. May help lower cholesterol

Select the best response.

21. Which herb would the nurse recognize as one that provides relief of digestive and gastrointestinal distress?
    a. Chamomile
    b. *Ginkgo biloba*
    c. Echinacea
    d. St. John's wort

22. A child of a parent with Alzheimer's disease asks about a complementary therapy that can improve memory. The nurse provides information knowing that which substance has been used in patients with Alzheimer's disease?
    a. Echinacea
    b. Ginger
    c. *Ginkgo biloba*
    d. Chamomile

23. Health teaching for a patient who was prescribed warfarin would include information on which product? **Select all that apply**.
    a. Bilberry
    b. Garlic
    c. Ginseng
    d. Licorice
    e. Turmeric

24. A patient with atrial fibrillation takes warfarin. During history intake, the nurse noticed the patient also has been taking ginseng. Which action would be appropriate for the nurse to take? **Select all that apply**.
    a. Discuss with the patient the potential interactions of ginseng with anticoagulants.
    b. Tell the patient to stop taking the anticoagulant.
    c. Advise the patient to continue taking the same brand of herbal therapy.
    d. Advise the patient to report signs and symptoms of bleeding.
    e. Discuss with the patient foods to avoid.

25. Which statement by the patient reflects the prudent use of herbs? **Select all that apply**.
    a. "Herbs are fine to use when breastfeeding."
    b. "Do not take a large quantity of any one herbal product."
    c. "Give the herb time to work for a persistent symptom before seeking care from a health care provider."
    d. "Do not give herbs to infants or young children."
    e. "Brands of herbal products are interchangeable."

26. The nurse is caring for a patient who takes a variety of herbal products and is starting a prescription antidiabetic drug. The nurse teaches the patient knowing that the effects of an antidiabetic drug are altered with which herbal product?
    a. Astragalus
    b. Echinacea
    c. Ginseng
    d. St. John's wort

27. Which drug class has negative interactions with St. John's wort? **Select all that apply**.
    a. Anticoagulants
    b. Anticonvulsants
    c. Antidepressants
    d. Birth control drugs
    e. Paralytic drugs

CASE STUDY: CRITICAL THINKING

Read the scenario and answer the following questions on a separate sheet of paper.

A patient reports having several episodes of "crying spells." The patient has a history of depression that has been controlled with fluoxetine. The patient started taking an herb that a friend provided to improve "mental health." Also at night, the patient has been using "nice smelling spray" on the bed to help with sleep.

1. Which herbal preparations would the nurse suspect the patient is taking?

2. For which potential complications would the nurse assess the patient?

6 Pediatric Considerations

Complete the following.

1. Infants have _____ protein sites than adults, resulting in _____ risk of toxicity.

2. The degree and rate of absorption of drugs in a pediatric patient are based on _____, _____, _____, and _____.

3. Gastric pH does not reach adult acidity until around _____ to _____ year(s) of age.

4. Distribution of a drug throughout the body is affected by _____, _____, _____, and effectiveness of various barriers to drug transport.

5. Until about the age of _____, the pediatric patient requires a(n) _____ dose of water-soluble drugs to achieve therapeutic levels.

Match the child's age group in Column I with a cognitive element in Column II to consider when administering drugs.

Column I

_____ 6. Infant

_____ 7. Toddler

_____ 8. Preschool

_____ 9. School-age

_____ 10. Adolescents

Column II

a. Allow some choice
b. Involve in the administration process
c. Collaborate regarding plan of care
d. Provide simple explanation
e. Use minimum restraint necessary

REVIEW QUESTIONS

Select the best response.

11. The nurse is administering an oral drug with a low pH to a 2-week-old infant. Which action describes the impact of the infant's age on the absorption? **Select all that apply**.
    a. Absorption may be slower.
    b. Absorption may be quicker.
    c. This drug will be absorbed at the same rate as an older child.
    d. Oral drugs should not be administered to this age group.

12. An 18-month-old child has been prescribed an oral drug that is water-soluble. Based on the nurse's knowledge of drug distribution, how may the dosage need to be modified to reach a therapeutic level?
    a. Alternate route
    b. Decreased
    c. Increased
    d. No change

13. Since the blood-brain barrier in infants is immature, which drug outcome would be more likely?
    a. Increased effect of drug
    b. More side effects from drug
    c. Quicker results of drug
    d. Higher toxicity risk

14. Which drug action would the nurse know about the rate of absorption for topical drugs to a 3-year-old child?
    a. The drug will absorb faster.
    b. The drug will absorb slower.
    c. There will be no difference.
    d. It depends on the sex of the child.

15. Which components are related to pharmacokinetics? **Select all that apply**.
    a. Absorption
    b. Distribution
    c. Excretion
    d. Metabolism
    e. Onset

16. A child has been admitted for nausea, vomiting, and diarrhea, and the health care provider has prescribed several drugs. Which concern would be appropriate for the nurse to have regarding drug administration? **Select all that apply**.
    a. Renal tubular function may be decreased.
    b. Dehydration may lead to toxicity.
    c. An alternate route should be considered.
    d. Rectal administration will promote quick absorption.
    e. Developmental levels must be considered.

17. The nurse is teaching a group of parents on how to administer drugs to their children. Which element of drug administration would be included in the teaching? **Select all that apply**.
    a. Allow the child to determine the time of drug administration.
    b. Lightly restrain the child as needed.
    c. Praise the child after successful administration.
    d. Never threaten the child into taking the drug.
    e. Never tell the child what to expect; just give the drug.
    f. Herbal preparations should not, in general, be given to children.

CASE STUDY: CRITICAL THINKING

Read the scenario and answer the following questions on a separate sheet of paper.

A 4-year-old child fell from a tree branch and fractured a forearm. An intravenous (IV) site needs to be established and analgesia administered.

1. What strategies would the nurse take to provide developmentally appropriate care?

2. Discuss the utilization of topical anesthetics before inserting an IV.

3. How may the caregiver be involved in the child's care while the IV is established?

7 Geriatric Considerations

STUDY QUESTIONS

Complete the following.

1. Age-related factors among older adults influence pharmacokinetic profile of the drug's _____, _____, _____, and excretion.

2. Drugs for older adults are prescribed at _____ dosages and _____ increase in dosage based on therapeutic _____.

3. Some of the characteristics in older adults that increase the risk for problems related to drugs include _____ and _____ changes associated with _____.

4. Pharmacodynamic responses to drugs are altered with aging because of the changes in the number of _____ sites, which affects the _____ of certain drugs.

5. Identify at least five drugs that nurses would avoid administering to older adults with stage 4 or 5 chronic kidney disease.

Match the physiologic changes in Column I with the pharmacokinetic phase in Column II.

Column I

a. Altered by the decline in renal function
b. Altered by a decline in muscle mass and an increase in fat
c. Altered by decreased small-bowel surface area, decreased gastric emptying, and reduced gastric blood flow
d. Altered by the decline in hepatic circulation, liver atrophy, and a reduction in hepatic enzyme activity

Column II

6. Absorption

7. Distribution

8. Metabolism

9. Excretion

Identify the drug class for each group of drugs.

_____ 10. Lisinopril, benazepril, enalapril, quinapril

_____ 11. Acebutolol, atenolol, sotalol

_____ 12. Lithium, gabapentin, duloxetine, bupropion, venlafaxine, pregabalin

_____ 13. Irbesartan, losartan, valsartan

Answer the following questions as true or false. If false, rewrite the statement into a true statement.

_____ 14. Risk factors associated with polypharmacy do not include advanced age.

_____ 15. Risk factors associated with polypharmacy include being female.

_____ 16. Risk factors associated with polypharmacy include having more than one health care provider.

_____ 17. Risk factors associated with polypharmacy do not include the use of OTC drugs or herbal agents.

_____ 18. Beers criteria is a document that lists drugs that have negative interactions in older adults when they drink alcohol.

_____ 19. Risk factors associated with polypharmacy include the use of vitamin and mineral supplements.

_____ 20. Polypharmacy increases the risk of falls among older adults.

Select the best response.

21. Which lab result is an indicator of normal renal function for an adult?
    a. Glomerular filtration rate: 100–125 mL/min
    b. Aspartate aminotransferase: 4–12 mL/min
    c. Troponin: 80–120 mL/min
    d. Urea: 1.2–4.5

22. The safest antihypertensive drugs for older adults have a low incidence of which side effect?
    a. Constipation
    b. Electrolyte imbalance
    c. Loss of appetite
    d. Vision disturbances

23. An older adult patient recently started on diphenhydramine for runny nose, headache, sneezing, and scratchy eyes. A list of drugs taken daily includes digoxin, fluoxetine, and a daily multivitamin. Which statement made by the patient indicates a need for further teaching?
    a. "I cannot work outside anymore because of the digoxin."
    b. "I think I need to find a different allergy drug to take."
    c. "I take fluoxetine because I have depression."
    d. "I should not take my wife's headache drug."

24. Which drug information would have fewer adverse and toxic effects while maintaining its therapeutic effect?
    a. Half-life of 50 hours
    b. 90% protein bound
    c. Half-life of 4 hours
    d. Fat-soluble

25. Which lab value would the nurse monitor in an older adult to assess kidney function? **Select all that apply.**
    a. BUN
    b. Creatinine clearance
    c. CBC
    d. Lipase
    e. Triglycerides

26. An older adult reports feeling dizzy every morning when getting out of bed. Which physiological effect does the nurse recognize the patient is most likely experiencing?
    a. Bradycardia
    b. Intermittent claudication
    c. Hyperventilation
    d. Orthostatic hypotension

27. Which action would the nurse recommend to a patient who experiences dizziness when arising from bed?
    a. Change positions slowly.
    b. Move a chair close to the bed.
    c. Take deep breaths.
    d. Measure pulse before standing.

28. Following hospitalization, the older adult patient receives a home visit from the nurse. The patient asks if the drugs taken before hospitalization should continue. Which response would be appropriate by the nurse?
    a. "Yes, you should continue to take the drugs that you took before going to the hospital."
    b. "You should take one-half the dosage of each drug that you took prior to hospitalization."
    c. "You should take only the drugs that have been prescribed on discharge and not drugs that you took prior to hospitalization unless you were told differently."
    d. "You should continue to take those drugs that have been helpful to you."

29. The older adult patient has difficulties opening the bottle of celecoxib. Which response would be most appropriate by the nurse?
    a. "Please ask your pharmacist to place your medicine in a bottle with a non-childproof cap."
    b. "You can keep your medicine in a glass cup in the medicine cabinet."
    c. "You could place your medicine in an envelope."
    d. "A family member could help you with your daily medication regimen."

30. An older adult patient is to take newly prescribed drugs at different times. Which suggestion by the nurse would be appropriate so that the patient can adhere with the drug regimen?
    a. "Line up the bottles of medications on a table and take them in that order."
    b. "Obtain a weekly pill container with multiple time slots from the drugstore and fill the container the day or week before with the drugs."
    c. "Ask a neighbor to give the daily drugs."
    d. "Write down the drugs that you have taken each day."

31. In older adults, drug dosages are adjusted based on which factor? **Select all that apply**.
    a. Amount of adipose tissue
    b. Height
    c. Nutritional status
    d. Laboratory results
    e. Response to drug

32. Before administering drugs to an older adult, which drug information would the nurse review beforehand? **Select all that apply.**
   a. Whether the drug is highly protein-bound
   b. Half-life of the drug
   c. Patient's last bowel movement
   d. Serum levels of drugs with a narrow therapeutic range
   e. Baseline vital signs

CASE STUDY: CRITICAL THINKING

Read the scenario and answer the following questions on a separate sheet of paper.

An older adult presents to the clinic for an annual checkup. The patient has a medical history of diabetes, insomnia, and hypertension. Vital signs are temperature 99.2°F, heart rate 83 beats/minute, respiratory rate 16 breaths/minute, blood pressure 142/90 mm Hg, and blood glucose 96 mg/dL. While obtaining the health history, the patient complains of having trouble falling and staying asleep, and having to get up several times per night to go to the bathroom. Medications the patient is currently taking include hydrochlorothiazide, triazolam, and chamomile tea. The patient states, "I try to remember to take my drugs, and sometimes I take an extra one, just in case I forgot one."

1. Which laboratory tests would the nurse anticipate for the patient?

2. Which suggestions would be appropriate for the nurse to make to help with the patient's sleeping difficulties?

3. What further teaching would the nurse provide about the patient's drug regimen?

8 Drugs in Substance Use Disorder

Match the therapy in Column I to its description in Column II.

Column I

_____ **1.** Cognitive behavioral therapy

_____ **2.** Motivational enhancement therapy

_____ **3.** Contingency management

Column II

a. Based on frequent behavior monitoring and removal of rewards for substance use

b. Recognize and stop negative patterns and enhance self-control

c. Develop motivation internally to commit to specific plan

Complete the following.

4. Misused drugs typically increase _____ and other _____ in the limbic system of the brain.

5. The _____ _____ is a structure within the brain that regulates the body's ability to feel pleasure.

6. The study of environmental influences on genetics is called _____.

7. Disulfiram _____ the enzyme involved in metabolizing alcohol.

8. Heroin addiction may be treated with _____.

9. Benzodiazepines are FDA approved to treat addiction to _____.

10. Opioids provide a sense of _____ and _____; methadone _____ these feelings.

11. _____ questionnaire can be used to screen for alcohol misuse.

12. Substance use disorder among nurses can be recognized by changes in _____, _____, _____, and _____.

Answer the following questions as true or false. If false, rewrite the statement into a true statement.

_____ **13.** Electronic cigarettes are safer than tobacco products.

_____ **14.** Dehydroepiandrosterone (DHEA) is found in many dietary supplements and is approved to slow aging.

_____ **15.** Discrepancies in controlled-drug handling and records among health care professionals may indicate drug diversion.

Match the term in Column I with the definition in Column II.

Column I

_____ **16.** Craving

_____ **17.** Impaired control

_____ **18.** Tolerance

_____ **19.** Withdrawal syndrome

Column II

a. Diminished ability to control the use of a drug in terms of onset, level, or termination

b. A strong desire for the drug effects

c. A group of signs and symptoms of physiologic disturbance upon cessation or reduction of a drug

d. Requiring a significantly increased amount of a drug to achieve the desired effect

REVIEW QUESTIONS

Select the best response.

20. A patient is seen in the emergency department for reportedly swallowing a small balloon full of cocaine. Which clinical manifestation would the nurse recognize if the balloon ruptured?
    a. Dilated pupils and restlessness
    b. Hypotension and tachycardia
    c. Insomnia and fine tremors
    d. Respiratory depression and pinpoint pupils

21. Which medication can be given to help a patient with opioid withdrawal?
    a. Disulfiram
    b. Lorazepam
    c. Methadone
    d. Naloxone

22. The patient has decided to quit smoking. Which key point would the nurse include in the teaching plan? **Select all that apply.**
    a. Assess that the patient is motivated to quit.
    b. Assist in setting a quit date of 1 month.
    c. Help the patient identify what increases the desire to smoke.
    d. Advise the patient to use chewing tobacco as a substitute.
    e. Provide the patient with a list of smoking cessation aids.

23. Which range of nurses abuse drugs and demonstrate impaired practice attributable to that abuse?
    a. 2 in 10
    b. 3 in 20
    c. 4 in 100
    d. 1 in 10

24. A family member finds the patient unconscious with a depressed respiratory rate. A bottle of fentanyl is found by the family. Which action would the family member, if available, is legally allowed to administer?
    a. Intravenous naloxone
    b. Sublingual flumazenil
    c. Intramuscular flumazenil
    d. Intranasal naloxone

CASE STUDY: CRITICAL THINKING

Read the scenario and answer the following questions on a separate sheet of paper.

An adult patient presents to the emergency department (ED). The patient is unresponsive to verbal and painful stimuli and smells strongly of alcohol. Vital signs include temperature of 96.8°F, heart rate of 104 beats/minute, respiratory rate of 6 breaths/minute, blood pressure of 90/68 mm Hg, and oxygen saturation of 88% on room air.

1. What would be the initial treatment?

2. What are the potential complications of alcohol toxicity?

3. Describe the pharmacokinetics of disulfiram and the side effects if taken with any alcohol.

4. Identify the drug-drug interactions that can occur when taken concomitantly with disulfiram that would have similar reactions as if the person had been ingesting alcohol.

9 Safety and Quality

STUDY QUESTIONS

Identify the Quality and Safety Education for Nurses Institute competency for the following definition.

1. Minimizing risk to patients. _____

2. Respecting the patient's rights. _____

3. Working collaboratively with inter-professional teams. _____

4. Improving patient's delivery of care. _____

5. Using technology to improve care. _____

6. Delivering safe care based on current research. _____

Match the correct "Right" in Column I with the nursing implication for drug administration in Column II.

Column I

_____ 7. Right route

_____ 8. Right patient

_____ 9. Right time

_____ 10. Right documentation

_____ 11. Right assessment

_____ 12. Right drug

_____ 13. Right dose

_____ 14. Right education

_____ 15. Right to refuse

_____ 16. Right to evaluation

Column II

a. Measurement of a patient's apical pulse
b. Amount of drug given as prescribed
c. Drug given intramuscularly (IM) as prescribed
d. Teaching a patient about possible side effects of the drug
e. The patient refuses to take drug
f. Verification of patient's identification (ID)
g. Nurse charts patient's pain was decreased after drug administration
h. Patient receives the prescribed drug
i. Nurse checks blood pressure following blood pressure drug administration
j. Drug given at the time prescribed

Match the situation in Column I with the instructions in Column II. Instructions in Column II will be used more than once.

Column I

_____ 17. Drugs poured by others

_____ 18. Patient states the drug is different than usual

_____ 19. Bad-tasting drugs first, then pleasant-tasting drugs

_____ 20. Drugs in an unlabeled container

_____ 21. An opened multidose vial with date and time it was opened and initialed

_____ 22. Drugs left with visitors

Column II

a. Do not administer
b. Do administer

23. Provide the meaning of each and determine if it is acceptable to use.
    a. ID
    b. MS
    c. q.o.d.
    d. gtt
    e. kg
    f. 1.0 mg
    g. 0.8 mg
    h. qd
    i. KVO
    j. IVPB
    k. OU
    l. D/C
    m. bid

24. Provide the meaning of the following abbreviations on the drug type.

Abbreviations	Meaning
CR	
ER	
IR	
XR	
XT	

REVIEW QUESTIONS

Select the best response.

25. A patient has been prescribed antibiotics that are scheduled for every 8 hours. Which statement by the patient indicates the need for more teaching regarding the drug regimen?
    a. "I take this drug every 8 hours around the clock."
    b. "I have to take the drug even if I feel better."
    c. "I just take it divided into three doses while I'm awake."
    d. "I cannot take it more often even if I don't feel better."

26. The patient has been prescribed a drug to be taken a.c. and HS. Which instruction would the nurse give the patient?
    a. "Take this drug every 6 hours."
    b. "Take this drug before meals and at bedtime."
    c. "Take this drug after meals and first thing in the morning."
    d. "Take this drug after meals and as needed."

27. Which statement describes the purpose of the "tall man" letters?
    a. To assist with drug reconciliation.
    b. To aid in labeling drug allergies.
    c. To promote safety between drugs with similar names.
    d. To label differences in dosage strength of the same drug.

28. The nurse is calculating an opioid dose for the patient. The dose seems "large." Which action would the nurse take initially?
    a. Check the patient's name band and administer the drug.
    b. Call the health care provider.
    c. Recalculate the dose.
    d. Withhold the drug and document as not given.

29. The older adult patient tells the nurse, "I'm not taking that pill. I don't want it, and I won't take it!" Which action would the nurse take first?
    a. Document the patient's refusal.
    b. Force the patient to take the drug.
    c. Educate the patient on the importance of the drug.
    d. Call the health care provider who prescribed the drug.

30. Which abbreviation is not allowed by The Joint Commission? **Select all that apply**.
    a. IM
    b. U
    c. IU
    d. q.d.
    e. MS

31. A patient tells the nurse the unused opioids were flushed down the toilet. Which response would be best by the nurse?
    a. "Flushing unused drugs is okay."
    b. "Be sure to crush the drugs before flushing them."
    c. "Crush the drugs and throw them in the trash."
    d. "Throw them in the trash after mixing the drugs with unpalatable nonfood substance."

CASE STUDY: CRITICAL THINKING

Read the scenario and answer the following questions on a separate sheet of paper.

A nurse is preparing to administer three of the patient's morning drugs. The nurse educates the patient that the drugs are for blood pressure, diabetes, and depression. When the patient looked at the drugs, the patient exclaims "these are not the pills I take."

1. Identify the "six rights" in drug administration?

2. Which methods can the nurse use to determine the "right patient" is receiving the drugs?

3. Determine the nurse's best action when the patient states "these are not the pills I take?"

10 Drug Administration

Complete the following.

1. _____ and _____ drugs must be swallowed whole.

2. Handheld nebulizers deliver a very _____ _____ in a spray of medication.

3. When giving patients a drug via a handheld nebulizer, the patient should be placed in _____ position.

4. A nasogastric tube should be flushed with _____ mL of water (or the prescribed amount) following drug administration.

5. Following insertion of a rectal suppository, the patient should remain in a side-lying position for at least _____ minutes.

Match the route in Column I with the correct length of the needle in Column II.

Column I

_____ **6.** Subcutaneous (SUBQ)

_____ **7.** Intradermal (ID)

_____ **8.** Intramuscular (IM)

Column II

a. ¼ to ½ inch in length

b. ⅝ to ½ inch in length

c. ⅜ to ⅝ inch in length

Complete the following.

9. The injection site that is away from major nerves and is a preferred site for Z-track injections is the _____.

10. The preferred site for immunizations for infants and children who are not ambulating is the _____.

11. The site that is easily accessible but is suitable for only small-volume doses is the _____.

12. The preferred site for intramuscular injections in infants and children of any age is the _____.

13. Label the landmarks for ventrogluteal injection.

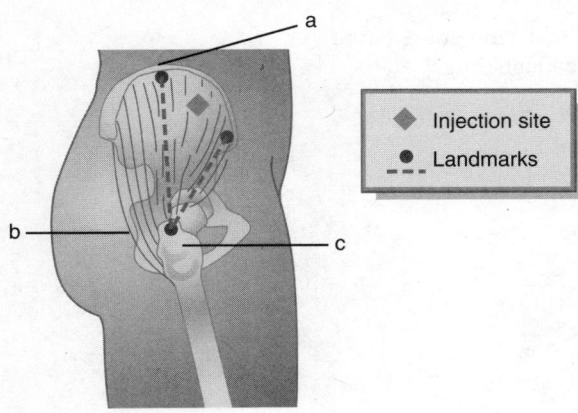

27

Select the best response.

14. A patient is vomiting and has been prescribed an antiemetic. Which route would be least preferred for this patient?
    a. Intradermal
    b. Intravenous
    c. Oral
    d. Rectal suppository

15. A 2-year-old child has been prescribed antibiotic eardrops. The nurse is providing education to the parents. Which instruction is correct in manipulating the auricle?
    a. Down and back
    b. Forward and back
    c. Forward and up
    d. Up and back

16. A patient has been prescribed an intramuscular (IM) injection. The drug is thick and must be administered deep IM. Which site would the nurse choose for the injection?
    a. Deltoid
    b. Dorsolateral
    c. Vastus lateralis
    d. Ventrogluteal

17. Which site is preferred for an immunization injection in an 8-week-old infant?
    a. Deltoid
    b. Dorsogluteal
    c. Vastus lateralis
    d. Ventrogluteal

18. A patient is being discharged on new drugs. Which statement made by the patient would indicate that more teaching is needed?
    a. "I can take any over-the-counter drug or herbal preparation that I think would be helpful."
    b. "I need to make sure I keep appointments with my health care provider."
    c. "I need to report any side effects to my health care provider."
    d. "I will contact my pharmacy if I am going out of town to ensure that I have enough drug."

19. The patient has been started on a new oral drug. Which information would the nurse include in the teaching? **Select all that apply**.
    a. Desired effect of the drug
    b. Dietary considerations
    c. Storage of all drugs in the refrigerator
    d. Research testing and development
    e. Written instructions on how to administer the drug

20. The patient has been prescribed a steroid metered-dose inhaler (MDI) for asthma. Which statement by the patient indicates understanding of how to use the MDI?
    a. "I can use it as often as I need it."
    b. "I need to rinse out my mouth after I use it."
    c. "I should direct the opening toward my tongue so that I can swallow it."
    d. "I can administer multiple puffs at one time."

CASE STUDY: CRITICAL THINKING

Read the scenario and answer the following questions on a separate sheet of paper.

An adult patient is prescribed promethazine 12.5 mg intramuscular (IM) for intractable nausea. The nurse prepares to administer the drug.

1. Identify the size of the needle and syringe needed for IM injection.

2. Determine the potential IM injection sites for this patient?

3. Analyze the best method the nurse would use for promethazine IM? Provide a rationale.

11 Drug Labels and Dosage Calculations

INTRODUCTION

This chapter in this study guide includes numerous drug labels to allow learners to become familiar with reading drug labels and calculating drug dosages from the information provided on the drug labels. In addition, many practice problems in this study guide include conversion factors with metric and household systems; drug reconstitutions for enteral and parenteral drugs; and dosage calculations for enteral and parenteral drugs, including insulin, and intravenous flow rates. It is highly recommended to read and study this chapter in the accompanying textbook prior to drug calculations in this study guide.

Practice reading drug labels and calculating dosages provides an opportunity to gain skill and competence in collecting and organizing the required data. Practice problems have examples of the administration of drugs via a variety of routes, including enteral (gastrointestinal) and parenteral (subcutaneous, intramuscular, and intravenous). Practice problems also include calculating dosages based on body weight and body surface area (BSA), intravenous heparin infusions, and other critical care drugs.

When calculating dosages, select one of the three methods (basic formula, ratio and proportion/fractional equation, or dimensional analysis) presented in the accompanying textbook. It is recommended that one becomes familiar with one method and to use that one method for all calculations. *Using two or more methods of dosage calculations can lead to an incorrect medication error*. After completing the required calculations, determine if the calculated answer is reasonable. In the event of a discrepancy, review both the thought process used in answering the problem and the actual mathematical calculation. It may be necessary to review the related section in this chapter. Practice problems provide reinforcement to gain expertise in the process of actually calculating drug dosages.

During each step in a multistep process of dosage calculation (except in dimensional analysis) round the numbers to the nearest *whole* number for drops; round to the nearest *tenth* for kilograms, pounds, milliliters, milligrams, micrograms, grams, milliequivalents and units; round to the nearest hundredths for BSAs (m^2); and round to the nearest *minute* for time. Final answers for all drug calculations: (1) round to the nearest *whole number* for milligrams, micrograms, grams, milliequivalents, units, and drops and (2) round to the nearest *tenth* for kilograms, pounds, and milliliters. When doing dimensional analysis, conversion factors are already built into the equation and the final answer is the only number that is rounded. All calculations, except for the BSA using the West Nomogram, can be accomplished using dimensional analysis. Therefore, dimensional analysis is the recommended method for dosage calculations.

The answers are in the back of the Study Guide. Some of the calculations will be illustrated in the Answer Key using dimensional analysis.

METRIC AND HOUSEHOLD SYSTEMS

Match the term in Column I with the appropriate abbreviation in Column II.

Column I		Column II	
_____ 1.	Gram	a.	T or tbsp
_____ 2.	Milligram	b.	g or G
_____ 3.	Liter	c.	mL
_____ 4.	Milliliter	d.	lb
_____ 5.	Kilogram	e.	fl oz
_____ 6.	Microgram	f.	mg
_____ 7.	Meter	g.	L or l
_____ 8.	Fluid ounce	h.	gtt
_____ 9.	Quart	i.	kg
_____ 10.	Pint	j.	mcg
_____ 11.	Pound	k.	t or tsp
_____ 12.	Cup	l.	c
_____ 13.	Tablespoon	m.	pt
_____ 14.	Teaspoon	n.	qt
_____ 15.	Drops	o.	m

Complete the following.

16. Convert the following frequently used conversions within the metric system:

   A. 1 g = _____ mg

   B. 1 L = _____ mL

   C. 1 mg = _____ mcg

Convert the following unit of measurement.

17. 3 g = _____ mg

18. 1.5 L = _____ mL

19. 0.1 g = _____ mg

20. 2500 mL = _____ L

21. 250 mL = _____ L

22. 500 mg = _____ g

23. 2 qt = _____ pt

24. 2 pt = _____ fl oz

25. 1½ qt = _____ fl oz

26. 32 fl oz = _____ pt

27. 3000 mcg = _____ mg

28. 3 t = _____ mL

29. 30 mL = _____ fl oz

30. 1 T = _____ t

31. 1 g = _____ mg

32. _____ g = 500 mg

33. 0.1 g = _____ mg

34. _____ L = 1000 mL, or _____ qt

35. 240 mL = _____ fl oz

36. 30 mL = _____ fl oz, or _____ T, or _____ t

37. 5 mL = _____ t

38. 3 T = _____ fl oz, or _____ t

39. 5 fl oz = _____ mL, or _____ T

For any drug calculations, use the basic formula, ratio, and proportion/fractional equation, or dimensional analysis. The recommended method is the dimensional analysis.
   Select the best response.

1. Before calculating drug dosages, all units of measurement must be converted to one system. Which system is the best method for the nurse to use?
   a. Any system the nurse prefers
   b. A system that fits with how the nurse will administer the drug
   c. A system that is converted easily
   d. The system on the drug label

2. Which method are for administering drugs by parenteral routes? **Select all that apply.**
   a. Via a nasogastric tube
   b. Subcutaneous
   c. Intramuscular
   d. Intradermal
   e. Intravenous
   f. Any liquid drug via all routes

3. Which route of administration can be used for insulin and heparin? **Select all that apply.**
   a. Oral
   b. Intramuscular
   c. Subcutaneous
   d. Intravenous
   e. Intradermal

4. Vials are glass containers with (self-sealing rubber tops/tapered glass necks). Vials are usually (discarded/reusable if properly stored). **Circle the correct answers.**

5. Before drug reconstitution, the nurse would check the drug circular and/or drug label for instructions. After a drug has been reconstituted and additional doses are available, which information would the nurse write on the drug label? **Select all that apply.**
   a. Date to discard
   b. Initials
   c. The health care provider's order
   d. Diluent

6. The nurse is preparing an intramuscular (IM) injection for an average adult. Which needle gauge and length could be used to administer the IM?
   a. 20 or 21 gauge; ½ or ⅜ in. in length
   b. 23 or 25 gauge; ½ or ⅝ in. in length
   c. 19, 20, or 21 gauge; 1, 1½ or 2 in. in length
   d. 25 or 26 gauge; 1 or 1½ in. in length

7. Which two parts of a syringe must remain sterile?
   a. Outside of syringe and plunger
   b. Tip of the syringe and plunger
   c. Both the tip and outside of the syringe
   d. Tip and outside of syringe and plunger

8. Subcutaneous injections can be administered at which degree angle(s)?
   a. 10-degree and 15-degree angles
   b. 45-degree, 60-degree, and 90-degree angles
   c. 45-degree angle only
   d. 90-degree angle only

9. The nurse calculates the drug dosage to be 0.25 mL. Which syringe size is most appropriate?
   a. 3-mL syringe
   b. Insulin syringe
   c. Tuberculin syringe
   d. 10-mL syringe

10. To mix 3 mL of sterile saline solution in a vial containing a powdered drug, which size syringe is most appropriate?
    a. Tuberculin syringe
    b. Insulin syringe
    c. 3-mL syringe
    d. 5-mL syringe

11. Solutions in drug A and drug B are compatible. To combine 5 mL of drug A with 8 mL of drug B to be administered via syringe pump, the nurse would use which syringe size(s)?
    a. One 5-mL syringe and one 10-mL syringe
    b. Two 10-mL syringes
    c. One 20-mL syringe
    d. Two 5-mL syringes and one 10-mL syringe

Interpreting Drug Labels

Note: When converting a unit of measurement from one system to another, convert to the unit on the *drug label*.
   Example:
   Order: Penicillin V 0.5 g PO q8h
   Available:

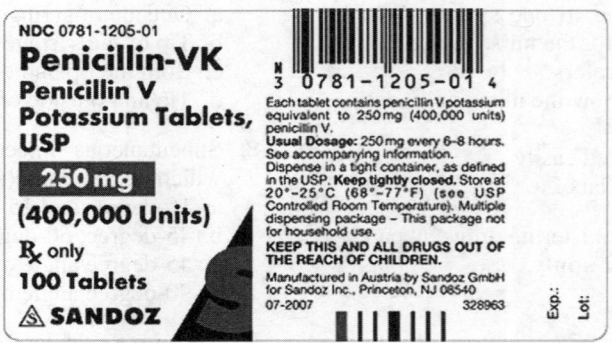

Convert gram to milligram (unit of measurement to unit of measurement)

12. Provide the information requested on the following drug label.

A. What is the brand name?_____

B. What is the generic name?_____

C. What is the formulation of this drug?_____

D. What is the form of this drug?_____

13. Provide the information requested on the following drug label.

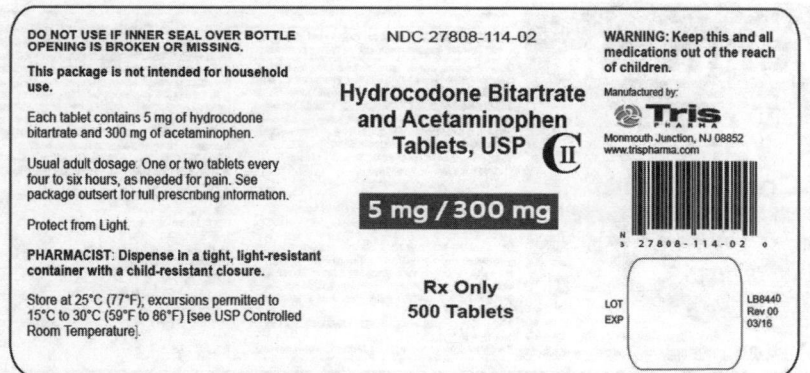

A. What is the name of the drug? _____

B. What is the formulation? _____

C. Is this drug a controlled substance? _____

D. Circle on the label the marking that indicates it is a controlled substance.

E. What is the form of the drug? _____

F. How should the drug be stored? _____

G. What company manufactured the drug? _____

14. Provide the information requested on the following drug label.

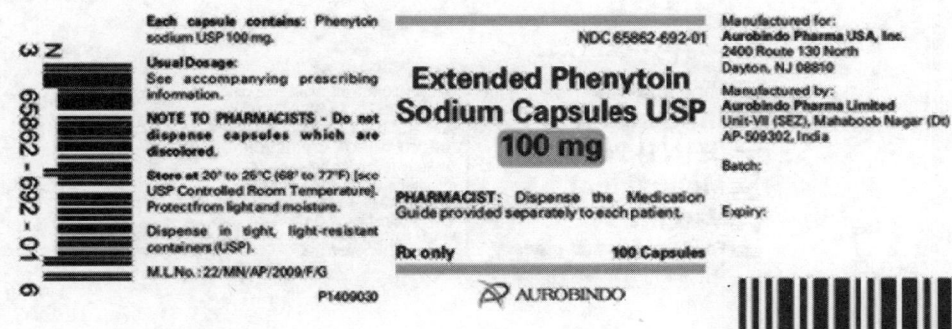

A. What is the generic name? _____

B. Is the drug a controlled substance? _____

C. What is the form of the drug? _____

D. How much of the drug is in each capsule? _____

E. Circle the marking on the label that indicates whether a prescription is required.

F. How should the drug be stored? _____

15. Provide the information requested on the following drug label.

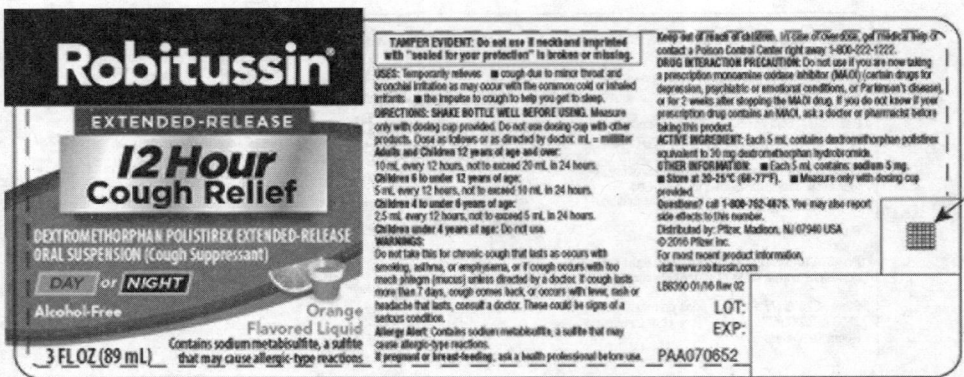

    A. What is the generic name? _____

    B. What is the trade name? _____

    C. Does this drug require a prescription? _____

    D. What is the form of the drug? _____

    E. What is the concentration of the drug? _____

    F. What is the total volume in milliliters? _____

    G. What is the usual dose for adults and children 12 years of age and over? _____

    H. How many adult dosages are available? _____

16. Provide the information requested on the following drug label.

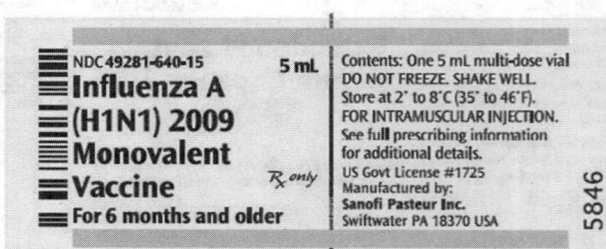

    A. What is the name of the drug? _____

    B. What is the form of the drug? _____

    C. Is the vial a single-dose vial or multidose vial? _____

    D. How should the drug be stored? _____

    E. How should this drug be administered? _____

17. Provide the information requested on the following drug label.

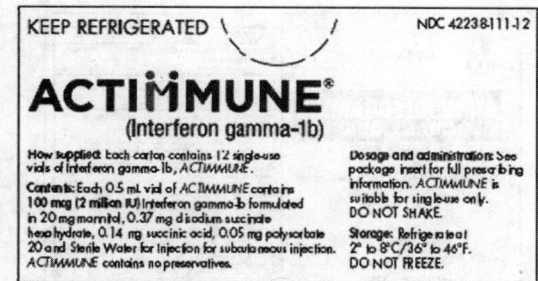

A. What is the generic name? _____

B. What is the trade name? _____

C. How should it be stored? _____

18. Order: ritonavir 0.5 g PO bid
Available:

A. Is conversion needed to give this drug?
   a. No; it may be administered in grams.
   b. No; the pill may be split if needed.
   c. Yes; it should be converted to grains.
   d. Yes; it should be converted to milligrams.

B. How many tablets of this drug would the nurse administer?
   a. ½ tablet
   b. 1 tablet
   c. 3 tablets
   d. 5 tablets

19. Order: diphenhydramine 25 mg PO q6h, PRN
Available: diphenhydramine 12.5 mg/5 mL

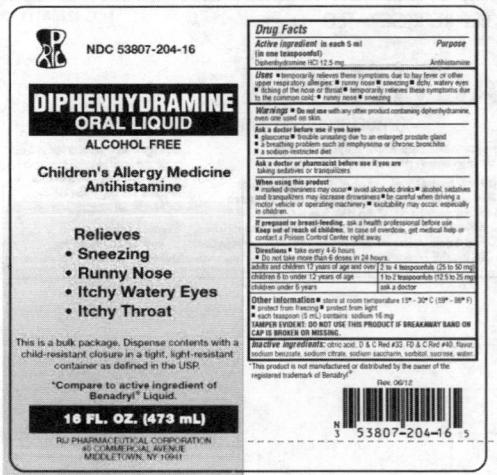

A. Is conversion needed to give this drug?
    a. No; it can be administered in milligrams as ordered.
    b. No; you cannot mix milligrams and milliliters.
    c. Yes; it should be converted to grains.
    d. Yes; it should be converted to grams.

B. How many milliliters would the nurse give?
    a. 5 mL
    b. 10 mL
    c. 15 mL
    d. 20 mL

20. Order: clarithromycin 0.25 g PO bid
Available:

NDC 0781-6022-52
Clarithromycin for Oral Suspension, USP
125 mg* per 5 mL
when reconstituted
*When mixed as directed, each teaspoonful
(5 mL) contains 125 mg of clarithromycin in
a fruit-punch flavored, aqueous vehicle.
R_x only
50 mL (when mixed)
⚠ SANDOZ

A. Is conversion needed to give this medication?
    a. No; it may be administered in grams.
    b. No; you cannot mix milligrams and milliliters.
    c. Yes; it should be converted to grains.
    d. Yes; it should be converted to milligrams.

B. How many milliliters would be administered?
    a. 5 mL
    b. 10 mL
    c. 15 mL
    d. 20 mL

21. Order: hydroxyzine 25 mg PO q6h
Available:

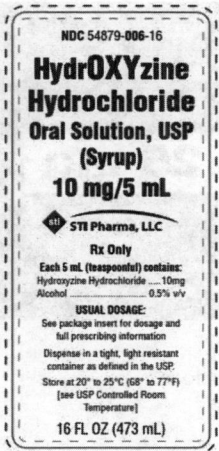

How many milliliters would be administered?
a. 5 mL
b. 7.5 mL
c. 10 mL
d. 12.5 mL

22. Order: ceftriaxone 500 mg IM
Available:

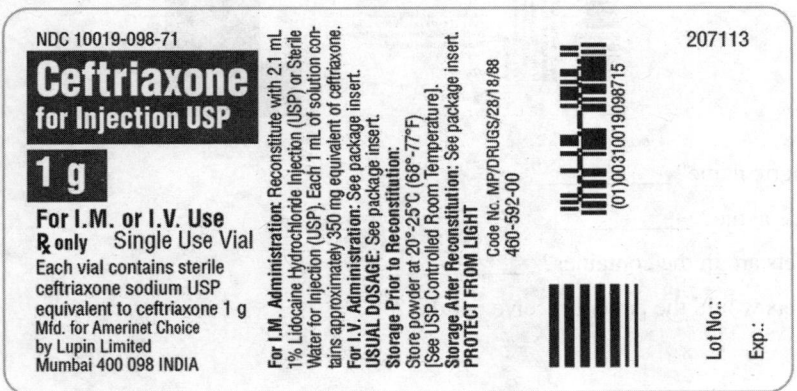

A. How many milliliters would be administered?
   a. 1 mL
   b. 1.4 mL
   c. 2 mL
   d. 2.4 mL

B. What size syringe would be most appropriate? _____

23. Order: acarbose 50 mg PO tid
    Available:

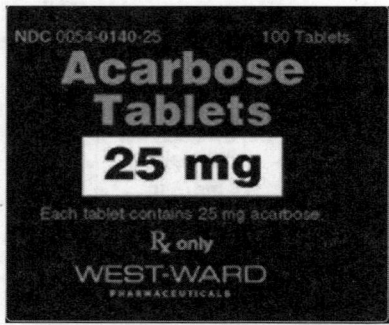

How many tablets would be administered per dose?
a. 1 tablet
b. 2 tablets
c. 3 tablets
d. 4 tablets

24. Order: losartan potassium 100 mg daily
    Available:

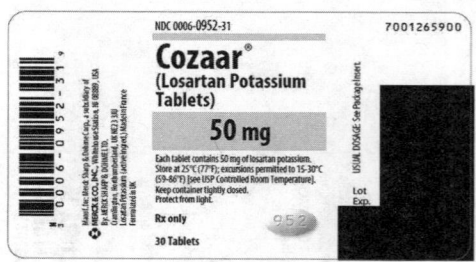

A. What is the generic name? _____

B. What is the trade name? _____

C. How many tablets are in the container? _____

D. How many tablets would the patient receive per day?
    a. 1 tablet
    b. 2 tablets
    c. 3 tablets
    d. 4 tablets

25. Order: propranolol 15 mg PO q6h
    Available: propranolol 10-mg and 20-mg scored tablets

A. Which tablet strength would be administered? Why?
    a. 10-mg tablets
    b. 20-mg tablets

B. How many tablets would be administered?
    a. 1 tablet
    b. 1½ tablets
    c. 2 tablets
    d. 2½ tablets

26. Order: furosemide 80 mg PO daily
Available:

A. What is the generic name? _____

B. What is the trade name? _____

C. How should the medication be stored? _____

D. How many tablets would be administered?
   a. 2 tablets
   b. 3 tablets
   c. 4 tablets
   d. 5 tablets

27. Order: potassium ER 40 mEq PO daily
Available:

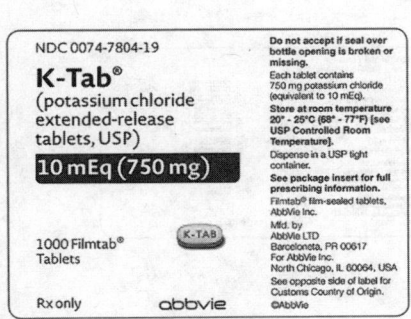
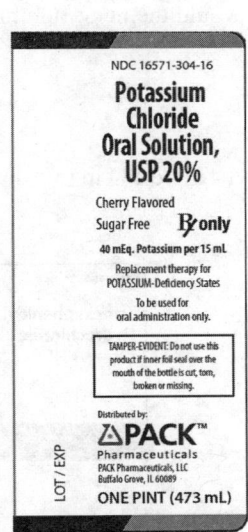

A. Which form is most appropriate? Why?

B. On assessment, the nurse discovers the patient has a nasogastric tube (NGT) and is unable to swallow. Which action would be correct for the nurse to do?
   a. Give the drug as ordered.
   b. Give the oral liquid.
   c. Call the prescriber.
   d. Give the drug intravenously.

C. After calling the prescriber, the order was changed to 20 mEq via an NGT bid.

   a. Which form should be used? Why? _____

   b. How many milliliters would the nurse give per dose? _____

Chapter **11** **Drug Labels and Dosage Calculations**

28. Order: verapamil 60 mg PO QID
Available:

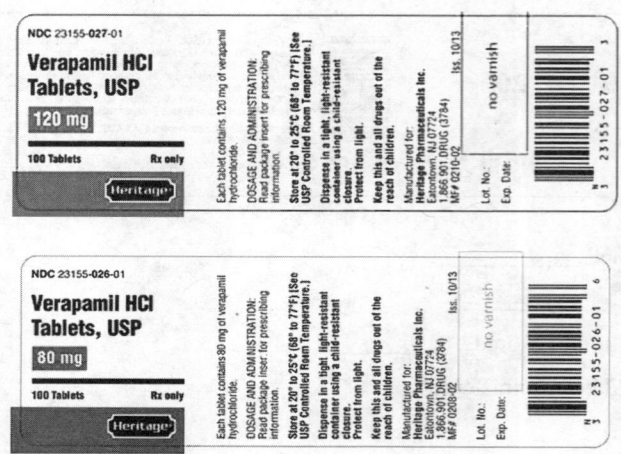

A. Which strength of verapamil is most appropriate?
   a. 120-mg tablets
   b. 80-mg tablets

B. How many tablets would the nurse administer?
   a. ½ tablet
   b. 1 tablet
   c. 1½ tablets
   d. 2 tablets

29. Order: trihexyphenidyl 4 mg/d PO in two divided doses q12h
Available:

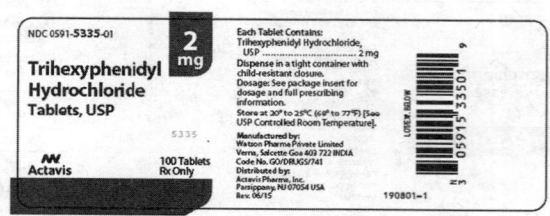

A. How many tablets per dose? _____

B. How many tablets per 24 hours? _____

30. Order: oxacillin 400 mg IM q6h
Available:

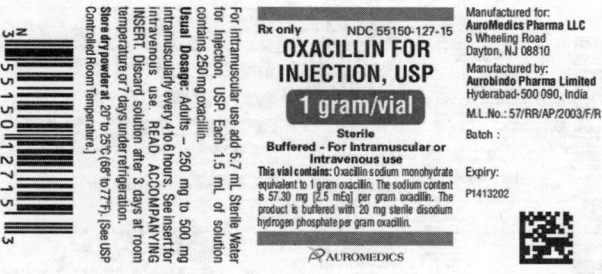

A. How much diluent should be added for an intramuscular injection? _____

B. How many milliliters would the patient receive?
   a. 0.5 mL
   b. 1.5 mL
   c. 2 mL
   d. 2.4 mL

31. Order: adalimumab 40 mg subcut every other week
Available:

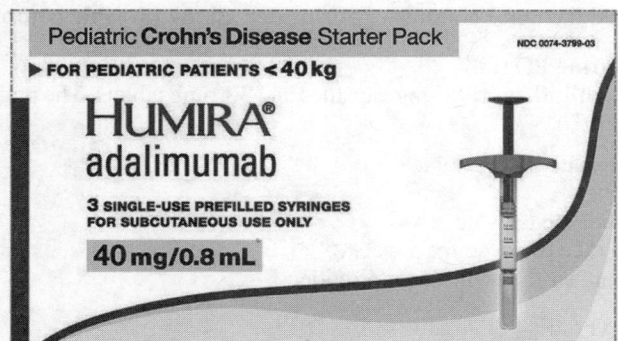

A. What is the route of administration? _____

B. What is the dosage strength?

C. How many milliliters would the patient receive?

D. What size syringe(s) is appropriate? **Select all that apply.**
   a. Tuberculin
   b. Insulin
   c. 1-mL syringe
   d. 3-mL syringe

32. Order: trazodone 150 mg PO daily
Available: trazodone in 50-mg tablets and 100-mg tablets

A. How many tablets would the nurse administer if the 50-mg tablet is used?
   a. 1 tablet
   b. 2 tablets
   c. 3 tablets
   d. 4 tablets

B. How many tablets would the nurse administer if the 100-mg tablet is used?
   a. ½ tablet
   b. 1 tablet
   c. 1½ tablets
   d. 2 tablets

33. Order: warfarin 7.5 mg PO daily
Available:

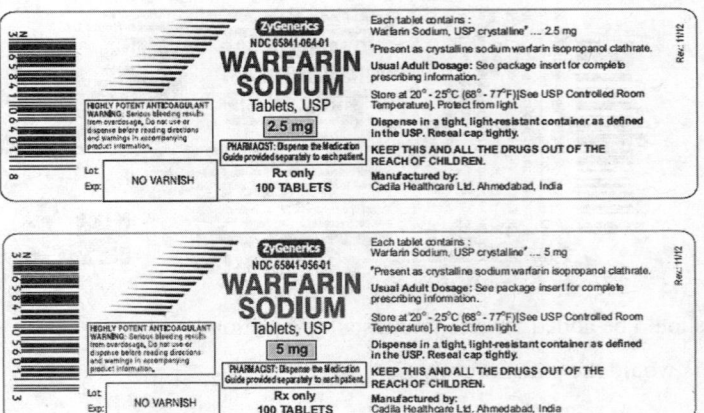

A. Which dosage strength should be selected?
  a. Warfarin 2.5 mg
  b. Warfarin 5 mg

B. How many tablet(s) would the nurse administer? **Consider all the possible combinations.**

34. Order: lithium carbonate 300 mg PO tid
Available: lithium carbonate in 150- and 300-mg capsules and 300-mg tablets. The patient's lithium level is 1.8 mEq/L (normal value is 0.5–1.5 mEq/L).

Which action is most appropriate by the nurse?
  a. Give 150 mg (half the dose).
  b. Give 300-mg tablet and not the capsule.
  c. Advise the patient not to take the dose for a week.
  d. Withhold the drug and contact the health care provider.

35. Order: carvedilol 6.25 mg PO bid
Available:

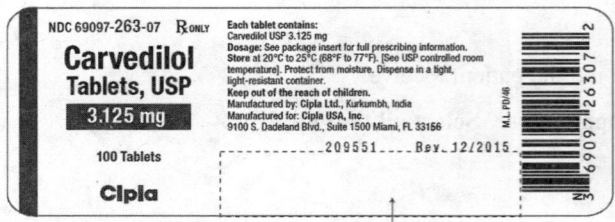

A. How many tablets would the nurse administer per dose?
  a. 1 tablet
  b. 2 tablets
  c. 3 tablets
  d. Call the pharmacy to bring 6.25 tablets

B. How many tablets would the patient receive in 24 hours?
  a. 4 tablets
  b. 6 tablets
  c. 8 tablets
  d. 10 tablets

36. Order: azithromycin 500 mg PO on day 1, then 250 mg PO daily for next 4 days
Available:

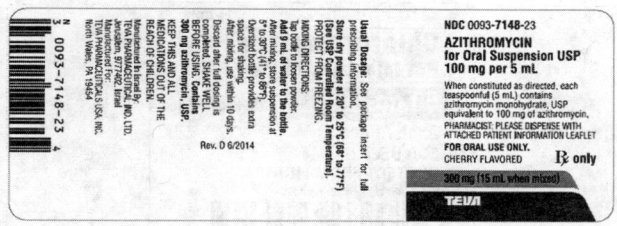

A. Circle the route on the label.
B. How many milliliters would the nurse administer the first day?
   a. 2.5 mL
   b. 6.5 mL
   c. 12.5 mL
   d. 25 mL
C. How many milliliters would the nurse administer per day for the next 4 days?
   a. 5 mL/day
   b. 6.25 mL/day
   c. 10 mL/day
   d. 12.5 mL/day

37. Order: trihexyphenidyl elixir 1 mg PO tid
Available: trihexyphenidyl 2 mg/5 mL

What amount would the nurse administer per dose?
a. 2 mL
b. 2.5 mL
c. 3 mL
d. 5 mL

38. Order: trimethobenzamide 200 mg IM STAT
Available: trimethobenzamide ampule, 100 mg/1 mL

How many milliliters would the nurse administer?
a. 0.5 mL
b. 0.8 mL
c. 1 mL
d. 2 mL

39. Order: chlorpromazine 20 mg deep IM tid
Available:

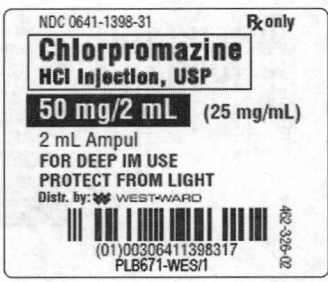

How many milliliters would the nurse administer?
a. 0.3 mL
b. 0.5 mL
c. 0.8 mL
d. 1 mL

40. A patient is scheduled to take digoxin 0.25 mg. The hospital is currently out of stock of digoxin 0.25 mg and has only 0.125-mg strength on hand. The patient was concerned when the pills were received because they were of a different color and a different amount from those normally taken at home. When the patient questions the tablets, which response by the nurse is most appropriate?
a. "Please don't worry; it is because we use generic drugs."
b. "Please don't worry; I calculated this carefully and it is your regular dose."
c. "We don't have the 0.25-mg tablets available, so I brought you two pills of 0.125 mg to equal your 0.25 mg dose."
d. "You are right, this is the wrong dosage. I will be right back with the correct one."

41. Order: carbidopa 12.5 mg/levodopa 125 mg PO bid
Available:

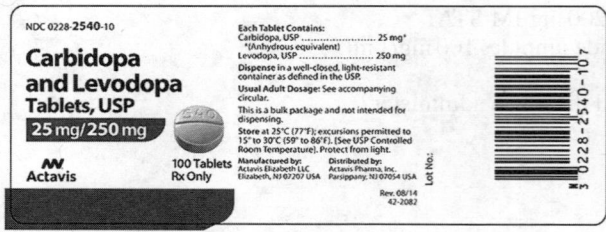

Which action by the nurse is most appropriate?
a. Administer ½ tablet.
b. Administer 1 tablet.
c. Administer 1½ tablets.
d. Do not administer the medication, and call the pharmacy for the correct dose.

42. Order: lactulose 25 g PO q6h
Available:

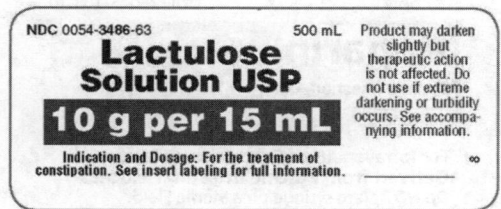

How many milliliters would the patient receive per dose?
a. 10 mL
b. 16.7 mL
c. 25 mL
d. 37.5 mL

43. Order: hydromorphone 2 mg subcut q4h PRN for pain
Available:

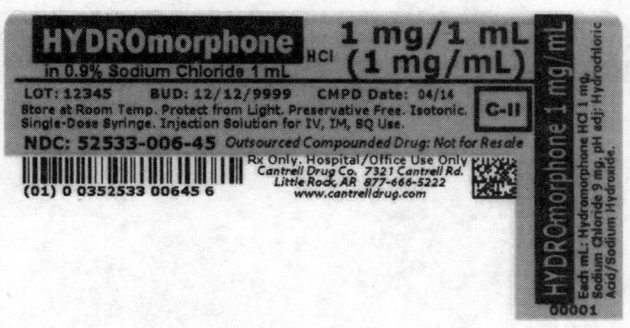 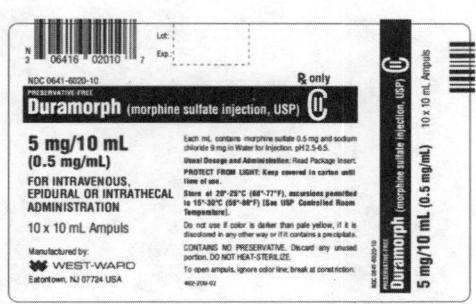

A. Are the drugs on the label interchangeable?

B. How many milliliters would the nurse administer of the correct drug?
a. 0.5 mL
b. 1 mL
c. 1.5 mL
d. 2 mL

44. Order: cyanocobalamin 1000 mcg IM daily for 5 days
Available: cyanocobalamin 10,000 mcg/10 mL

How many milliliters would the nurse administer?
a. 0.4 mL
b. 0.6 mL
c. 0.8 mL
d. 1 mL

45. Order: heparin 3000 units subcut q6h
Available:

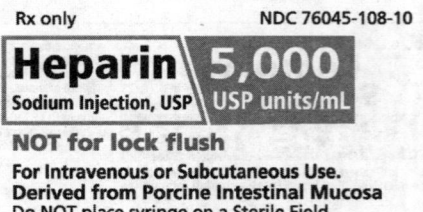

Rx only   NDC 76045-108-10

Heparin **5,000**
Sodium Injection, USP USP units/mL

NOT for lock flush

For Intravenous or Subcutaneous Use.
Derived from Porcine Intestinal Mucosa
Do NOT place syringe on a Sterile Field.

How many milliliters would the nurse administer?
a. 0.2 mL
b. 0.4 mL
c. 0.6 mL
d. 0.8 mL

46. Order: insulin regular 15 units subcut before breakfast.
Available:

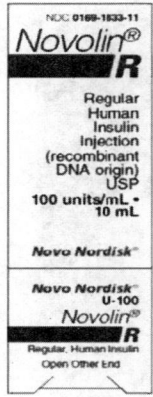

NDC 0169-1833-11
Novolin®
R
Regular
Human
Insulin
Injection
(recombinant
DNA origin)
USP
100 units/mL •
10 mL

Novo Nordisk®

Novo Nordisk®
U-100
Novolin®
R
Regular, Human Insulin
Open Other End

Shade in the dosage on the syringe.

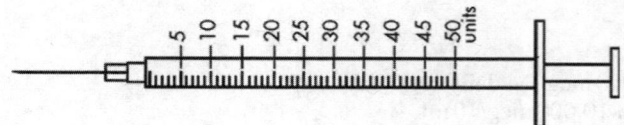

47. Order: topiramate 50 mg per day PO administered in two equally divided doses
Available:

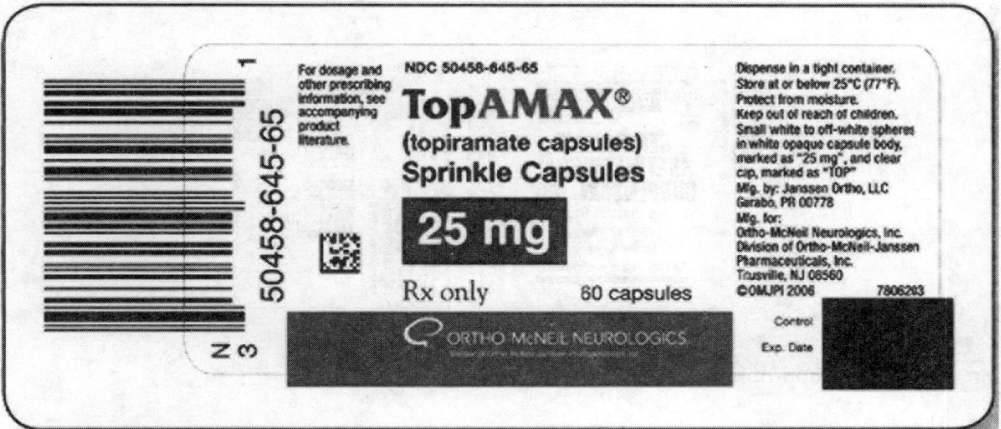

A. What is the trade name? _____

B. What is the generic name? _____

C. What is the form? _____

D. How many capsules per dose? _____

DRUG CALCULATIONS USING BODY WEIGHT

48. Order: penicillin V potassium 200,000 units PO q6h
Child weighs 46 lb
Recommended child's drug dosage: 25,000–90,000 units/kg/day in 3–6 divided doses.
Available: (NOTE: The dosage per 5 mL is in milligrams and units.)

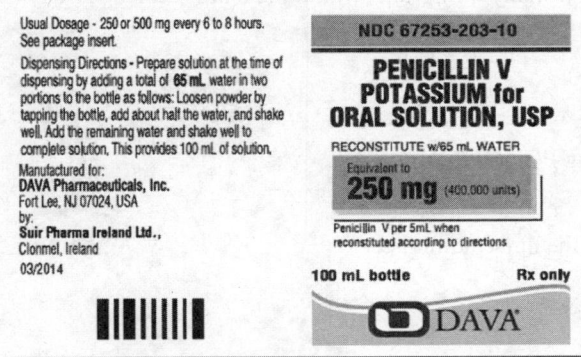

A. Is the prescribed dose in a safe range?
  a. No
  b. Yes

B. How many milliliters would the child receive for each dose?
  a. 1 mL
  b. 1.5 mL
  c. 2 mL
  d. 2.5 mL

49. Order: cefuroxime axetil 200 mg PO q12h
Child's age: 8 years; weight: 75 pounds
Recommended dosage (3 months–12 years): 10–15 mg/kg/day
Available:

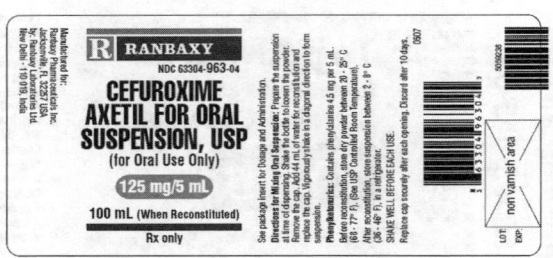

A. Is the prescribed dose appropriate?
  a. No
  b. Yes

B. If the 200 mg dose is given, how many milliliters would the child receive per dose?
  a. 2 mL
  b. 4 mL
  c. 6 mL
  d. 8 mL

50. Order: amoxicillin 75 mg PO q8h
Child weighs 5 kg
Recommended child's drug dosage: 80–90 mg/kg/day in divided doses

A. Is the prescribed dose appropriate?
  a. No
  b. Yes

B. According to the order, how many milligrams would the child receive per day (24 hours)?
  a. 225 mg
  b. 400 mg
  c. 450 mg
  d. 600 mg

51. Order: acetaminophen 250 mg PO q6h PRN
Available: 160 mg/5 mL

How many milliliters would the nurse administer?
  a. 3.2 mL
  b. 6 mL
  c. 7.8 mL
  d. 10 mL
  e. 12 mL

52. Order: ceftriaxone 50 mg/kg IM daily
Child weighs 8 kg
Available:

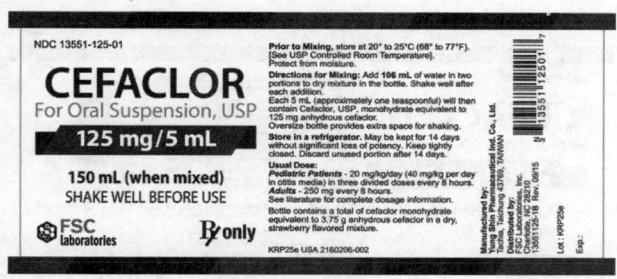

A. How much diluent is needed? _____

B. What is the final concentration? _____

C. How many milliliters would the child receive per dose?
    a. 0.5 mL
    b. 1.1 mL
    c. 1.5 mL
    d. 2 mL
    e. 2.4 mL

53. Order: erythromycin suspension 160 mg PO q6h
Child weighs 25 kg
Recommended child's drug dosage: 30–50 mg/kg/day in divided doses q6h
Available:

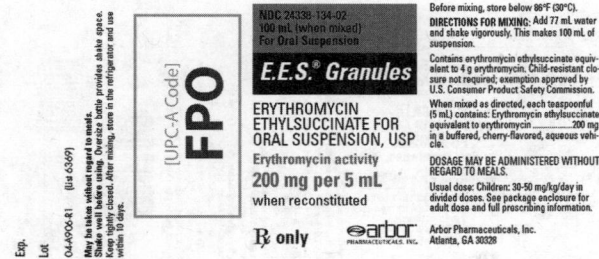

A. Is the prescribed dosage within dose parameters?
    a. Yes, the dosage is safe.
    b. No, the dosage is too low.
    c. No, the dosage is too high.

B. How many milliliters would the child receive for the ordered dosage?
    a. 0.25 mL
    b. 2 mL
    c. 3 mL
    d. 4 mL

54. Order: cefaclor 75 mg PO q8h
Child weighs 22 pounds
Recommended child's drug dosage: 20–40 mg/kg/day in three divided doses
Available:

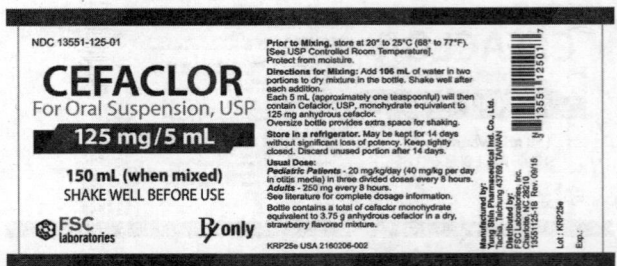

A. Calculate the minimum and maximum recommended dosage range per dose. _____

B. Is the ordered dosage appropriate? _____

C. How many milliliters per dose would be given?

    a. 2 mL
    b. 3 mL
    c. 4 mL
    d. 5 mL
    e. 6 mL

55. Order: amoxicillin/clavulanate potassium 150 mg (amoxicillin component) PO q8h
Child weighs 26 pounds
Recommended child's drug dosage: 45 mg/kg/day in three divided doses
Available:

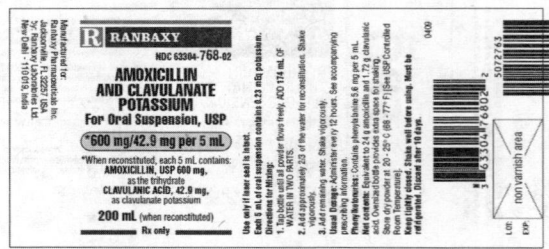

A. How many kilograms does the child weigh?
    a. 10 kg
    b. 12 kg
    c. 14 kg
    d. 15 kg

B. Is the prescribed dosage within dose parameters?
    a. Yes, the dosage is safe.
    b. No, the dosage is too low.
    c. No, the dosage is too high.

C. How many milliliters of the ordered dosage would the child receive per dose?
    a. 1.3 mL
    b. 1.5 mL
    c. 2 mL
    d. 3.5 mL

56. Order: acetaminophen 135 mg PO q6h PRN for fever
Child weighs 25 pounds
Recommended dosage range: 10–15 mg/kg/dose q4–6h PRN

  a. What is the child's weight in kilograms? _____

  b. What are the minimum and maximum safe dosage ranges? _____

  c. Is the ordered dose safe? _____

57. A 3-year-old is ordered ticarcillin/clavulanic acid 50 mg/kg (ticarcillin component) IV q6h. The child weighs 23 pounds. How many milligrams would the child receive per dose? _____

58. A child with meningitis is ordered ceftriaxone 100 mg/kg/day IV divided q12h. The child weighs 65 pounds.

  A. How many milligrams would the child receive per day? _____

  B. How many milligrams would the child receive per dose? _____

DRUG CALCULATIONS USING BODY SURFACE AREA
USE THE WEST NOMOGRAM AS INDICATED IN THE FOLLOWING DRUG CALCULATIONS

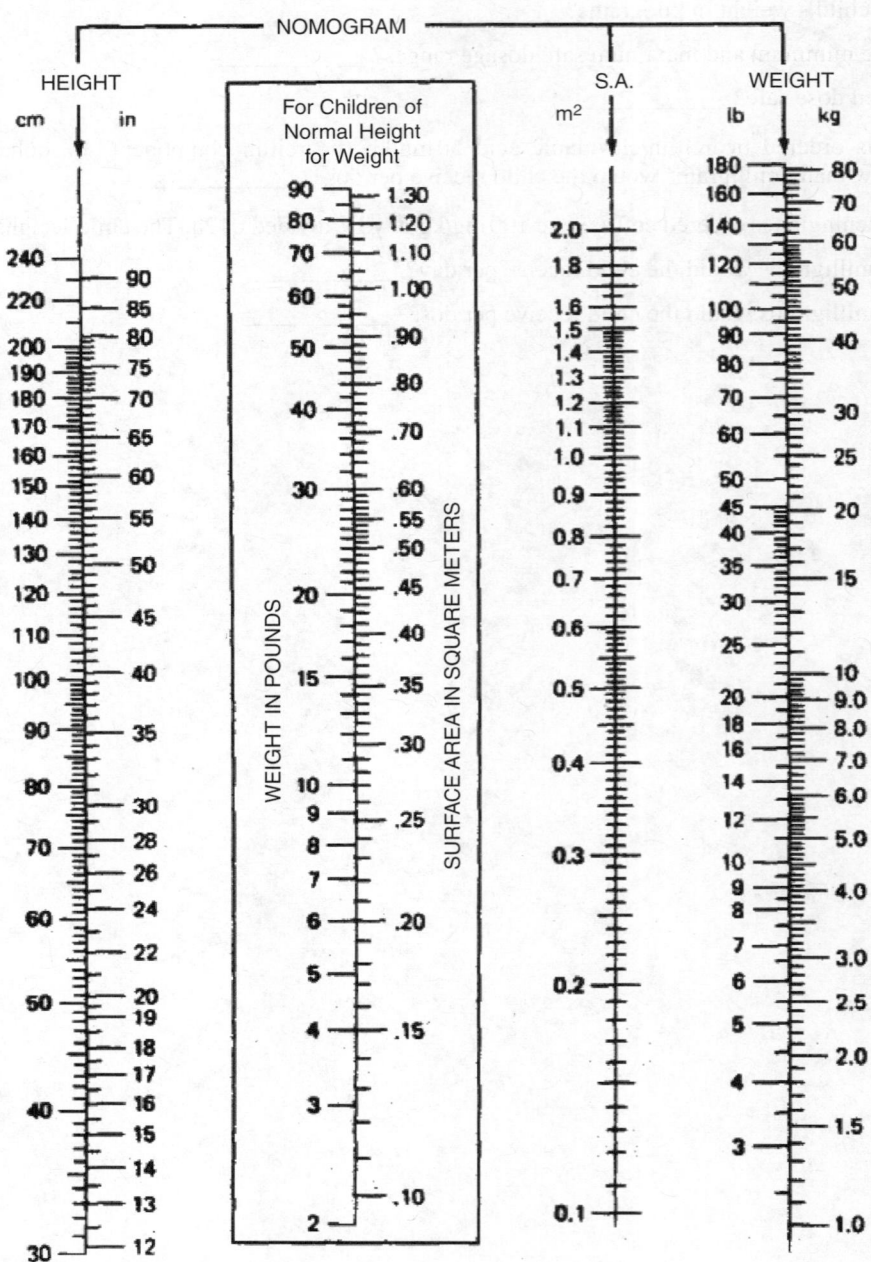

NOMOGRAM

HEIGHT · S.A. · WEIGHT

For Children of Normal Height for Weight

WEIGHT IN POUNDS

SURFACE AREA IN SQUARE METERS

59. Refer to the West nomogram and determine the BSA for the following children of normal height and weight.

A. Child weighs 5 pounds _____

B. Child weighs 25 pounds _____

C. Child weighs 53 pounds _____

60. Refer to the West nomogram to determine the following BSAs.

A. A child who is 43 in. tall and weighs 54 pounds _____

B. A child who is 39 in. tall and weighs 60 pounds _____

C. A child who is 56 cm tall and weighs 15 kg _____

61. Calculate the following BSA using the square root method for inches and pounds.

A. A child weighs 25 pounds and is 32 in. tall _____

B. A child weighs 58 pounds and is 48 in. tall _____

C. A child is 40 in. tall and weighs 34 pounds _____

62. Calculate the following BSAs using the square root method for centimeters and kilograms.

A. A child weighs 8 kg and is 28.2 cm long _____

B. A child weighs 28.1 kg and is 133.4 cm tall _____

C. A child is 85.5 cm tall and weighs 25 kg _____

63. Order: lomustine $100 \, mg/m^2$
Child's weight is 80 pounds; height is 40 in. tall.

A. Calculate the BSA using the West nomogram. _____

B. Calculate the BSA using the square root method. _____

C. Using the calculated answer from B, determine the milligrams the child would receive per dose. _____

64. Drug X $50 \, mg/m^2$ is ordered for a child who weighs 70 pounds and is 54 in. tall.

A. What is the BSA using the square root method? _____

B. How many milligrams would the child receive? _____

65. Drug X $35 \, mg/m^2$ is ordered for a child who weighs 43 pounds and is 52 in. tall.

A. What is the BSA using the square root method? _____

B. What is the dosage? _____

66. Drug X $500 \, mg$ is ordered for a child who is 100 pounds and 54 in. tall.

A. What is the BSA using the square root method? _____

B. What is the child's dose? _____

67. Carmustine $350 \, mg$ IV as a single dose every 4 weeks. The child weighs 71 pounds and is 60 in. tall.

A. What is the BSA using the square root method? _____

B. How many milligrams would the child receive? _____

68. Methotrexate $3.3 \, mg/m^2$ IV daily every 4 weeks is ordered for an adolescent who is 104 pounds and 64 in. tall.

A. What is the BSA using the square root method? _____

B. How many milligrams would the adolescent receive? _____

69. Order: cyclophosphamide 350 mg/m^2
    Child's weight: 36.9 kg; height: 59 cm

    A. What is the child's BSA using the square root method? _____

    B. How many milligrams would the child receive? _____

70. Order: imatinib 340 mg/m^2/day PO divided into two doses.
    Child weighs 47.5 kg and is 160 cm tall

    A. What is the BSA using the square root method? _____

    B. How many milligrams would the child receive per dose? _____

DRUG CALCULATIONS FOR DRUGS REQUIRING RECONSTITUTION

71. Order: oxacillin sodium 300 mg IM q6h
    Available:

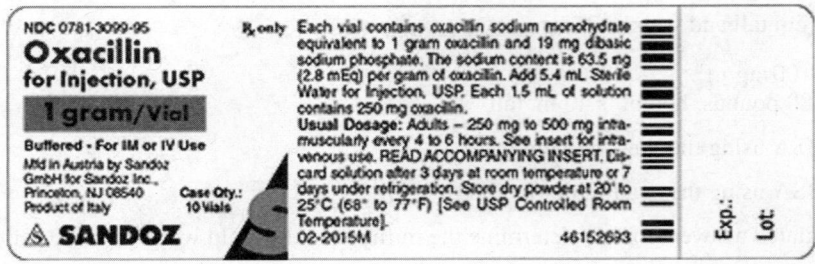

A. The nurse must add _____ mL of sterile water to yield _____ mg/_____ mL of drug solution.
B. How many milliliters would the nurse administer?
   a. 0.5 mL
   b. 1 mL
   c. 1.8 mL
   d. 2 mL

72. Order: nafcillin 500 mg IM q4h
    Available:

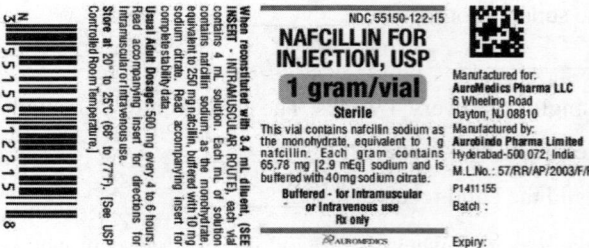

A. The nurse must add _____ mL of diluent to yield _____ mg/mL of drug solution.
B. How many milliliters would the nurse administer?
   a. 1 mL
   b. 2 mL
   c. 3 mL
   d. 4 mL

73. Order: cefotetan disodium 500 mg IM q12h
Available: (NOTE: Mix 2 mL of diluent. Once reconstituted, each milliliter of solution contains cefotetan of 400 mg.)

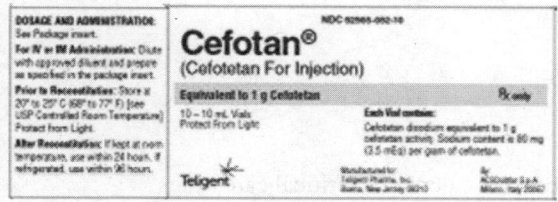

How many milliliters would the nurse administer per dose?
a. 1 mL
b. 1.3 mL
c. 2 mL
d. 2.3 mL

74. Order: ampicillin sodium 350 mg IM q6h
Available:

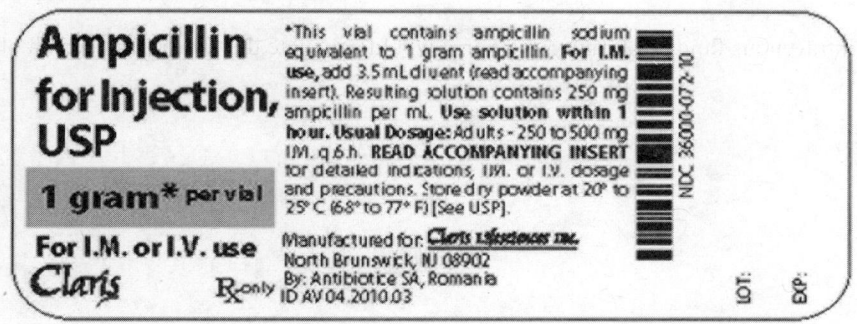

How many milliliters would the nurse administer per dose?
a. 0.8 mL
b. 1 mL
c. 1.4 mL
d. 2 mL

75. Order: tobramycin 3 mg/kg IM in three divided doses
Patient's weight: 184 pounds
Available:

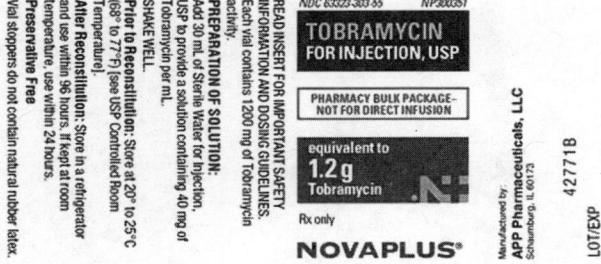

How many milliliters would the nurse administer per dose?
a. 1.5 mL
b. 2.8 mL
c. 4.2 mL
d. 6.3 mL

76. The health care provider orders heparin infusion. The nurse would calculate the dosage for infusion in which of the following units of measurement?
    a. mL/h
    b. gtt/min
    c. units/h
    d. units/kg/h

77. Which calculation method is best for calculating critical care drugs?
    a. Ratio and proportion method because they contain multiple steps.
    b. Fractional equation method because conversion factors are not needed.
    c. Basic formula method because it is the easiest.
    d. Dimensional analysis because all the units of measurement and conversion factors are included in one equation.

78. When an electronic infusion device is used to deliver intravenous fluids or drugs, the nurse would calculate the flow rate in which of the following units of measurement?
    a. gtt/min
    b. units/h
    c. gtt/mL
    d. mL/h

79. When infusing intravenous fluids by gravity, the nurse would calculate the flow rate in which of the following units of measurement?
    a. gtt/min
    b. gtt/mL
    c. units/h
    d. mL/h

Match the common fluid abbreviation in Column I to the appropriate IV solution bags in Column II.

Column I

_____ **80.** D_5 1/2NS

_____ **81.** LR or RL

_____ **82.** D_5W

_____ **83.** D_5NS

Column II

a.

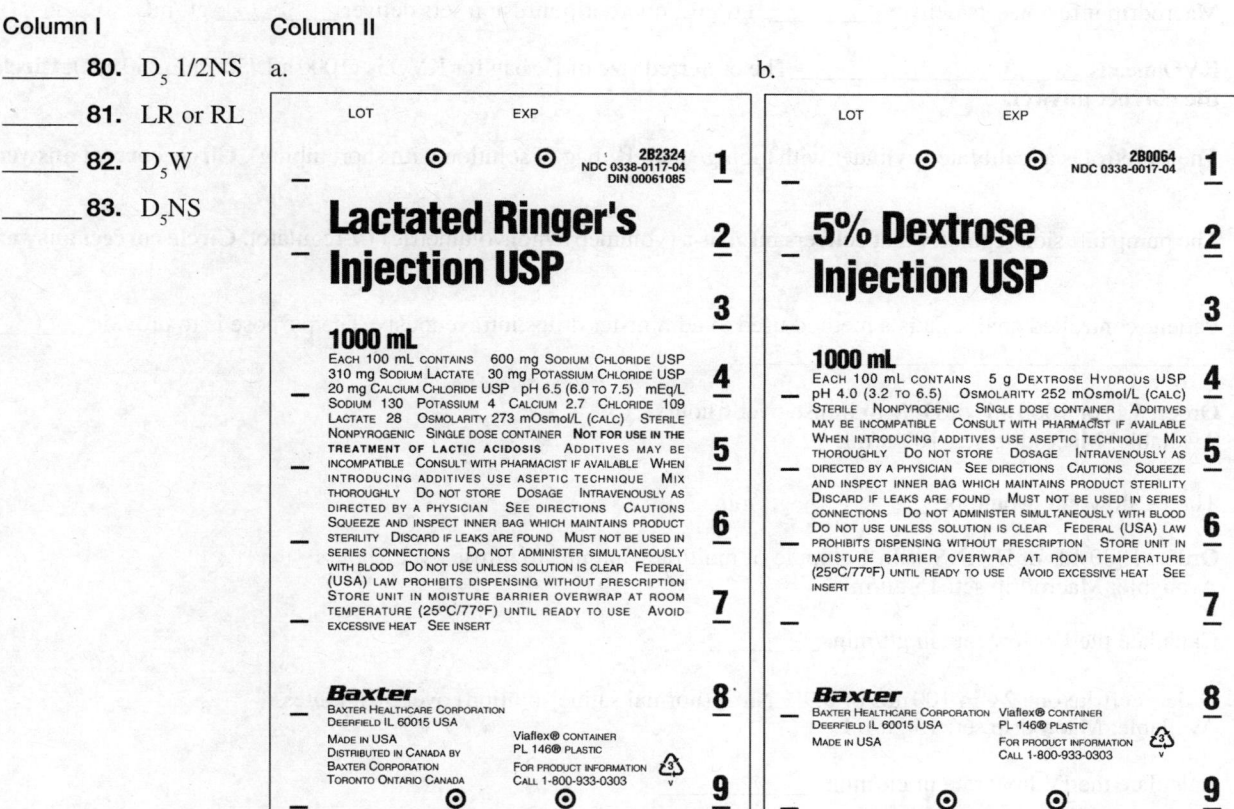

LOT   EXP

2B2324
NDC 0338-0117-04
DIN 00061085

Lactated Ringer's Injection USP

1000 mL

EACH 100 mL CONTAINS   600 mg SODIUM CHLORIDE USP 310 mg SODIUM LACTATE   30 mg POTASSIUM CHLORIDE USP 20 mg CALCIUM CHLORIDE USP   pH 6.5 (6.0 TO 7.5)   mEq/L SODIUM 130 POTASSIUM 4 CALCIUM 2.7 CHLORIDE 109 LACTATE 28 OSMOLARITY 273 mOsmol/L (CALC) STERILE NONPYROGENIC SINGLE DOSE CONTAINER **NOT FOR USE IN THE TREATMENT OF LACTIC ACIDOSIS** ADDITIVES MAY BE INCOMPATIBLE CONSULT WITH PHARMACIST IF AVAILABLE WHEN INTRODUCING ADDITIVES USE ASEPTIC TECHNIQUE MIX THOROUGHLY DO NOT STORE DOSAGE INTRAVENOUSLY AS DIRECTED BY A PHYSICIAN SEE DIRECTIONS CAUTIONS SQUEEZE AND INSPECT INNER BAG WHICH MAINTAINS PRODUCT STERILITY DISCARD IF LEAKS ARE FOUND MUST NOT BE USED IN SERIES CONNECTIONS DO NOT ADMINISTER SIMULTANEOUSLY WITH BLOOD DO NOT USE UNLESS SOLUTION IS CLEAR FEDERAL (USA) LAW PROHIBITS DISPENSING WITHOUT PRESCRIPTION STORE UNIT IN MOISTURE BARRIER OVERWRAP AT ROOM TEMPERATURE (25ºC/77ºF) UNTIL READY TO USE AVOID EXCESSIVE HEAT SEE INSERT

Baxter
BAXTER HEALTHCARE CORPORATION
DEERFIELD IL 60015 USA
MADE IN USA
DISTRIBUTED IN CANADA BY
BAXTER CORPORATION
TORONTO ONTARIO CANADA

Viaflex® CONTAINER
PL 146® PLASTIC

FOR PRODUCT INFORMATION
CALL 1-800-933-0303

b.

LOT   EXP

2B0064
NDC 0338-0017-04

5% Dextrose Injection USP

1000 mL

EACH 100 mL CONTAINS   5 g DEXTROSE HYDROUS USP pH 4.0 (3.2 TO 6.5) OSMOLARITY 252 mOsmol/L (CALC) STERILE NONPYROGENIC SINGLE DOSE CONTAINER ADDITIVES MAY BE INCOMPATIBLE CONSULT WITH PHARMACIST IF AVAILABLE WHEN INTRODUCING ADDITIVES USE ASEPTIC TECHNIQUE MIX THOROUGHLY DO NOT STORE DOSAGE INTRAVENOUSLY AS DIRECTED BY A PHYSICIAN SEE DIRECTIONS CAUTIONS SQUEEZE AND INSPECT INNER BAG WHICH MAINTAINS PRODUCT STERILITY DISCARD IF LEAKS ARE FOUND MUST NOT BE USED IN SERIES CONNECTIONS DO NOT ADMINISTER SIMULTANEOUSLY WITH BLOOD DO NOT USE UNLESS SOLUTION IS CLEAR FEDERAL (USA) LAW PROHIBITS DISPENSING WITHOUT PRESCRIPTION STORE UNIT IN MOISTURE BARRIER OVERWRAP AT ROOM TEMPERATURE (25ºC/77ºF) UNTIL READY TO USE AVOID EXCESSIVE HEAT SEE INSERT

Baxter
BAXTER HEALTHCARE CORPORATION
DEERFIELD IL 60015 USA
MADE IN USA

Viaflex® CONTAINER
PL 146® PLASTIC

FOR PRODUCT INFORMATION
CALL 1-800-933-0303

c.

LOT   EXP

2B1073
NDC 0338-0085-03

5% Dextrose and 0.45% Sodium Chloride Injection USP

500 mL

EACH 100 mL CONTAINS   5 g DEXTROSE HYDROUS USP   450 mg SODIUM CHLORIDE USP   pH 4.0 (3.2 TO 6.5)   mEq/L SODIUM 77 CHLORIDE 77 HYPERTONIC OSMOLARITY 406 mOsmol/L (CALC) STERILE NONPYROGENIC SINGLE DOSE CONTAINER ADDITIVES MAY BE INCOMPATIBLE CONSULT WITH PHARMACIST IF AVAILABLE WHEN INTRODUCING ADDITIVES USE ASEPTIC TECHNIQUE MIX THOROUGHLY DO NOT STORE DOSAGE INTRAVENOUSLY AS DIRECTED BY A PHYSICIAN SEE DIRECTIONS CAUTIONS SQUEEZE AND INSPECT INNER BAG WHICH MAINTAINS PRODUCT STERILITY DISCARD IF LEAKS ARE FOUND MUST NOT BE USED IN SERIES CONNECTIONS DO NOT USE UNLESS SOLUTION IS CLEAR FEDERAL (USA) LAW PROHIBITS DISPENSING WITHOUT PRESCRIPTION STORE UNIT IN MOISTURE BARRIER OVERWRAP AT ROOM TEMPERATURE (25ºC/77ºF) UNTIL READY TO USE AVOID EXCESSIVE HEAT SEE INSERT

Baxter
BAXTER HEALTHCARE CORPORATION
DEERFIELD IL 60015 USA
MADE IN USA

Viaflex® CONTAINER
PL 146® PLASTIC

FOR PRODUCT INFORMATION
CALL 1-800-933-0303

d.

LOT   EXP

2B1064
NDC 0338-0089-04

5% Dextrose and 0.9% Sodium Chloride Injection USP

1000 mL

EACH 100 mL CONTAINS   5 g DEXTROSE HYDROUS USP 900 mg SODIUM CHLORIDE USP   pH 4.0 (3.2 TO 6.5) mEq/L SODIUM 154 CHLORIDE 154 HYPERTONIC OSMOLARITY 560 mOsmol/L (CALC) STERILE NONPYROGENIC SINGLE DOSE CONTAINER ADDITIVES MAY BE INCOMPATIBLE CONSULT WITH PHARMACIST IF AVAILABLE WHEN INTRODUCING ADDITIVES USE ASEPTIC TECHNIQUE MIX THOROUGHLY DO NOT STORE DOSAGE INTRAVENOUSLY AS DIRECTED BY A PHYSICIAN SEE DIRECTIONS CAUTIONS SQUEEZE AND INSPECT INNER BAG WHICH MAINTAINS PRODUCT STERILITY DISCARD IF LEAKS ARE FOUND MUST NOT BE USED IN SERIES CONNECTIONS DO NOT USE UNLESS SOLUTION IS CLEAR FEDERAL (USA) LAW PROHIBITS DISPENSING WITHOUT PRESCRIPTION STORE UNIT IN MOISTURE BARRIER OVERWRAP AT ROOM TEMPERATURE (25ºC/77ºF) UNTIL READY TO USE AVOID EXCESSIVE HEAT SEE INSERT

Baxter
BAXTER HEALTHCARE CORPORATION
DEERFIELD IL 60015 USA
MADE IN USA

Viaflex® CONTAINER
PL 146® PLASTIC

FOR PRODUCT INFORMATION
CALL 1-800-933-0303

Complete the following.

84. Macrodrip infusion sets deliver _____ gtt/mL; microdrip infusion sets deliver _____ gtt/mL.

85. KVO means _____The preferred size of IV bag for KVO is (1000 mL/500 mL/250 mL). **Circle the correct answer.**

86. The Buretrol is a (calibrated cylinder with tubing/small IV bag of solution with short tubing). **Circle correct answer.**

87. The pump infusion regulator that delivers mL/h is a (volumetric/nonvolumetric) IV regulator. **Circle correct answer.**

88. Patient-controlled analgesia is a method used to administer drugs intravenously. The purpose is to provide _____ _____.

89. Order: 1 L or 1000 mL of D_5W to infuse over 6 hours
    Available: Macrodrip set: 10 gtt/mL

    The IV flow rate would be _____ gtt/min.

90. Order: 1000 mL of $D_5½NS$ with 1 ampule of multiple vitamins to infuse over 8 hours
    Available: Macrodrip set: 15 gtt/mL

    Calculate the IV flow rate in gtt/min. _____

91. Order: ceftriaxone 2 g in 100 mL of 0.9% NaCl (normal saline solution) over 30 minutes
    Available: Macrodrip set: 15 gtt/mL

    Calculate the IV flow rate in gtt/min. _____

92. Order: The following IV fluids to infuse over 24 hours are ordered. They include 1 L of D_5W, 1 L of $D_5½NS$, and 500 mL of D_5LR.
    Available:

    A. One liter is equal to _____ milliliters.

    B. Total number of milliliters of IV solutions to infuse in 24 hours is _____.

    C. What is the flow rate? _____

93. A liter of IV fluid was started at 7:00 a.m. and was to infuse for 8 hours. The IV set delivers 10 gtt/mL. At 12:00 p.m., only 500 mL were infused.

    A. How much IV fluid is left?
       a. 100 mL
       b. 200 mL
       c. 300 mL
       d. 400 mL
       e. 500 mL

    B. Recalculate the flow rate for the remaining IV fluids in gtt/min. _____

94. Order: cimetidine 200 mg IV q6h
Set and solution: Buretrol with drop factor 60 gtt/mL; primary IV fluid of 500 mL of 0.9% NaCl

Instruction: Dilute cimetidine 200 mg in 50 mL of normal saline and infuse in 15 minutes.

A. How much cimetidine will be infused per milliliter?
   a. 2 mg
   b. 3 mg
   c. 4 mg
   d. 5 mg

B. Calculate the flow rate in gtt/min.
   a. 50 gtt/min
   b. 100 gtt/min
   c. 150 gtt/min
   d. 200 gtt/min

95. Order: cefazolin 1000 mg IV q8h
Available:

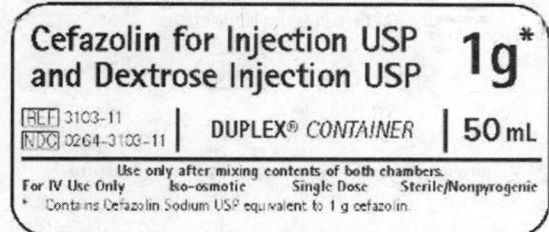

IV tubing with drop factor, 15 gtt/mL
Which flow rate to be infused over 1 hour is correct?
a. 6.5 gtt/min
b. 7 gtt/min
c. 12.5 gtt/min
d. 13 gtt/min

96. Order: nafcillin 1000 mg IV q4h
Available:

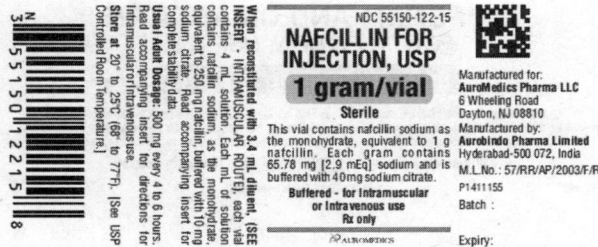

IV tubing available: Secondary set with drop factor 15 gtt/mL

Instruction: Dilute nafcillin 1000 mg in 100 mL of D_5W and infuse in 40 minutes.

A. How many mL of diluent should be added? _____

B. What is the drug's concentration? _____

C. Which flow rate is correct?
   a. 22 gtt/min
   b. 38 gtt/min
   c. 53 gtt/min
   d. 69 gtt/min

97. Order: fluconazole 400 mg IV daily
Available:

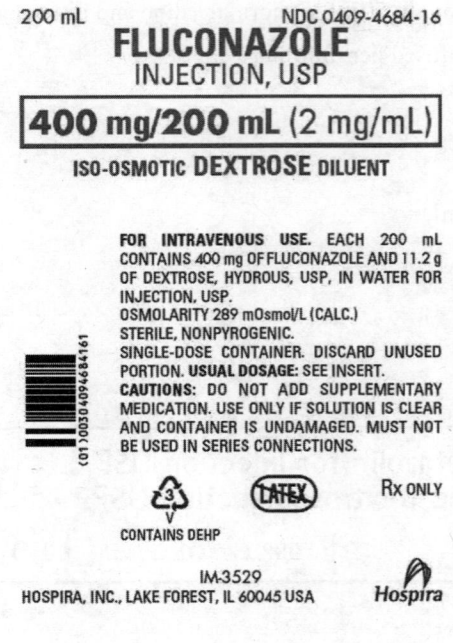

IV tubing available: Secondary set with drop factor 15 gtt/mL

Instruction: Infuse over 2 hours.

What is the flow rate? _____

98. Order: imipenem; cilastatin 500 mg IV q8h
Available: imipenem; cilastatin 500 mg in 100-mL solution

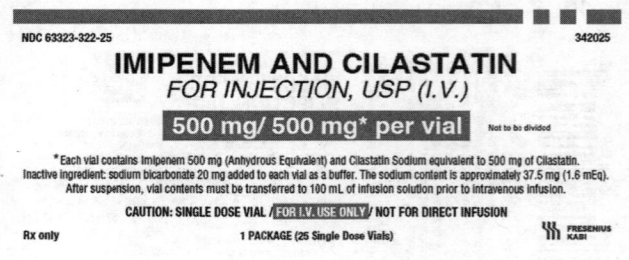

Instruction: Infuse over 30 minutes.

Calculate the gtt/min with an infusion set with 20 gtt/mL. _____

99. Order: sulfamethoxazole/trimethoprim 10 mcg/kg/d (trimethoprim component), IV divided in two doses. Patient weighs 135 pounds.
Available: sulfamethoxazole/trimethoprim 400 mg/80 mg per 5 mL

Instruction: Further dilute in 250 mL of D5W and infuse over 2 hours.

A. What is the total dosage in micrograms for the day? _____

B. How many micrograms for each dose? _____

C. What is the flow rate? _____

D. The hospital is experiencing a power failure after 20 minutes of infusion. Recalculate the flow rate in gtt/min with IV tubing 20 gtt/mL to be infused over 1 hour and 40 minutes.

100. Order: metronidazole 500 mg IV q6h

Available:

100 mL   NDC 0409-7811-27

► METRONIDazole ◄
Injection, USP
500 mg/100 mL (5 mg/mL)

EACH mL CONTAINS METRONIDAZOLE 5 mg; SODIUM
CHLORIDE 7.9 mg; DIBASIC SODIUM PHOSPHATE,
ANHYDROUS 0.48 mg; CITRIC ACID, ANHYDROUS
0.23 mg. SODIUM 14 mEq/100 mL. 314 mOsmol/LITER
(CALC.). pH 5.8 (4.5 to 7.0).
ADDITIVES SHOULD NOT BE MADE TO THIS SOLUTION.
DO NOT REFRIGERATE
SINGLE-DOSE CONTAINER. FOR I.V. USE. USUAL DOSAGE:
SEE INSERT. STERILE, NONPYROGENIC. PROTECT FROM
LIGHT. USE ONLY IF SOLUTION IS CLEAR AND CONTAINER
IS UNDAMAGED. MUST NOT BE USED IN
SERIES CONNECTIONS.

Rx ONLY   ®N: LATEX   △3 ▽ V
IM-2347   CONTAINS DEHP
MANUFACTURED BY HOSPIRA, INC., LAKE FOREST, IL 60045 USA
N+ AND NOVAPLUS ARE REGISTERED TRADEMARKS
OF NOVATION, LLC.

Instruction: Infuse in 30 minutes.

What is the flow rate?_____

101. Order: amikacin sulfate 7.5 mg/kg q12h
Adult weight: 64 kg
Available:

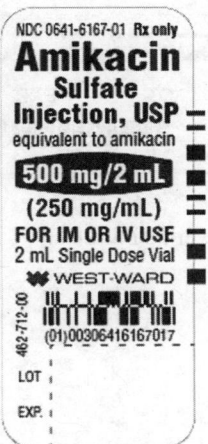

NDC 0641-6167-01 Rx only
Amikacin
Sulfate
Injection, USP
equivalent to amikacin
500 mg/2 mL
(250 mg/mL)
FOR IM OR IV USE
2 mL Single Dose Vial
WEST-WARD

(01)00306416167017

LOT
EXP.

A. How many milliliters would equal amikacin 400 mg?_____

Instruction: Dilute amikacin 400 mg in 100 mL of D_5W and infuse in 30 min.

B. What is the flow rate?_____

Chapter **11**   **Drug Labels and Dosage Calculations**

102. Order: minocycline 100 mg IV q12h
Available: Add 5 mL of sterile water.

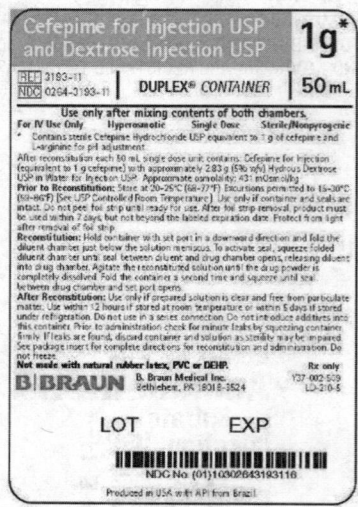

Instruction: Further dilute minocycline 100 mg in 500 mL of D5W and infuse in 6 hours.

What is the flow rate? _____

103. Order: cefepime hydrochloride 1 g IV q12h
Available:

Instruction: Drop factor, 60 gtt/mL. Infuse over 30 minutes.

What is the flow rate?_____

104. Order: ampicillin sodium/sulbactam sodium 1.5 g IV q6h
Available: (NOTE: ADD-Vantage vials do not need further dilution.)

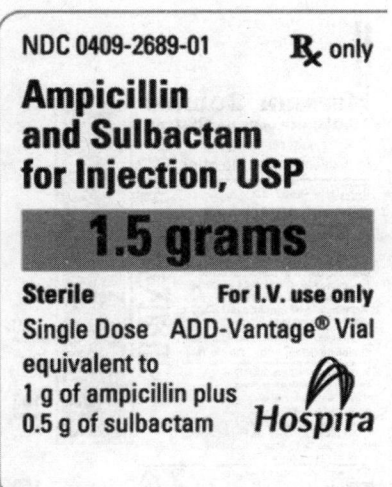

NDC 0409-2689-01   **R** only

**Ampicillin
and Sulbactam
for Injection, USP**

1.5 grams

Sterile   **For I.V. use only**
Single Dose   ADD-Vantage® Vial
equivalent to
1 g of ampicillin plus
0.5 g of sulbactam   *Hospira*

Set and solution: IV tubing with drop factor of 15 gtt/mL

Instruction: Infuse ampicillin sodium/sulbactam sodium 1.5 g solution in 100 mL of D5W over 30 minutes.

What is the flow rate? _____

105. Order: heparin 30,000 units/day continuous infusion
Available:

250 mL SINGLE-DOSE CONTAINER   NDC 0409-7794-52
HEPARIN   RX ONLY
**12,500 USP Units/250 mL
(50 USP Units/mL)**

**HEPARIN SODIUM IN
5% DEXTROSE INJECTION**   50
WARNING: CONTAINS SULFITES
EACH 100 mL CONTAINS
HEPARIN SODIUM 5,000 USP
UNITS (PORCINE INTESTINAL   100
MUCOSA); DEXTROSE,
HYDROUS 5 g; CITRIC ACID,
ANHYDROUS 51 mg; SODIUM
CITRATE, DIHYDRATE
334 mg; SODIUM METABISULFITE
20 mg; ELECTROLYTES: SODIUM   150
38 mEq/L; CITRATE 42 mEq/L.
STERILE. USUAL DOSAGE: SEE
INSERT. ADDITIVES SHOULD
NOT BE MADE TO THIS
SOLUTION. LATEX-FREE. SINGLE
DOSE CONTAINER. DISCARD
UNUSED PORTION. FOR   200
INTRAVENOUS USE ONLY.

IM-3490
HOSPIRA, INC., LAKE FOREST, IL 60045 USA   *Hospira*

A. How many units per hour is the patient receiving? _____

B. What is the flow rate?_____

106. Order: heparin bolus 80 units/kg, then maintenance infusion of 18 units/kg/h
Patient's weight: 180 pounds
Available:

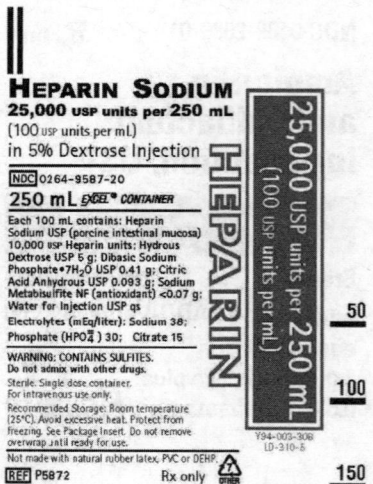

A. What is the patient's weight in kilograms? _____

B. How many units for the bolus? _____

C. Calculate the maintenance infusion flow rate. _____

107. A patient was prescribed heparin sodium 18 units/kg/h; titrate according to the weight-based heparin protocol. The patient's weight is 123 pounds. Heparin 25,000 units/250 mL (100 unit/mL) is available.

A. Calculate the flow rate in milliliters per hour. _____

B. Activated partial thromboplastin time (aPTT) is 40 sec, and the protocol states to rebolus with 40 units/kg and increase the infusion rate by 2 units/kg/h.

How many more units did the patient receive? _____ What is the new flow rate? _____

108. A patient was prescribed heparin sodium 18 units/kg/h; titrate according to the weight-based heparin protocol for a patient with pulmonary embolus. The patient's weight is 63 kg. Heparin 25,000 units/250 mL (100 units/mL) is available.

A. Calculate the flow rate in milliliters per hour. _____

B. aPTT is 45 sec, and the protocol states to rebolus with 40 units/kg and increase infusion by 2 units/kg.

How many more units did the patient receive? _____ What is the new flow rate? _____

109. A patient was prescribed heparin sodium 18 units/kg/h; titrate according to the weight-based heparin protocol. The patient's weight is 70 kg. Heparin 12,500/250 mL (50 unit/mL) is available.

A. Calculate the flow rate in milliliters per hour. _____

B. aPTT is >90 sec, and the protocol states to hold the infusion for 1 hour and decrease rate by 3 units/kg/h.

What is the new flow rate? _____

110. Order: diltiazem 0.25 mg/kg bolus over 2 minutes, then 15 minutes later, rebolus with 0.35 mg/kg IV, then start maintenance infusion at 10 mg/h.
Weight: 65 kg
Available:
For bolus:

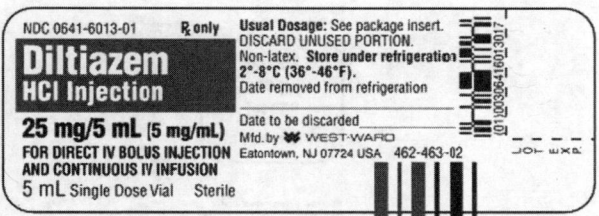

For maintenance infusion:

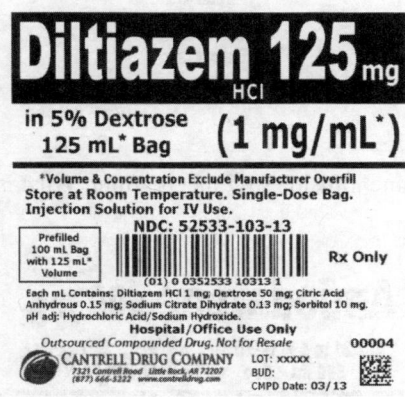

A. What is the total bolus in milligrams? _____

B. What is the flow rate for the maintenance infusion? _____

111. Order: dobutamine 2 mcg/kg/min as a continuous infusion. Titrate according to patient's hemodynamic response.
Weight: 63 kg
Available:

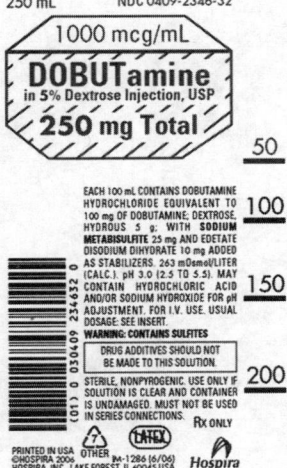

What is the flow rate? _____

112. Order: dobutamine 5 mcg/kg/min as a continuous infusion. Titrate according to patient's hemodynamic response.
Weight: 78 kg
Available:

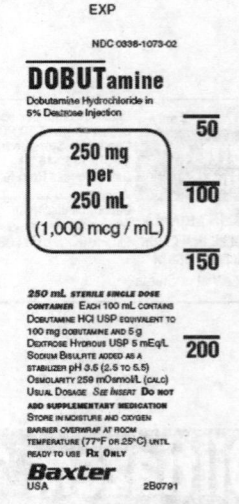

A. What is the flow rate? _____

B. Nurse is to increase the dobutamine infusion by 2 mcg/kg/min. What is the new flow rate? _____

113. Order: amiodarone 0.5 mg/min
Available:

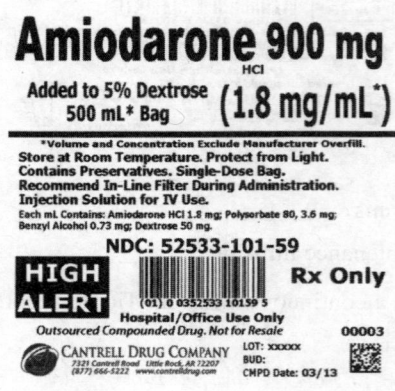

What is the flow rate? _____

114. Patient is receiving nitroglycerin 0.25 mg/min for unstable angina.
Available:

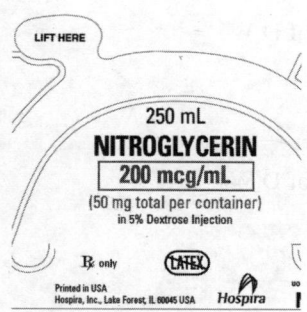

What is the flow rate? _____

115. Patient is receiving nitroglycerin 55 mcg/min.
Available:

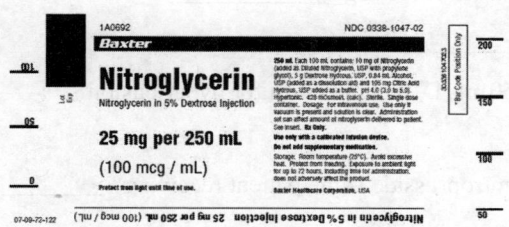

What is the flow rate? _____

116. Order: dobutamine 5 mcg/kg/min

Patient's weight: 152 lb

Available: dobutamine 500 mg in 250 mL D5W

What is the flow rate? _____

117. Order: dobutamine 10 mcg/kg/min

Patient's weight: 95 kg

Available: dobutamine 1000 mg in 250 mL D_5W

What is the flow rate? _____

118. Order: dopamine 5 mcg/kg/min

Patient weighs 130 lb

Available: dopamine 800 mg in 500 mL of D_5W

What is the flow rate? _____

119. Order: dopamine 300 mcg/min

Available: dopamine 400 mg in 250 mL of D_5W

What is the flow rate? _____

120. Order: heparin at 800 units/h

Available: heparin 25,000 units in 250 mL of D_5W

What is the flow rate? _____

121. Order: lidocaine 2 g in 250 mL of D_5W at 30 mL/h

A. How many mg/min is the patient receiving? _____

B. What is the flow rate? _____

122. Order: nitroprusside 100 mg/250 mL D_5W at 29 mL/h for hypertension

The patient weighs 143 lb

A. How many mcg/kg/min of nitroprusside is the patient receiving? _____

B. What is the flow rate? _____

12 Fluid Volume and Electrolytes

STUDY QUESTIONS

Match the electrolyte in Column I with its normal value in Column II.

Column I

_____ **1.** Magnesium

_____ **2.** Calcium

_____ **3.** Sodium

_____ **4.** Potassium

_____ **5.** Chloride

_____ **6.** Phosphorus

Column II

a. 96–106 mEq/L
b. 135–145 mEq/L
c. 2.4–4.4 mEq/L
d. 1.5–2.5 mEq/L
e. 3.5–5 mEq/L
f. 8.6–10.2 mg/dL

Match the description in Column I with its term in Column II.

Column I

_____ **7.** Similar to plasma concentration

_____ **8.** Based on milliosmoles per kilogram of water

_____ **9.** Solutions containing fewer particles and more water

_____ **10.** Solutions having a higher solute/particle concentration

Column II

a. Osmolality
b. Isoosmolar
c. Hypoosmolar
d. Hyperosmolar

REVIEW QUESTIONS

11. The nurse provided education to a patient on oral potassium supplement. Which statement by the patient indicates that more education is required?
a. "I can take this with a few sips of water."
b. "It may upset my stomach."
c. "I should drink at least six ounces of water or juice when I take it."
d. "I must not chew up the tablet."

12. A patient who has been diagnosed with hypokalemia is admitted to the hospital for potassium replacement intravenously (IV). Which nursing action is appropriate when preparing this drug?
a. Prepare the syringe to give IV push.
b. Push the potassium into the IV bag and do not mix before administration.
c. Push the potassium into the IV bag and shake vigorously.
d. Obtain an IV pump and pump tubing.

13. The nurse notices that the patient's intravenous (IV) site has become erythematous and edematous while IV potassium was infusing. Which action is most appropriate by the nurse?
a. Flush the IV site with normal saline and continue the infusion.
b. Flush the IV site with heparin.
c. Stop the IV and check for blood return.
d. Discontinue the current IV site and restart in another site.

14. A patient has been receiving intravenous potassium. The nurse notices the patient is now tachycardic. What other symptom might the nurse expect to see if the patient is becoming hyperkalemic? **Select all that apply.**
a. Abdominal distention
b. Nausea
c. Numbness in extremities
d. Polyuria
e. Hypoglycemia

15. A patient is found to be hyperkalemic. Which medication would the nurse anticipate administering?
    a. Magnesium mixed in 250 mL of normal saline
    b. 0.9% sodium chloride (NS) bolus of 500 mL
    c. A fluid challenge of 250 mL of 10% dextrose in water ($D_{10}W$).
    d. Sodium bicarbonate

16. A patient has been started on an enteral potassium supplement. Which teaching would be included for this patient? **Select all that apply**.
    a. List the signs and symptoms of both hypokalemia and hyperkalemia.
    b. Regular testing of serum potassium levels is required.
    c. The patient should increase his intake of potassium-rich foods.
    d. The drug must be taken on a full stomach or with a glass of water.
    e. The patient should sit up for 30 minutes after taking the drug.

17. Which value indicates normal range for serum osmolality?
    a. 175–195 mOsm/kg
    b. 275–295 mOsm/kg
    c. 330–350 mOsm/kg
    d. 475–495 mOsm/kg

18. Which term is used to describe the body fluid when the serum osmolality is 285 mOsm/kg?
    a. Hypoosmolar
    b. Hyperosmolar
    c. Isoosmolar
    d. Dehydrated

19. A patient with severe head trauma is receiving 3% sodium chloride. It has an osmolality of 900 mOsm/kg. This is considered to be which type of solution?
    a. Hypotonic
    b. Hypertonic
    c. Isotonic
    d. Neotonic

20. By which route is the majority of potassium excreted?
    a. Feces
    b. Kidneys
    c. Liver
    d. Lungs

21. A patient has pancreatitis. The nurse knows the patient is at risk for which electrolyte abnormality? **Select all that apply**.
    a. Hypocalcemia
    b. Hypernatremia
    c. Hypomagnesemia
    d. Hyperkalemia

22. The nurse is teaching the patient about calcium absorption and includes the health teaching that vitamin D is needed for calcium absorption. Which area of the body does vitamin D help in calcium absorption?
    a. Large intestine
    b. Small intestine
    c. Kidneys
    d. Liver

23. Calcium is distributed bound and unbound to proteins in which proportions?
    a. 25%:75%
    b. 50%:50%
    c. 75%:25%
    d. 90%:10%

24. A patient is prescribed 2 liters of intravenous (IV) fluids: 1000 milliliters (mL) of 5% dextrose in water (D_5W) followed by 1000 mL of 5% dextrose in 0.45% sodium chloride ($D_5$1/2 NS). Which term classifies these fluids?
    a. Colloids
    b. Crystalloids
    c. Lipids
    d. Parenteral nutrition

25. A patient is in the hospital overnight after having surgery and the patient was prescribed 5% dextrose in 0.45% sodium chloride ($D_5$1/2 NS) intravenously. $D_5$1/2 NS is considered which type of fluid?
    a. Hypotonic
    b. Hypertonic
    c. Isotonic
    d. Normotonic

26. A patient is receiving high-molecular-weight dextran after an explosion has burned over 50% of the body. Which action describes the purpose of dextran?
    a. Temporarily restore circulating volume
    b. Serve as a line to infuse blood into
    c. Piggyback fluid for antibiotics
    d. Whole blood substitute

27. Which body fluid has a similar electrolyte composition to lactated Ringer solution?
    a. Plasma
    b. Skin
    c. Tears
    d. White blood cells

28. A patient is taking potassium chloride and hydro-chlorothiazide. The patient's serum potassium level is 2.4 mEq/L. Which clinical manifestation would the nurse expect to see in this patient? **Select all that apply**.
    a. Bradycardia
    b. Headache
    c. Muscle weakness
    d. Nausea
    e. Anorexia

29. Magnesium deficiencies are frequently associated with which other electrolyte imbalance?
    a. Hypocalcemia
    b. Hyperkalemia
    c. Hyponatremia
    d. Hyperphosphatemia

30. A patient with a serum potassium level of 3.2 mEq/L asks why potassium supplement was prescribed. Which response by the nurse is most appropriate?
    a. "Your potassium level is 3.2 mEq/L which is low and should be corrected."
    b. "You will only be on the drug for a few days, so don't worry."
    c. "You obviously aren't taking enough in your diet, so you have to take this."
    d. "Have you been constipated lately? Constipation will cause a low potassium level."

31. A patient has the following lab results: Na^+ 150 mEq/L, K^+ 4.2 mEq/L, Cl^- 100 mEq/L, Ca^{++} 9.8 mEq/L, Mg^{++} 1.8 mg/dL, PO_4^- 3.1 mEq/L. Which electrolyte imbalance is the patient exhibiting?
    a. Hypocalcemia
    b. Hyperkalemia
    c. Hypernatremia
    d. Hypomagnesemia

32. A patient with a serum potassium level of 6.1 mEq/L will exhibit which clinical manifestation? **Select all that apply**.
    a. Abdominal cramps
    b. Muscle weakness
    c. Oliguria
    d. Paresthesia of the face
    e. Tachycardia and later bradycardia

33. Which drugs are used to treat hyperkalemia? **Select all that apply**.
    a. Digoxin and furosemide
    b. Glucagon and magnesium
    c. Glucose and insulin
    d. Sodium polystyrene sulfonate and sorbitol
    e. Sodium bicarbonate and calcium gluconate

34. A patient has had diarrhea for several days and has a serum calcium level of 7.2 mg/dL. Which clinical manifestation would the nurse expect to see in this patient? **Select all that apply**.
    a. Hyperactive deep tendon reflexes
    b. Irritability
    c. Numbness of the fingers
    d. Pathologic fractures
    e. Tetany

CASE STUDY: CRITICAL THINKING

Read the scenario and answer the following questions on a separate sheet of paper.

A 28-year-old patient presents to the emergency room with multiple stab wounds to the chest and abdomen. Vital signs on arrival include blood pressure 84/62 mm Hg, heart rate 118 beats/minute, respiratory rate 30 breaths/minute, pulse oximetry 94% on room air, and temperature 96.4°F.

1. Which assessment would be a priority for this patient?

2. Which fluid(s) would the nurse anticipate in being prescribed?

3. Explain the advantage of using whole blood versus packed red blood cells.

13 Vitamin and Mineral Replacement

Match the appropriate word or phrase in Column I with the letter of the fat- or water-soluble vitamins in Column II. The vitamins listed in Column II will be used more than once.

Column I

_____ 1. Vitamin A

_____ 2. Vitamin B complex

_____ 3. Vitamin C

_____ 4. Vitamin D

_____ 5. Vitamin E

_____ 6. Vitamin K

_____ 7. Toxic in excessive amounts

_____ 8. Metabolized slowly

_____ 9. Minimal protein binding

_____ 10. Readily excreted in urine

_____ 11. Slowly excreted in urine

Column II

a. Fat-soluble vitamins

b. Water-soluble vitamins

Match the appropriate vitamin in Column I with the letter of the common food sources in Column II.

Column I

_____ 12. Vitamin A

_____ 13. Vitamin B_{12}

_____ 14. Vitamin C

_____ 15. Vitamin D

_____ 16. Vitamin E

Column II

a. Salmon, egg yolk, milk

b. Wheat germ, egg yolk, avocado

c. Fish, liver, egg yolk

d. Green and yellow vegetables

e. Tomatoes, pepper, citrus fruits

Label the *ChooseMyPlate* diagram with the appropriate food groups.

17.

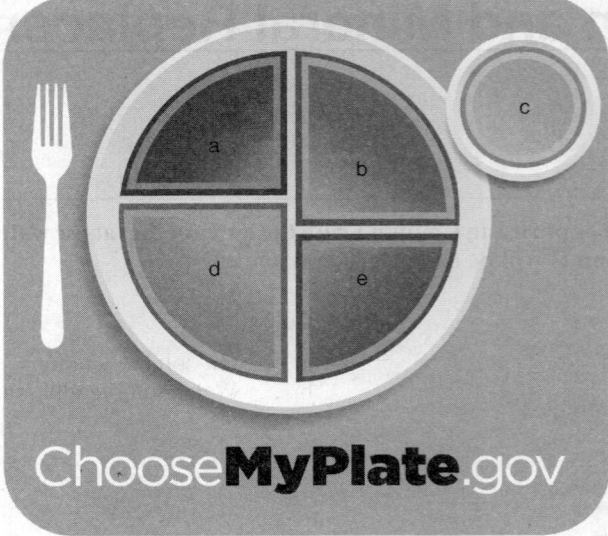

a. _____
b. _____
c. _____
d. _____
e. _____

REVIEW QUESTIONS

Select the best response.

18. Regulation of calcium and phosphorous metabolism and calcium absorption from the intestine is a major role of which vitamin?
   a. A
   b. B₁₂
   c. C
   d. D

19. A patient who just gave birth wants to know why the baby needs vitamin K. Which response would be appropriate by the nurse?
   a. "It will help the baby's digestive tract work better."
   b. "Vitamin K helps a baby maintain its temperature."
   c. "Vitamin K helps the blood to clot."
   d. "This will help prevent infections for the first month."

20. Protection of red blood cells from hemolysis is a role of which vitamin?
   a. A
   b. D
   c. E
   d. K

21. During a well-woman exam, a young female patient is interested in becoming pregnant and asks the nurse which supplements she should take. Which response would be best by the nurse?
   a. "Folic acid supplements are recommended in women who may become pregnant to prevent neural tube defects."
   b. "Vitamin A 8000 units should be taken to promote bone growth."
   c. "Mega doses of iron are important for blood formation."
   d. "Vitamin C 1600 mg should be taken to prevent colds, which are more common in pregnancy."

22. The patient has been involved in a motorcycle collision and has lost 1500 mL of blood from a pelvic fracture. Which mineral is essential for the regeneration of hemoglobin?
   a. Chromium
   b. Copper
   c. Iron
   d. Selenium

23. The patient has a history of heavy alcohol abuse. The patient presents to the emergency department confused, combative, and complaining of double vision. The family states the patient has become very forgetful recently. The nurse would anticipate that the prescriber will order which substance for this patient?
   a. Vitamin C
   b. Vitamin B_1
   c. Dextrose
   d. Vitamin B_6

24. Which vitamin or mineral is responsible for collagen synthesis?
   a. Vitamin C
   b. Vitamin D
   c. Iron
   d. Zinc

25. The patient takes an antacid for reflux and an iron supplement for anemia. Which information would the nurse include in patient education regarding these drugs?
   a. "The drugs help each other do its job."
   b. "Iron and antacids must be taken on alternate days."
   c. "Antacids will decrease iron absorption."
   d. "Iron will decrease the effectiveness of the antacids."

26. A patient is advised to drink a liquid iron preparation through a straw because it may cause which side effect?
   a. Bleeding gums
   b. Esophageal varices
   c. Corroded tooth enamel
   d. Tooth discoloration

27. Which patient might be at the most risk for vitamin A deficiency?
   a. A 36-year-old pregnant patient
   b. An 18-year-old patient with celiac disease
   c. A 74-year-old patient with a urinary tract infection
   d. A 33-year-old patient with sickle cell anemia

28. Vitamin A is stored in the liver, kidneys, and fat. By which route is it excreted?
   a. Rapidly through the bile and feces
   b. Slowly through the urine and feces
   c. Rapidly through the bile only
   d. Slowly through the feces only

29. A 24-year-old patient has been prescribed large doses of vitamin A as treatment for acne. Which advice would the nurse provide to this patient? **Select all that apply**.
   a. Contact the health care provider concerning drug dosing.
   b. Report peeling skin, anorexia, or nausea and vomiting to the health care provider.
   c. Do not exceed the recommended dosage without consulting the health care provider.
   d. Avoid alcohol consumption.
   e. Mega doses of vitamin A are necessary for several months to alleviate acne.

30. The patient has a history of tuberculosis and is on isoniazid therapy. The patient presents to the clinic with complaints of numbness and weakness to the hands and feet. Which vitamin supplement might be considered for this patient?
   a. Niacin
   b. Pyridoxine
   c. Riboflavin
   d. Thiamine

31. The patient with sustained burns to 40% of his body and is receiving long-term parenteral nutrition would be at risk for which mineral deficiency?
   a. Copper
   b. Iron
   c. Selenium
   d. Zinc

32. Chromium is thought to be helpful in control of which condition?
   a. Alzheimer disease
   b. Common cold
   c. Type 2 diabetes
   d. Raynaud phenomenon

33. Which food is high in copper?
   a. Broccoli
   b. Grapefruit
   c. Lamb
   d. Shellfish

34. The patient presents to the emergency department with an overdose of the oral anticoagulant warfarin. The nurse would anticipate the administration of which vitamin for this patient?
   a. B_2
   b. C
   c. E
   d. K

Read the scenario and answer the following questions on a separate sheet of paper.

A patient with a history of atrial fibrillation and on an anticoagulant warfarin is seen in the clinic for routine blood work to monitor the international normalized ratio. While obtaining patient's medication history, it was discovered that the patient has been taking various vitamins, including vitamins A, C, and E. The patient also has been on a "health conscious" diet, consuming large amounts of fresh fruits, vegetables, and fresh fish.

1. Describe the mechanisms of action for vitamins A, C, and E and the potential complications of hypervitaminosis.

2. Discuss the drug-drug and drug-food interactions that can occur with warfarin.

3. Explain the education the nurse would provide.

14 Nutritional Support

STUDY QUESTIONS

Complete the following.

1. Adequate nutritional support is needed for the body's _____ _____.

2. A critically ill person requires _____ more than the normal energy requirement.

3. In addition to nutritional support, _____ and _____ balance must be considered.

4. A _____ _____ _____ should be used when considering enteral nutrition.

5. The gastrostomy tube, also known as a _____ tube, is placed _____, _____, or _____.

Answer the following questions as true or false. If the statement is false, reword the sentence to make it true.

_____ **6.** Early enteral nutrition restores intestinal motility and maintains gastrointestinal (GI) function.

_____ **7.** Nutritional support is considered if the patient has had little or no nutrition for more than 5 days.

_____ **8.** Parenteral and enteral nutrition are synonymous and are delivered through the same route.

_____ **9.** Nasoduodenal, nasojejunal, and jejunostomy enteral nutrition deliver food below the pyloric sphincter.

Label the following

10. Label the types of GI tubes for enteral feedings.

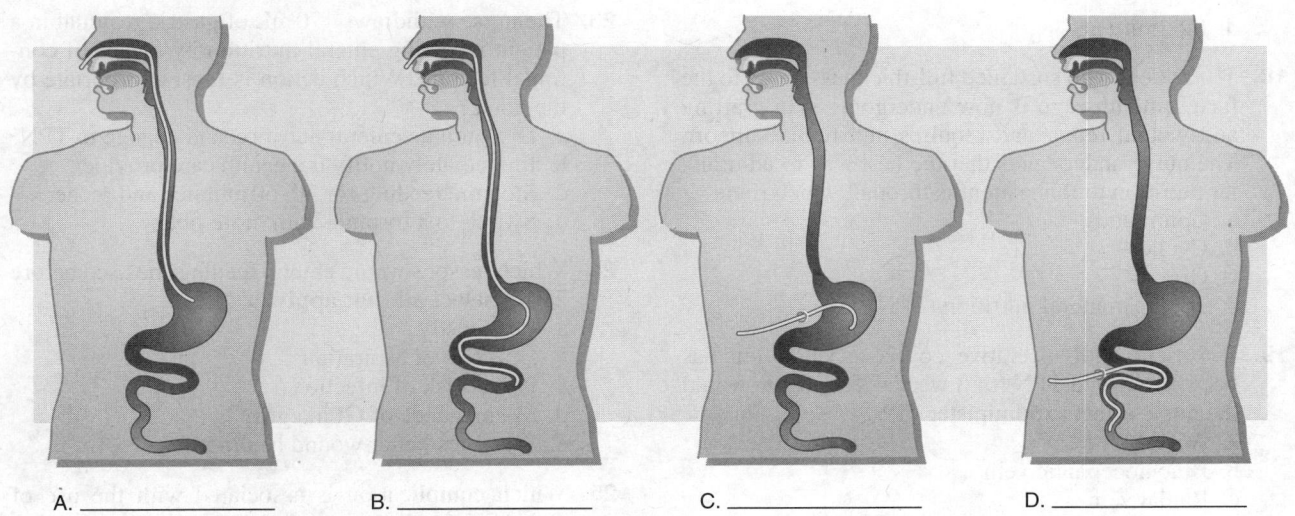

A. _____   B. _____   C. _____   D. _____

Match the terms in Column I with the descriptions in Column II.

Column I

_____ **11.** Bolus

_____ **12.** Intermittent

_____ **13.** Continuous

_____ **14.** Cyclic

Column II

a. Feeding given every 3–6 hours for 30–60 minutes
b. Feeding given continuously into the small intestine
c. Feeding infused over 8–16 hours per day
d. 250–400 mL given at one time; used for ambulatory patients

REVIEW QUESTIONS

Select the best response.

15. An older adult patient has a history of hypertension, arthritis, and diabetes. Which category of formula for enteral feeding would the nurse anticipate?
    a. Specialty
    b. Polymeric
    c. Semielemental
    d. Modular

16. The patient with a functional GI system is at risk for aspiration because of difficulty swallowing. Which supplemental nutrition would the nurse anticipate will be prescribed?
    a. Enteral via nasogastric tube
    b. Parenteral via peripheral IV
    c. Parenteral via central IV
    d. Enteral via jejunostomy tube

17. Which enteral feeding is administered over 30–60 minutes by pump infusion?
    a. Bolus
    b. Continuous
    c. Gravity
    d. Intermittent

18. The patient who sustained full-thickness burns to the face 2 months ago is now undergoing skin grafting and wound repair and requires nutritional support. The nurse understands that the best way to administer nutrition to this patient is through which route?
    a. Continuous
    b. Cyclic
    c. Gravity
    d. Total parenteral nutrition (TPN)

19. A patient with ulcerative colitis exacerbation has been prescribed TPN for 8 weeks. Which site would the nurse select to administer TPN?
    a. Accessory vein
    b. Brachiocephalic vein
    c. Radial vein
    d. Subclavian vein

20. Which percentage of carbohydrates is provided by TPN?
    a. <10%
    b. 10%–20%
    c. 25%–50%
    d. 60%–70%

21. The patient sustained a severe head injury and is on continuous enteral tube feedings. These feedings are commonly administered over which time frame?
    a. over 30–60 minutes
    b. over 24 hours
    c. over 15 minutes
    d. over 8–16 hours

22. Which side effect is commonly associated with enteral nutrition? **Select all that apply**.
    a. Constipation
    b. Diarrhea
    c. Urinary retention
    d. Yeast infection

23. The nurse withdraws 170 mL of gastric residual in a patient receiving enteral nutrition by means of continual feeding. Which action is most appropriate by the nurse?
    a. Discontinue enteral nutrition and change to TPN.
    b. Immediately notify the health care provider.
    c. Stop the feeding for 30–60 minutes and recheck.
    d. Switch to a formula with more fiber.

24. Which reasons would enteral feedings be used before TPN? **Select all that apply**.
    a. Less costly
    b. Less risk of aspiration
    c. Lower risk of infection
    d. Maintenance of GI integrity
    e. Promotes better wound healing

25. Which complication is associated with the use of TPN? **Select all that apply**.
    a. Air embolism
    b. Aspiration
    c. Hyperglycemia
    d. Pneumothorax

Read the scenario and answer the following questions on a separate sheet of paper.

A young adult sustained severe trauma from a rollover motor vehicle collision. The patient has been on TPN for several weeks and is being transitioned to enteral feeding through a nasogastric tube before a gastrostomy tube is placed.

1. Describe the steps a nurse would consider when transitioning a patient from TPN to enteral nutrition?

2. Describe the precautions a nurse would take to prevent aspiration?

 **Adrenergic Agonists and Antagonists**

Match the term in Column I with the letter of the description in Column II.

Column I

_____ **1.** Alpha₁ blocker

_____ **2.** Beta-blocker

_____ **3.** Selectivity

_____ **4.** Sympathomimetic

_____ **5.** Sympatholytic

Column II

a. Blocks action of sympathetic nervous system
b. Has a greater affinity for certain receptors
c. Causes vasodilation
d. Causes decreased heart rate
e. Similar in action to stimulation of the sympathetic nervous system

Complete the following.

6. Adrenergic receptors are located on the _____ cells of smooth muscles.

7. Bladder relaxation and urinary sphincter constriction resulting in urinary retention may occur with high doses of _____ agonists.

8. Sympathomimetics (do/do not) pass into the breast milk. *(Circle correct answer.)*

9. Adrenergic blockers are also called _____.

10. The antidote for infiltration intravenously (IV) of alpha- and beta-adrenergic drugs such as norepinephrine and dopamine is _____.

11. A beta-adrenergic blocker that can be given for migraine or hypertension is _____.

12. Mood changes such as depression and suicidal tendencies are possible when taking which type of adrenergic blocker? _____

13. Carvedilol, penbutolol, and pindolol are examples of selective/nonselective beta blockers. *(Circle the correct answer.)*

14. Nonselective beta-blockers, such as propranolol, are contraindicated in patients with _____ and _____.

15. A patient is taking albuterol 2 mg tablet by mouth to maintain pulmonary function. The patient was prescribed carvedilol 3.125 mg twice daily for heart failure. Identify the drug-drug interaction(s). _____

Match the letter of the adrenergic response in Column I to the associated receptor in Column II (Receptors in Column II may be used more than once, and response may affect more than one receptor type.)

Column I

_____ **16.** Increases gastrointestinal relaxation

_____ **17.** Increases force of heart contraction

_____ **18.** Dilates pupils

_____ **19.** Decreases salivary secretions

_____ **20.** Inhibits release of norepinephrine

_____ **21.** Dilates bronchioles

_____ **22.** Increases heart rate

_____ **23.** Promotes uterine relaxation

_____ **24.** Dilates blood vessels

Column II

a.   Alpha$_1$
b.   Alpha$_2$
c.   Beta$_1$
d.   Beta$_2$

REVIEW QUESTIONS

Select the best response.

25. A patient with asthma asks the nurse how the albuterol inhaler will work to help breathe better. Which response by the nurse best explains the action of the drug?
   a. "Albuterol will increase your heart rate so you will feel like you are able to breathe better."
   b. "Albuterol causes the airways to open up more in the lungs, improving function."
   c. "Albuterol will cause an increase in urinary output to remove extra fluid from the lungs."
   d. "Albuterol causes bronchial smooth muscle contraction that forces air into the lungs."

26. A patient presents to the clinic with a swollen face and tongue, difficulty breathing, and audible wheezes after eating a peanut butter sandwich for lunch. Which action would the nurse first take?
   a. Ensure a patent airway.
   b. Obtain an electrocardiogram (ECG).
   c. Administer 1 mg of 1:1000 epinephrine subcutaneously.
   d. Start an intravenous (IV) normal saline.

27. A patient calls the home health agency to tell the nurse about shaking and trembling after using the albuterol inhaler. Which question would the nurse first ask the patient?
   a. "Are you having any other symptoms?"
   b. "How long ago did this start?"
   c. "When was the last time you used your inhaler?"
   d. "How many puffs on the inhaler did you take?"

28. Which drug is classified as beta blockers? **Select all that apply**.
   a. Albuterol
   b. Atenolol
   c. Propranolol
   d. Amphetamine
   e. Acebutolol

29. The nurse discovers an intravenous (IV) site has infiltrated on a patient receiving IV dopamine. The nurse prepares to administer which drug as an antidote.
   a. Dobutamine
   b. Epinephrine
   c. Phentolamine
   d. Reserpine

30. When completing the patient health history, the nurse finds a history of narrow-angle glaucoma. When performing the drug reconciliation, which drug would concern the nurse? **Select all that apply**.
   a. Pseudoephedrine
   b. Midodrine
   c. Albuterol
   d. Carvedilol

31. Some over-the-counter drugs for cold symptoms contain substances that have sympathetic properties. These drugs are contraindicated in patients with which disease process?
   a. Allergic rhinitis
   b. Hypertension
   c. Orthostatic hypotension
   d. Chronic bronchitis

82

Chapter **15** **Adrenergic Agonists and Antagonists**

Copyright © 2026 Elsevier Inc. All rights are reserved, including those for text and data mining, AI training, and similar technologies.

32. Which adrenergic drug used in emergency settings does not decrease renal function?
    a. Norepinephrine
    b. Dopamine
    c. Phenylephrine
    d. Dobutamine

33. Beta$_1$ receptors are located in which area of the body? **Select all that apply**.
    a. Gastrointestinal tract
    b. Lungs
    c. Kidneys
    d. Brain
    e. Heart

34. A patient tells the nurse during the admitting history that alternative and complementary therapies are used to help manage medical conditions. Which drug would raise a concern in a patient taking St. John's wort?
    a. Reserpine
    b. Albuterol
    c. Propranolol
    d. Pseudoephedrine

35. A nurse received an order for timolol 100 mg b.i.d. Which action would be most appropriate by the nurse?
    a. Give the patient the drug after proper identification.
    b. Hold the drug, and contact the health care provider regarding the dosage.
    c. Give the drug now, and request a new order during patient rounds.
    d. Assess the patient's vital signs, and give the drug.

36. Catecholamine can be best defined by which statement?
    a. A substance that can produce a sympathomimetic response
    b. Another name for a beta blocker
    c. A type of decongestant
    d. A receptor site in the lungs

CLINICAL JUDGMENT UNFOLDING CASE STUDY

Phase 1:
Question 1:
SLO: Apply knowledge of the mechanisms of action and adverse drug reactions for adrenergic agonists
NGN Item Type: Highlight Text
Cognitive Skills: Recognize Cues

A 58-year-old male patient, who presented to the emergency department (ED) unresponsive and in cardiac arrest, received two ampules of epinephrine intravenously (IV). The patient became responsive. Patient continued with hypotension and bradycardia and received additional epinephrine in addition to starting dopamine 5 mcg/kg/min IV to be titrated by 2 mcg/kg/min every 15 minutes until the patient's systolic blood pressure is

90 mm Hg or higher and the heart rate is at least 70 beats per minute. After being in the ED for 3 hours, the patient became responsive and more aware and was transferred to the intensive care unit (ICU) with 0.9% sodium chloride infusing at 125 mL/hr and dopamine at 25 mcg/kg/min. Upon receiving the patient, the ICU nurse documents the following findings:

- Blood pressure 88/48 mm Hg
- Cardiac monitor showing sinus rhythm
- Heart rate 62 beats per minute
- Heart without murmurs, rubs, or gallops
- IV site to left forearm with redness and pain
- Lungs with faint crackles to the bases on auscultation
- Patient's complaint of "difficulty breathing"
- Peripheral pulses palpable but weak
- Respiratory rate 20 breaths per minute
- Urine output in urine drainage bag with 20 mL of amber-colored urine

Highlight the above information the nurse recognizes requiring immediate attention.

Question 2:
SLO: Identify appropriate nursing actions for patients receiving adrenergic agonists
NGN Item Type: Drop-Down Cloze
Cognitive Skills: Analyze Cues

A 58-year-old male patient who presented to the ED unresponsive and in cardiac arrest received two ampules of epinephrine intravenously (IV) resulting in the patient becoming responsive. Patient continued with hypotension and bradycardia and received additional epinephrine in addition to starting dopamine 5 mcg/kg/min IV to be titrate by 2 mcg/kg/min every 15 minutes until patient's systolic blood pressure is 90 mm Hg or higher and the heart rate is at least 70 beats per minute. After being in the ED for 3 hours, the patient was transferred to the ICU with 0.9% sodium chloride infusing at 125 mL/hr and dopamine at 25 mcg/kg/min. Upon receiving the patient, the ICU nurse documents the following findings:

- Blood pressure 88/48 mm Hg
- Cardiac monitor showing sinus rhythm
- Heart rate 62 beats per minute
- Heart without murmurs, rubs, or gallops
- IV site to left forearm with redness and pain
- Lungs with faint crackles to the bases on auscultation
- Patient's complaint of "difficulty breathing"
- Peripheral pulses palpable but weak
- Respiratory rate 20 breaths per minute
- Urine output in urine drainage bag with 20 mL of amber-colored urine

Choose the most likely options for the missing information from the statements below by selecting from the list of options provided.

Based on the blood pressure, the nurse would most likely ___1___ the rate of dopamine to ___2___ after moving the IV site to another location. To treat extravasation due to dopamine infiltration, the nurse would anticipate instilling ___3___ 5 mg that is diluted in 10–15 mL of normal saline. The nurse determines that the patient could be experiencing ___4___ because of crackles to the lung's bases and complaint of "difficulty breathing."

Options for 1	Options for 2	Options for 3	Options for 4
Decrease	23 mcg/kg/min	Protamine sulfate	Fluid overload
Increase	25 mcg/kg/min	Phytonadione	Pneumonia
Not change	27 mcg/kg/min	Phentermine	Collapsed lung
		Phentolamine mesylate	

Phase 2:
Question 3:
SLO: Prioritize nursing care for patients receiving adrenergic agonists
NGN Item Type: Multiple Response Select All That Apply
Cognitive Skills: Prioritize Hypotheses

A 58-year-old male patient has been in the ICU for 3 days postcardiac arrest receiving an infusion of dopamine at 27 mcg/kg/min and sodium chloride at 75 mL/hr. The patient continues to report "difficulty breathing" and "chest discomfort." Vital signs include blood pressure 102/64 mm Hg, heart rate 98 beats per minute, respiratory rate 22 breaths per minute. The nurse also auscultated crackles to the bases of the lungs. Cardiac monitor shows patient to be in sinus rhythm with occasional unifocal premature ventricular contractions. Urine output for the last 8 hours was 120 mL.

Which *priority* assessment findings would the nurse further review for potential complications of adrenergic agonist? Select all that apply.

____ **a.** Complaints of "difficulty breathing" and "chest discomfort"

____ **b.** Decreased renal function

____ **c.** Blood pressure 102/64 mm Hg

____ **d.** Heart rate 98 beats per minute

____ **e.** Oliguria

____ **f.** Respiratory rate of 22 breaths per minute

____ **g.** Crackles to the bases of the lungs on auscultation

Question 4:
SLO: Plan nursing actions for a patient receiving adrenergic agonists
NGN Item Type: Matrix Multiple Choice
Cognitive Skills: Generate Solutions

A 58-year-old male patient has been in the ICU for 3 days postcardiac arrest receiving an infusion of dopamine at 27 mcg/kg/min and sodium chloride at 75 mL/hr. The patient continues to report "difficulty breathing" and "chest discomfort." Vital signs include blood pressure 132/70 mm Hg, heart rate 100 beats per minute, respiratory rate 20 breaths per minute. The nurse also auscultated crackles to the bases of the lungs. Cardiac monitor shows patient to be in sinus rhythm with occasional unifocal premature ventricular contractions. Urine output for the last 8 hours were 120 mL. Further assessment revealed 1+ pedal and ankle edema and oxygen saturation of 92% on room air. The nurse notified the attending health care provider to report the assessment findings.

Use an X for the potential order below that is Indicated (appropriate or necessary), or Contraindicated (could be harmful) for a patient receiving adrenergic agonist.

Potential Order	Anticipated	Contraindicated
12-lead electrocardiogram (ECG)		
Chest x-ray		
Decrease sodium chloride infusion to 30 mL/hr		
Furosemide 10 mg IV once		
Increase intravenous fluids		
Monitor blood pressure and heart rate every 5 minutes		
Oxygen 2 L per nasal cannula		
Titrate dopamine down		

Phase 3:
Question 5:
SLO: Select the appropriate teaching to patients who are taking adrenergic antagonist
NGN Item Type: Drop-Down Table
Cognitive Skills: Take Action

A 58-year-old male patient, who is 7 days postcardiac arrest, is being transferred to a step-down unit. The nurse reviews the transfer orders that include metoprolol 50 mg twice daily. **Indicate which nurse's response listed in the first column is appropriate for each patient's question. Note not all the nurse's response will be used.**

Nurse's Response	Patient's Questions	Appropriate Nurse's Response
"When getting out of bed, change your position slowly to prevent a sudden drop in blood pressure."	"Can I stop taking this medicine if my blood pressure is good?"	
"Take the medicine twice daily, one in the morning and one just before you go to bed."	"Will the medicine prevent me from enjoying sex?"	
"Place ice pack to your genitalia to prevent long-term erection."	"Can I take my nasal decongestant when I get home?"	
"Stopping the medicine abruptly can cause severe high blood pressure or severe chest pain."	"What do I need to do if I become dizzy when getting out of bed?"	
"Metoprolol can cause erectile dysfunction."	"My job requires me to work odd hours. Can I take both doses when I first wake up?"	
"If your blood pressure is normal for five days, you can stop taking the medicine."		
"Nasal decongestants can decrease the effectiveness of metoprolol."		

Question 6:
SLO: Evaluate the effectiveness of an adrenergic antagonist
NGN Item Type: Multiple Response Select All That Apply
Cognitive Skills: Evaluate Outcomes

A 58-year-old male patient is being prepared for discharge from the hospital postcardiac arrest. Current vital signs are the following: blood pressure 138/84 mm Hg, pulse 98 beats per minute, respiratory rate 16 breaths per minute, temperature 97.5°F. The patient is prescribed nitroglycerin sublingual spray as needed and metoprolol twice daily. **For each statement, highlight the patient's correct understanding of the adrenergic antagonist. Select all that apply.**

a. "I can take my nose spray to decrease congestion."
b. "I need to stand from a sitting a position slowly."
c. "I am able to take ibuprofen for headaches."
d. "The medicine increases oxygen to the heart."
e. "I will call my doctor if I have trouble breathing."
f. "I can take an extra dose of metoprolol if I have chest pain."
g. "My blood pressure can decrease if I take a nitroglycerin."

16 Cholinergic Agonists and Antagonists

STUDY QUESTIONS

Match the term in Column I with the mechanism of action in Column II.

Column I

_____ **1.** Acetylcholine (ACh)

_____ **2.** Anticholinergic

_____ **3.** Anticholinesterase

_____ **4.** Cholinergic agonists

_____ **5.** Cholinesterase

_____ **6.** Muscarinic receptor

_____ **7.** Nicotinic receptor

_____ **8.** Direct-acting parasympathomimetic

Column II

a. Stimulates smooth muscle and slows heart rate

b. Impacts skeletal muscles

c. Stimulates muscarinic and nicotinic receptors

d. Stimulate the parasympathetic system

e. Blocks the action of acetylcholine

f. Mimics cholinergic actions

g. Blocks the breakdown of acetylcholine

h. Causes the breakdown of acetylcholine

Labeling

9. Identify cholinergic effects on the different organs affected by the parasympathetic nervous system.

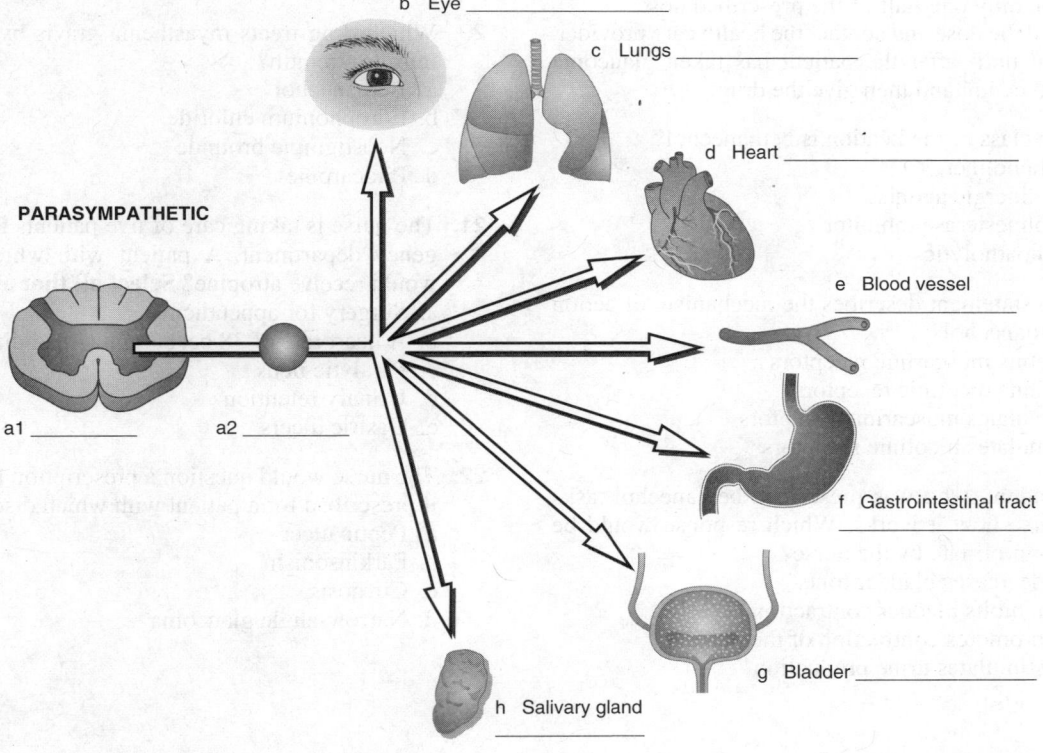

b Eye _____

c Lungs _____

PARASYMPATHETIC

d Heart _____

e Blood vessel _____

f Gastrointestinal tract _____

a1 _____   a2 _____

g Bladder _____

h Salivary gland _____

Select the best response.

10. Which drug would the nurse anticipate administering to a patient who ingested an organophosphate poison?
    a. Bethanechol
    b. Edrophonium chloride
    c. Metoclopramide
    d. Pralidoxime chloride

11. The pediatric patient has urinary retention. Which cholinergic drug would the nurse anticipate will be prescribed to increase urination?
    a. Bethanechol
    b. Edrophonium chloride
    c. Metoclopramide
    d. Neostigmine bromide

12. Anticholinergic eyedrops are used for which purpose?
    a. Constrict the pupils
    b. Dilate the pupils
    c. Decrease the intraocular pressure
    d. Detect astigmatism

13. A patient with narrow-angle glaucoma is prescribed an anticholinergic drug. Which action would be a priority by the nurse?
    a. Administer the medication as ordered after verifying the patient's identity.
    b. Give only one-half of the prescribed dose.
    c. Hold the dose and contact the health care provider.
    d. Wait until after the patient has taken glaucoma medication and then give the drug.

14. Which class of medication is bethanechol?
    a. Anticholinergic
    b. Cholinergic agonist
    c. Cholinesterase inhibitor
    d. Sympatholytic

15. Which statement describes the mechanism of action for bethanechol?
    a. Inhibits muscarinic receptors
    b. Inhibits nicotinic receptors
    c. Stimulates muscarinic receptors
    d. Stimulates nicotinic receptors

16. The patient, who was prescribed bethanechol, asks the nurse how it works. Which response would be most appropriate by the nurse?
    a. "It decreases bladder tone."
    b. "It inhibits bladder contraction."
    c. "It promotes contraction of the bladder."
    d. "It stimulates urine production."

17. Which outcome to the body would occur from receiving large doses of cholinergic drugs? **Select all that apply**.
    a. Decreased blood pressure
    b. Decreased salivation
    c. Increased bronchial secretions
    d. Mydriasis
    e. Urinary retention

18. The patient has been prescribed bethanechol and is experiencing decreased urinary output. Which action would be a priority by the nurse?
    a. Catheterize the patient to drain the bladder and measure output.
    b. Encourage the patient to increase fluid intake to increase urinary output.
    c. Encourage the patient to relax when urinating.
    d. Notify the health care provider with current intake and output values.

19. The patient has been taking bethanechol and is experiencing flushing, sweating, nausea, and abdominal cramps. Which action would be best for the nurse to take?
    a. Document the patient manifestations.
    b. Give the patient a laxative.
    c. Increase the patient's fluid intake.
    d. Obtain an order to administer atropine.

20. Which drug treats myasthenia gravis by increasing muscle strength?
    a. Bethanechol
    b. Edrophonium chloride
    c. Neostigmine bromide
    d. Pilocarpine

21. The nurse is taking care of five patients in the emergency department. A patient with which disorder would receive atropine? **Select all that apply**.
    a. Surgery for appendicitis
    b. A heart rate of 38 beats/minute and dizziness
    c. Paralytic ileus
    d. Urinary retention
    e. Gastric ulcers

22. The nurse would question a prescription for atropine if prescribed for a patient with which disorder?
    a. Peptic ulcer
    b. Parkinsonism
    c. Cirrhosis
    d. Narrow-angle glaucoma

23. The patient with a new diagnosis of peptic ulcers was prescribed propantheline. Which substance would the nurse teach that is a priority?
   a. Calcium
   b. Fat
   c. Fiber
   d. Protein

24. Which teaching point would the nurse include for a patient taking hyoscyamine for irritable bowel syndrome? **Select all that apply**.
   a. Ensure adequate fluid intake.
   b. Do not drive until you are aware of how this drug will affect your vision.
   c. Sucking on hard candy may help with dry mouth.
   d. Increased sweating is a common side effect.
   e. Report a rapid heart rate to your health care provider.

25. Anticholinergic drugs are contraindicated in patients with which disorder? **Select all that apply**.
   a. Coronary artery disease
   b. Diabetes mellitus
   c. Gastrointestinal obstruction
   d. Supraventricular tachycardia

26. A specific group of anticholinergics may be prescribed in the early treatment of which neuromuscular disorder?
   a. Multiple sclerosis
   b. Muscular dystrophy
   c. Myasthenia gravis
   d. Parkinsonism

27. The older adult patient is taking benztropine for symptoms associated with Parkinsonism. The nurse would instruct the patient to report which clinical manifestation(s) to the health care provider? **Select all that apply**.
   a. Diarrhea
   b. Dizziness
   c. Hallucinations
   d. Hyperthermia
   e. Palpitations

CASE STUDY: CRITICAL THINKING

Read the scenario and answer the following questions on a separate sheet of paper.

A 65-year-old patient received a prescription for tolterodine tartrate for the treatment of urinary incontinence.

1. Describe the mechanism of action for tolterodine?

2. Identify some of the major side effects of tolterodine.

3. Discuss some of its contraindications for tolterodine tartrate.

4. Discuss key teaching points for the nurse to provide when educating the patient.

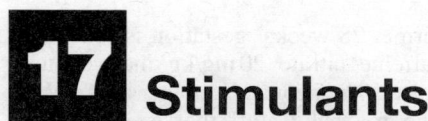

17 Stimulants

Complete the following.

1. The central nervous system (CNS) involves the _____ and the _____.

2. Attention-deficit/hyperactivity disorder (ADHD) can be caused by a _____ of neurotransmitters.

3. Amphetamines stimulate the release of neurotransmitters _____ and _____, and can lead to cardiovascular problems.

4. Anorexiants have a/an _____ effect on the brain to _____ _____.

5. CNS stimulants, also referred to as _____, stimulate respiration.

REVIEW QUESTIONS

Select the best response.

6. Which medical condition is CNS stimulant approved to treat? **Select all that apply**.
   a. ADHD
   b. Anorexia
   c. Narcolepsy
   d. Obesity
   e. Posttraumatic stress disorder

7. An adult patient has been prescribed methylphenidate for the treatment of narcolepsy. Which priority teaching would be included for this patient? **Select all that apply**.
   a. Avoid operating hazardous equipment.
   b. Caffeine should be avoided.
   c. Nervousness and tremors may occur.
   d. Take the medication before meals.
   e. Report any weight gain.

8. Which drug group acts on the brainstem and medulla to stimulate respiration?
   a. Amphetamine
   b. Analeptic
   c. Anorexiant
   d. Triptan

9. An adolescent patient is being treated with methylphenidate for ADHD. Which common effect would the nurse inform the patient and caregivers might occur? **Select all that apply**.
   a. Euphoria
   b. Headache
   c. Hypertension
   d. Irritability
   e. Hypotension
   f. Vomiting

10. To maintain the half-life of immediate-release methylphenidate, how often would this drug be taken?
    a. Daily
    b. 2–3 times a day
    c. 4 times a day
    d. Every other day

11. The patient has been prescribed phentermine hydrochloride for obesity. The patient also has Parkinson's disease and takes selegiline. Which nursing action would the nurse do before the patient starts the new drug?
    a. Contact the patient's primary health care provider to verify the prescription.
    b. Have baseline lab work drawn to assess liver function.
    c. Tell the patient to immediately stop taking the selegiline.
    d. Tell the patient to increase fluid intake with the next meal.

12. An overweight patient has a history of migraines, depression, and hypertension and has been started on phentermine-topiramate. For which condition is phentermine-topiramate used?
    a. ADHD
    b. Asthma
    c. Narcolepsy
    d. Short-term weight management

13. The pediatric patient has been started on methylphenidate for ADHD. Which information would the nurse include in the health teaching?
    a. Constipation is a common side effect.
    b. Counseling should be combined with drug.
    c. This drug will only be used for a few weeks.
    d. Weight gain is to be expected.

14. Which statement is true of methylphenidate? **Select all that apply**.
    a. If taken with monoamine oxidase inhibitors, it may increase a hypertensive crisis.
    b. The effects of anticoagulants may increase.
    c. Hyperglycemia may occur.
    d. Insulin will be more effective.
    e. There may be increased effects if taken with caffeinated beverages.

15. An 18-year-old patient is brought to the emergency department by the roommates. Blood pressure is 220/136 mm Hg, heart rate 142 beats/minute, and respiratory rate 26 breaths/minute. The patient is responsive only to deep pain. The patient's roommates report the patient was trying to lose weight and has been taking "these pills obtained over the Internet." Which medical condition would the nurse consider as the most likely cause for this patient's symptoms?
    a. Cardiac arrest
    b. Food poisoning
    c. Hemorrhagic stroke
    d. Pregnancy-induced hypertension

16. Central nervous system stimulants are absolutely contraindicated for patients with a history of which condition? **Select all that apply**.
    a. Coronary artery disease
    b. Diabetes
    c. Hypothyroidism
    d. Uncontrolled hypertension
    e. Glaucoma

17. A neonate born at 28 weeks' gestation is scheduled to receive caffeine citrate 20 mg/kg intravenously shortly after birth. The neonate's mother asks, "Why are you giving my baby stuff that is in coffee?" Which statement made by the nurse would be most appropriate?
    a. "Caffeine can help your baby breathe better."
    b. "It will help your baby gain weight faster."
    c. "The baby's temperature will be warmer with caffeine."
    d. "This is not the same substance that is in coffee."

CASE STUDY: CRITICAL THINKING

Read the scenario, and answer the following questions on a separate sheet of paper.

A new nurse started at a school where more than 75 students take methylphenidate for ADHD. The majority of the students come in between 11:30 am and 12:30 pm for their medication.

1. Describe the pharmacokinetic and pharmacodynamics profile for methylphenidate.

2. Discuss the nursing implications for giving methylphenidate at school regarding timing, monitoring, and health teaching for the students, family members, and teachers?

18 Depressants

STUDY QUESTIONS

Identify the induction time for the following anesthetics—slow or rapid:

1. Halothane _____

2. Enflurane _____

3. Midazolam _____

4. Propofol _____

5. Nitrous oxide _____

Complete the following.

6. The broad classification of CNS depressants includes the following seven groups: _____, _____, _____, _____, _____, _____, and _____.

7. The two phases of sleep are _____ and _____.

8. The mildest form of CNS depression is _____.

9. Anesthesia (may/may not) be achieved with high doses of sedative-hypnotics. *(Circle correct answer.)*

10. Procaine hydrochloride is used in local anesthesia as a short/moderate/long-acting anesthetic. *(Circle correct answer.)*

11. General anesthesia depresses the _____ system, alleviates _____, and causes a loss of _____.

12. Surgery is performed during the _____ stage of anesthesia. The other three stages are _____, _____, and _____.

13. Bupivacaine and tetracaine are drugs commonly used for _____ anesthesia.

14. A major potential adverse effect of spinal anesthesia is _____.

15. A type of spinal anesthesia used for patients in labor is a(n) _____.

16. Muscle relaxants (are/are not) part of balanced anesthesia. *(Circle correct answer.)*

17. Barbiturates that are used to induce sleep in those who have difficulty falling sleep are _____-acting.

18. One example of a nonbarbiturate, nonbenzodiazepine drug for the treatment of insomnia includes _____ and _____. *(Answers may vary.)*

19. The drug of choice for the management of benzodiazepine overdose is _____.

20. Local anesthetics are divided into two groups: _____ and _____.

Match the common side effects of sedative-hypnotics in Column I with the description in Column II.

Column I

_____ 21. Hangover

_____ 22. REM rebound

_____ 23. Dependence

_____ 24. Tolerance

_____ 25. Respiratory depression

_____ 26. Hypersensitivity

Column II

a. Need to increase dosage to get desired effect
b. Suppression of respiratory center in the medulla
c. Skin rashes
d. Residual drowsiness
e. Results in withdrawal symptoms
f. Vivid dreams and nightmares

REVIEW QUESTIONS

Select the best response.

27. Which class of drug is the most commonly prescribed drug to assist patients with sleep disorders?
    a. Analeptic
    b. Anesthetic
    c. Sedative-hypnotic
    d. Triptan

28. Which drugs would most likely be prescribed to control seizures?
    a. Intermediate-acting barbiturates
    b. Long-acting barbiturates
    c. Short-acting barbiturates
    d. Ultrashort-acting barbiturates

29. A patient returns to the unit after having surgery with spinal anesthesia. Which action would the nurse take to decrease the possibility of spinal headache? **Select all that apply.**
    a. Administer morphine 1–2 mg intravenously (IV).
    b. Ambulate the patient as soon as she regains sensation.
    c. Encourage the patient to stay flat in bed.
    d. Increase fluid intake.
    e. Position the patient in high-Fowler's position.

30. The patient who will be receiving spinal anesthesia for surgery is positioned with the back arched. The patient asks "Why do I have to sit a certain way? Why can't I just be comfortable?" Which statement would be best for the nurse to provide to the patient?
    a. "It is easier for the anesthesiologist if you sit this way."
    b. "Because of your age, you have to sit straight up."
    c. "The anesthesia is injected in a specific area so it distributes evenly."
    d. "You can sit however you like."

31. The patient is postoperative day 3 from major orthopedic surgery and is unable to sleep. If nonpharmacologic measures have not been effective, which drug would the nurse anticipate may be prescribed?
    a. Flumazenil
    b. Phenobarbital
    c. Triazolam
    d. Zolpidem

32. Which type(s) of anesthesia is/are administered using lidocaine? **Select all that apply.**
    a. General
    b. Inhaled
    c. Intravenous
    d. Local
    e. Spinal

33. The patient works 12-hour night shifts 1 week and 12-hour day shifts the following week. The patient tells the nurse that "some kind of sleeping pill from the drugstore" is used to help with sleep. Which main ingredient would the nurse suspect is contained in the over-the-counter medication to facilitate sleep?
    a. Antihistamines
    b. Barbiturates
    c. Benzodiazepines
    d. Opioid agonists

34. The 71-year-old patient presents to the healthcare provider with complaints of inability to go to sleep and inability to stay asleep. Which question would the nurse ask to further evaluate the complaint? **Select all that apply.**
    a. "What is your bedtime routine?"
    b. "How many caffeinated beverages do you drink per day?"
    c. "Do you take naps?"
    d. "Do you sleep with the windows open?"
    e. "Are you taking diuretics?"

CASE STUDY: CRITICAL THINKING

Read the scenario and answer the following questions on a separate sheet of paper.

A 42-year-old patient is scheduled for a laparoscopic cholecystectomy. The patient has had bad experiences with anesthesia before and is very anxious.

1. Identify the drugs the patient might be prescribed for anxiety before the patient's surgery?

2. Explain the principles of balanced anesthesia.

19 Antiseizure Drugs

Match the seizure type in Column I with its definition in Column II.

_____ **1.** Absence seizure

_____ **2.** Partial seizure

_____ **3.** Generalized seizure

_____ **4.** Myoclonic seizure

_____ **5.** Simple seizure

a. Involves one hemisphere of the brain with no loss of consciousness

b. Can be focal or massive with jerky movements lasting 10 seconds or less

c. No loss of consciousness and can have a motor, sensory, autonomic, or psychic form

d. Loss of consciousness usually lasts less than 10 seconds; also called petit mal seizures

e. A seizure that involves both hemispheres of the brain with loss of consciousness

Complete the following.

6. To diagnose epilepsy, results of a(n) _____ are useful.

7. Seventy-five percent of all epilepsy is primary or _____.

8. The International Classification of Seizures describes the two categories of seizures as _____ and _____.

9. Antiseizure drugs suppress abnormal electrical impulses, thus _____ the seizure, but they (do/do not) eliminate the cause. *(Circle the correct answer.)*

10. Antiseizure drugs (are/are not) used for all types of seizures. *(Circle the correct answer.)*

11. The first anticonvulsant used to treat seizures was _____, discovered in 1938, and continues to be the most commonly used drug for seizures.

12. It is strongly recommended that the patient check with the healthcare provider before taking _____ products.

13. Administration of phenytoin via the (oral/intramuscular/intravenous) route is not recommended because of its erratic absorption rate. *(Circle the correct answer.)*

REVIEW QUESTIONS

Select the best response.

14. The patient with a history of bipolar disorder recently experienced tonic-clonic seizures. Which drug would the nurse expect to be prescribed for this patient? **Select all that apply**.
    a. Carbamazepine
    b. Pregabalin
    c. Diazepam
    d. Ethosuximide
    e. Acetazolamide

15. The patient, who has a seizure disorder, just discovered that she is pregnant. At her first prenatal visit, she tells the nurse, "I quit taking all of my drugs because I don't want anything to be wrong with my baby." Which response would be most appropriate by the nurse?
    a. "You can't do that. You have to take your medications."
    b. "What drugs have been prescribed for you?"
    c. "How long have you had seizures?"
    d. "When was your last seizure?"

16. Which anticonvulsant is appropriate for status epilepticus? **Select all that apply**.
    a. Fosphenytoin
    b. Carbamazepine
    c. Phenobarbital
    d. Diazepam
    e. Topiramate

17. The patient has just been diagnosed with epilepsy and will be starting phenytoin. The patient's spouse asks how this drug works in the body. Which response is most appropriate by the nurse?
    a. "It inhibits the enzyme that destroys one of the neurotransmitters."
    b. "It helps stop the entry of sodium into the cell."
    c. "It has not been determined exactly how it prevents seizures."
    d. "It increases the amount of calcium that enters the cell."

18. The patient has just been diagnosed with a seizure disorder and has been started on valproic acid. Which statement by the patient indicates more instruction regarding the drug is needed? **Select all that apply**.
    a. "I just have to remember to take it once a day."
    b. "I do not have to worry about labs."
    c. "I need to take it at the same time every day."
    d. "This drug will cure my seizures."
    e. "I can take the drug with food."

19. The nurse has received an order to administer an initial dose of intravenous (IV) phenytoin to a patient with new-onset seizures. Which assessment would the nurse check before administering the first dose? **Select all that apply**.
    a. Hourly urine output
    b. Blood glucose levels
    c. Cardiac rhythm
    d. Blood pressure
    e. IV site

20. The patient receiving intravenous (IV) phenytoin for grand mal seizures complains of burning at the IV site. Which nursing action would be most appropriate?
    a. Call the health care provider immediately to change the drug to oral.
    b. Continue the infusion and reassure the patient.
    c. Flush the line with 10 mL of normal saline and continue the infusion.
    d. Discontinue the IV and restart the IV infusion at a different site.

21. A patient was started on an antiseizure drug for a seizure disorder of unknown cause and asks how long the drug will need to be taken. Which response would be appropriate by the nurse?
    a. "You will need to take an anticonvulsant of some type for your lifetime."
    b. "This drug should be taken until you haven't had a seizure for a month."
    c. "Seizures are unpredictable and so is the duration of the treatment."
    d. "You will only need to take it for a short period of time because antiseizures will cure the seizure disorder."

22. Which result is within the therapeutic range for phenytoin?
    a. 8 mcg/mL of bound phenytoin
    b. 18 mcg/mL of bound phenytoin
    c. 28 mcg/mL of unbound phenytoin
    d. 38 mcg/mL of unbound phenytoin

23. Which information would the nurse document after witnessing a patient having seizure? **Select all that apply**.
    a. Types of movements
    b. Duration of movements
    c. Ability to stop movements
    d. Progression of movements
    e. Preceding events

24. The nurse is preparing discharge teaching for a patient who has been started on phenytoin for a seizure disorder. Which information about the side effects of this drug would the nurse provide to the patient and family member?
    a. "There may be a green discoloration of the patient's urine."
    b. "It is best to use a hard-bristle toothbrush for dental care."
    c. "Nosebleeds and sore throats should be reported to the health care provider."
    d. "The patient should get up slowly to prevent fainting."

25. Which effect would the nurse expect to see if the patient is experiencing a common side effect of phenytoin?
    a. Gingival hyperplasia
    b. Excessive thirst
    c. Weight gain
    d. Muscle tremors

26. A patient presents to the emergency department in status epilepticus. Which drug would the nurse anticipate being prescribed first?
    a. Diazepam
    b. Midazolam
    c. Propofol
    d. Phenobarbital

27. Which statement is true about seizures and antiseizure uses in pregnancy? **Select all that apply**.
    a. Seizures may increase up to 33% in women with history of seizures.
    b. Many antiseizure drugs have teratogenic properties.
    c. Antiseizure drug use increases the loss of folic acid.
    d. Antiseizure drugs increase the effects of vitamin K.
    e. Valproic acid causes malformation in 40%–80% of fetuses.

28. Which antiseizure drug may also be used as prophylaxis for migraine headaches?
    a. Diazepam
    b. Phenytoin
    c. Valproic acid
    d. Clorazepate

CLINICAL JUDGMENT UNFOLDING CASE STUDY

Phase 1
Question 1:
SLO: Apply knowledge of abnormal test results in patients experiencing seizure activity
NGN Item Type: Highlight Text
Cognitive Skills: Recognize Cues

A 30-year-old female who has a history of type 1 diabetes and emphysema was found unconscious in a swimming pool. Cardiopulmonary resuscitation (CPR) was initiated and continued enroute to the emergency department (ED). With each chest compression, water was expelled from the lungs. After 20 minutes of CPR, the patient's cardiopulmonary status was restored While having blood drawn for labs, the patient started having sustained dysrhythmic bilateral muscle contractions. Diazepam 5 mg and phenytoin 30 mg/kg intravenously was administered. Patient weighs 174 pounds. Test results are as follows:

- CT of the head was unremarkable
- 12-lead electrocardiogram (ECG) showed atrial fibrillation with ventricular rate of 135 beats per minute
- Hemoglobin 14 g/dL
- Hematocrit 40%
- White blood cells 5000 cells/mcL
- Serum sodium 130 mEq/L
- Serum potassium 3.8 mEq/L
- Chest x-ray with ground-glass opacities bilaterally
- Abdomen distended
- Arterial blood gas revealed pH 7.28, pCO$_2$ 52 mm Hg, HCO$_3$ 18 mEq/L

Highlight the assessment findings that require follow-up by the nurse.

Question 2:
SLO: Compare the different seizure classifications and their treatment
NGN Item Type: Cloze
Cognitive Skills: Analyze Cues

A 30-year-old female who has a history of type 1 diabetes and emphysema was found unconscious in a swimming pool. Cardiopulmonary resuscitation (CPR) was initiated and continued enroute to the emergency department (ED). With each chest compression, water was expelled from the lungs. After 20 minutes of CPR, the patient's cardiopulmonary status was restored. While having blood drawn for labs, the patient started having sustained dysrhythmic bilateral muscle contractions. Diazepam 5 mg and phenytoin 30 mg/kg intravenously was administered. Patient weighs 174 pounds. Test results are as follows:

- CT of the head was unremarkable
- 12-lead electrocardiogram (ECG) showed atrial fibrillation with ventricular rate of 135 beats per minute
- Hemoglobin 14 g/dL
- Hematocrit 40%
- White blood cells 5000 cells/mcL
- Serum sodium 130 mEq/L
- Serum potassium 3.8 mEq/L
- Chest x-ray with ground-glass opacities bilaterally
- Abdomen distended
- Arterial blood gas revealed pH 7.28, pCO$_2$ 52 mm Hg, HCO$_3$ 18 mEq/L, O$_2$ saturation 86%

Choose the most likely options for the missing information from the statements below by selecting from the lists of options provided. Note that not all the responses will be used.

Based on the scenario, the patient's abnormal test results are most likely related to her ___1___. Muscle contractions that are dysrhythmic bilaterally indicates the patient is experiencing __2____ seizure activities. ___3___ is an example of a benzodiazepine and __3____ is a hydantoin. The total amount of phenytoin the patient would receive is ___4___ mg.

Options for 1	Options for 2	Options for 3	Options for 4
Emphysema	Tonic-clonic	Phenytoin	30
Diabetes	Partial	Clonidine	2373
Drowning	Myoclonic	Morphine	2610
Cardiopulmonary resuscitation efforts	Atonia	Diazepam	

Phase 2
Question 3:
SLO: Prioritize patient care in persons who have seizure disorder
NGN Item Type: Multiple Response Select All That Apply
Cognitive Skills: Prioritize Hypotheses

A 30-year-old female who has a history of type 1 diabetes and emphysema was found unconscious in a swimming pool. After a successful cardiopulmonary resuscitation (CPR), she experienced a tonic-clonic seizure activity in which she was given diazepam 5 mg and fosphenytoin 1186 mg intravenously. Initial CT of the head was unremarkable, and her arterial blood gas revealed acidemia. She is "weak and tired" and complains of "hurting all over." She also has productive cough. She experienced two more episodes of bilateral dysrhythmic muscular contractions and was given additional diazepam and phenytoin IV. Which **priority** potential complications would the nurse monitor?

a. Acute pain
b. Anxiety
c. Aspiration
d. Chronic obstructive pulmonary disease
e. Falls
f. Hyperglycemia
g. Myocardial infarction
h. Respiratory depression
i. Sepsis
j. Tissue hypoxia

Question 4:
SLO: Determine appropriate actions for patients taking antiseizure drugs
NGN Item Type: Matrix Multiple Choice
Cognitive Skills: Generate Solutions

A 30-year-old female who has a history of type 1 diabetes and emphysema was treated for seizure disorder. She is now 2 days without seizure activity. Phenytoin is converted to oral preparation. The patient tells the nurse that she is getting married in 2 weeks and wants to have children.
For each patient's concern/question, select the appropriate nurse's response from the first column. Note that not all responses will be used.

Nurse's Response	Patient's Question	Appropriate Nurse's Response
"Phenytoin can cause blood sugars to increase, not decrease. You may need to increase your insulin dose."	"I really do not want to take more medicine for the seizures."	
"Yes, you will need to decrease your insulin since phenytoin can cause hypoglycemia."	"How long will I need to be taking the medicine?"	
"I'm glad you told me about your urine. Tests need to be done to see where you are bleeding."	"Will I be able to get pregnant while on the medicine?"	
"Yes you can become pregnant while on this drug. It should not affect your baby."	"Will I need to decrease my insulin while on this medicine?"	
"Usually, persons with seizures are on antiseizure medicines for the rest of their life. But, if the person has been seizure free for 3–5 years, the doctor may stop the medicine."	"My urine is reddish in color. Does this medicine cause me to bleed?"	
"Be sure to discuss this with your doctor. Phenytoin can harm the fetus so a different antiseizure medication may be needed."		

Nurse's Response	Patient's Question	Appropriate Nurse's Response
"Phenytoin can cause your urine to turn pinkish-red or reddish-brown in color. This is normal and does not indicate you are bleeding."		
"As long as you are without seizures, you do not need to take the medicine."		
"The antiseizure medications help prevent abnormal electrical impulses in your brain."		

Phase 3

Question 5:

SLO: Select the appropriate nursing actions for patients receiving antiseizure drugs

NGN Item Type: Matrix Multiple Choice

Cognitive Skills: Take Action

A 30-year-old female has been in the hospital for 5 days for drowning incident and acute seizure activities. She also has type 1 diabetes and emphysema. The patient is to be discharged and the nurse is planning discharge teaching. The patient is prescribed phenytoin 100 mg orally three times a day. She is to resume her medications prior to hospitalization, which include insulin, albuterol/ipratropium metered dose inhaler, and oral contraceptive. **Use an X for the discharge teaching below that is Indicated (appropriate or necessary) or Contraindicated (could be harmful).**

Discharge Teaching	Indicated	Contraindicated
"Decrease your insulin dosage by 4 units since phenytoin can cause hypoglycemia."		
"Have dental checkups on a regular basis. Phenytoin can cause overgrowth of your gums."		
"You will need routine labs to monitor the drug level."		
"It is normal if you develop nose bleeds."		
"You will need to eat a high-fat diet while you are on phenytoin for better drug action."		
"Check your blood sugars more frequently."		

Question 6:

SLO: Evaluate patient's assessment findings to determine the effectiveness of antiseizure drug

NGN Item Type: Matrix Multiple Choice

Cognitive Skills: Evaluate Outcomes

A 30-year-old female has been in the hospital for 5 days for drowning incident and acute seizure activities. She also has type 1 diabetes and emphysema. The patient is to be discharged and the nurse is planning discharge teaching. The patient is prescribed phenytoin 100 mg orally 3 times a day. She is to resume her medications prior to hospitalization, which include insulin, albuterol/ipratropium metered dose inhaler, and oral contraceptive. **For each assessment finding, use an X to indicate whether nursing and collaborative interventions were Effective (helped meet expected outcomes) or Ineffective (did not meet expected outcomes).**

Assessment Finding	Effective	Ineffective
Fingerstick blood sugar 98 mg/dL		
Patient states "I do not need to worry about getting pregnant since I am on the pill."		
Blood pressure 94/50 mm Hg		
Phenytoin drug level 17 mcg/mL		
Abdomen nondistended, active bowel sounds, and nontender		
Gait even, smooth, and controlled		

20 Drugs for Parkinsonism and Alzheimer Disease

STUDY QUESTIONS

Match the description in Column II with the letter of the reference in Column I.

Column I

_____ **1.** Acetylcholinesterase (AChE) inhibitor

_____ **2.** Dopamine agonist

_____ **3.** Dystonic movement

_____ **4.** Bradykinesia

_____ **5.** Pseudo parkinsonism

Column II

a. Stimulates dopamine receptors
b. Drug-induced parkinsonism
c. Allows more acetylcholine in the neuron receptors
d. Involuntary abnormal movements
e. Slowed movements

Complete the following.

6. The two neurotransmitters within the neurons of the striatum of the brain that have opposing effects are _____ and _____.

7. Which neurotransmitters are deficient in Parkinson disease? _____

8. A drug used in a combination therapy to treat Parkinson disease by replacing the neurotransmitter is _____.

9. The substance that inhibits the enzyme dopa decarboxylase and allows more levodopa to reach the brain is _____.

10. An example of an acetylcholinesterase inhibitor is _____.

11. Acetylcholinesterase inhibitors _____ transmission at the cholinergic synapses.

12. The drug _____ prolongs action of levodopa and can decrease "on-off" fluctuations in patients with parkinsonism.

13. The drugs that are a combination of dopaminergic and a catechol-*O*-methyltransferase (COMT) inhibitor that provides the greatest dosing flexibility include _____, _____, and _____.

14. An example of a Food and Drug Administration (FDA)-approved anticholinergic drug used for Parkinson disease is _____.

15. Alzheimer disease is reversible/irreversible. (*Circle the correct response.*)

16. Patients with Alzheimer disease have deficient neurotransmitter _____.

17. Donepezil and rivastigmine are examples of _____ _____.

18. Aducanumab and lecanemab are examples of _____ _____ _____.

Select the best response.

19. A patient taking carbidopa-levodopa tablets for parkinsonism is complaining of dizziness, diarrhea, anxiety, and nasal stuffiness. Which complaints would the nurse recognize as a possible side effect of carbidopa-levodopa?
    a. Dizziness
    b. Diarrhea
    c. Anxiety
    d. Nasal stuffiness

20. The nurse is teaching a patient with parkinsonism about extended-release carbidopa-levodopa. Which statement by the patient indicates the need for further teaching? **Select all that apply.**
    a. "This drug may make my movements smoother."
    b. "My skin may turn yellow if I miss too many doses."
    c. "If I have trouble swallowing, I can crush my drug and mix it with applesauce."
    d. "I must take this medicine on an empty stomach."
    e. "I need to check my blood sugar regularly while taking this drug."

21. The nurse is helping a family prepare for a grocery shopping trip for a patient who has been prescribed selegiline for Parkinson disease. Which food item would the family avoid purchasing? **Select all that apply.**
    a. Aged cheeses
    b. Chocolate
    c. Peanut butter
    d. Wheat bread
    e. Yogurt

22. A patient with Alzheimer disease is taking rivastigmine and has also been started on a drug for depression. Which medication would the nurse question before administering the new drug?
    a. Atypical antidepressant
    b. Monoamine oxidase inhibitor (MAOI) antidepressant
    c. Selective serotonin reuptake inhibitor (SSRI) antidepressant
    d. Tricyclic antidepressant

23. A patient with parkinsonism currently takes carbidopa-levodopa, and the patient's health care provider adds entacapone to the drug regimen. Which change in the dosing of carbidopa-levodopa would the nurse expect to occur?
    a. There should be no change in the drug dosage.
    b. Both carbidopa and levodopa dosages should be decreased.
    c. Only the levodopa dosage should decrease.
    d. Only the carbidopa dosage should decrease.

24. Anticholinergics are contraindicated for patients with which disorder?
    a. Glaucoma
    b. Shingles
    c. Urinary frequency
    d. Diabetes
    e. Angina

25. A patient who was prescribed antiparkinson medication is brought into the emergency department after the family reports the patient is talking to "rabbits coming out of the walls" at home. Which drug would the nurse suspect may be causing this symptom? **Select all that apply.**
    a. Bromocriptine
    b. Selegiline
    c. Pramipexole
    d. Tolcapone

26. A patient's wandering and hostility levels have increased per family reports. Which dosing information would concern the nurse in this patient who is taking memantine 10 mg/day?
    a. The dose is too high a daily dose to maintain mental status.
    b. The patient has taken an overdose of the drug.
    c. The patient is not taking enough of the drug.
    d. A combination of memantine and amantadine may be needed.

27. Which statement by the patient indicates an understanding of how to relieve some of the side effects associated with the use of benztropine mesylate?
    a. "I can suck on hard candy or chew sugarless gum to prevent dry mouth."
    b. "I need to take my drug every 6 hours so I don't get constipated."
    c. "I should decrease the doses of all of my other drugs so I don't get dizzy."
    d. "I should urinate after meals so I do not retain urine."

CLINICAL JUDGMENT UNFOLDING CASE STUDY

Phase 1
Question 1:
SLO: Differentiate between Parkinson and Alzheimer disease
NGN Item Type: Highlight Text
Cognitive Skills: Recognize Cues

An 88-year-old male, who lives alone in an assisted living facility, told his daughter that he fell but did not "hurt anything." Because of the daughter's concerns of her father's fall, she accompanies him to his appointment with his healthcare provider. The nurse documents the following assessment:

- Awake, alert, oriented
- Blood pressure 123/72 mm Hg
- Heart rate 87 beats per minute
- History of 3 falls in the last 6 months with ecchymoses in various stages of healing to legs and arms
- Masked facial expressions
- Mild resting tremors to hands bilaterally
- Patient reports his feet "drags the floor"
- Positive for cogwheel rigidity

Highlight the assessment finding that would require follow-up by the nurse.

Question 2:
SLO: Apply knowledge of Parkinson disease and its neurotransmitters causing changes to patient's physical movement.
NGN Item Type: Drop-Down Cloze
Cognitive Skills: Analyze Cues

An 88-year-old male, who lives alone in an assisted living facility, told his daughter that he fell but did not "hurt anything." Because of the daughter's concerns of her father's fall, she accompanies him to his appointment with his health care provider. The nurse documents the following assessment:

- Awake, alert, oriented
- Blood pressure 123/72 mm Hg
- Heart rate 87 beats per minute
- History of 3 falls in the last 6 months with ecchymoses in various stages of healing to legs and arms
- Masked facial expressions
- Mild resting tremors to hands bilaterally
- Patient reports his feet "drags the floor"
- Positive for cogwheel rigidity

Based on the assessment, the nurse determines the patient's symptoms are related to an imbalance of the neurotransmitters _____1_____ (inhibitory) and ____2_____ (excitatory). The levels of dopamine are____3____ and acetylcholine are ____4___, which stimulates the release of ____5____.

Options for 1	Options for 2	Options for 3	Options for 4	Options for 5
Acetylcholine	Acetylcholine	Absent	Absent	Acetylcholine
Dopamine	Dopamine	Decreased	Decreased	Dopamine
Gamma-aminobutyric acid	Gamma-aminobutyric acid	Increased	Increased	Gamma-aminobutyric acid
Levodopa	Levodopa			Levodopa

Phase 2
Question 3:
SLO: Prioritize nursing care for patients with Parkinson Disease
NGN Item Type: Multiple Response Select All That Apply
Cognitive Skills: Prioritize Hypotheses

An 88-year-old male, who lives alone in an assisted living facility, had multiple falls due to movement disorders. The patient is diagnosed with Parkinson disease and was started on carbidopa-levodopa 25/100 mg daily. His medical history includes hypertension and diabetes type 2. Medications he routinely takes include lisinopril/hydrochlorothiazide 10/12.5 mg daily, calcium/vitamin D supplements, and metformin ER 500 mg daily. His blood pressure is 123/72 mm Hg and his heart rate is 87 beats per minute. Labs which include complete blood count and chemistry panel were unremarkable except for mild anemia and serum glucose of 110 mg/dL.

When teaching the patient and his daughter about the new medication, the nurse would place a *priority* to which potential complications? Select all that apply.

- Diarrhea
- Falls
- Functional ability
- Gastrointestinal distress
- Hyperglycemia
- Hypotension

Questions 4:
SLO: Plan actions when caring for patients prescribed antiparkinson drugs
NGN Item Type: Multiple Response Select All That Apply
Cognitive Skills: Generate Solutions

An 88-year-old male, who lives alone in an assisted living facility, had multiple falls due to movement disorders. The patient is diagnosed with Parkinson disease and was started on carbidopa-levodopa 25/100 mg daily. While preparing the medication, the patient reports having "nausea 30 minutes after taking the medicine" and that his "sweat seems to be darker."

Which nursing action would be indicated for patients taking carbidopa-levodopa? **Select all that apply**.

- Administer antinausea medication 30 minutes prior to administering antiparkinson drug
- Administer the medication with small amount of food

- Assess for orthostatic hypotension
- Instruct the patient to notify the nurse if urine becomes dark
- Monitor blood pressure for hypertension
- Observe patient's ability to perform activities of daily living, such as brushing teeth
- Obtain a finger stick blood sugar prior to administering the medicine
- Place patient as "high fall risk"

Phase 3
Question 5:
SLO: Determine appropriate nursing actions for patients prescribed antiparkinson drugs

NGN Item Type: Matrix Multiple Response
Cognitive Skills: Take Action

An 88-year-old male, who lives alone in an assisted living facility, had multiple falls due to movement disorders. The patient is diagnosed with Parkinson disease and was started on carbidopa-levodopa 25/100 mg daily. His home medications he routinely takes include lisinopril/hydrochlorothiazide 10/12.5 mg daily, calcium/vitamin D supplements, and metformin ER 500 mg daily.
For each potential complication in the second column, select the appropriate nursing action from the first column. Note that not all responses will be used.

Nursing Action	Potential Complication	Appropriate Nursing Action for Complication
Administer medicine with high protein food	Patient reports increased dizziness	
Administer antinausea medication	Falls	
Inform the patient this is harmless	Darkened area to clothing around the axillary region	
Check glucose for hyperglycemia	Patient report of increased head bobbing	
Consult case worker to assess home environment	Increased nausea with medicine	
Notify healthcare provider		
Provide small low-protein snack		
Check blood pressure with position changes (orthostasis)		

Question 6:
SLO: Evaluate the effectiveness of nursing interventions for patients on antiparkinson drugs
NGN Item Type: Highlight Text
Cognitive Skills: Evaluate Outcomes
Progress Notes:

An 88-year-old male patient is seen in the clinic for a 2-week follow-up post hospitalization due to frequent falls. The patient was prescribed carbidopa-levodopa 25/100 mg daily. Routine home medications of lisinopril/hydrochlorothiazide 10/12.5 mg daily, calcium/vitamin D supplements, and metformin ER 500 mg daily were resumed upon discharge. Daughter is present during the visit. Daughter reports patient with decreased appetite and has been "preparing protein shakes." Patient denies any dizziness or unusual weakness. Denies difficulty sleeping. Sitting blood pressure 132/88 mm Hg and pulse 64 beats per minute; standing blood pressure 110/62 mm Hg and pulse 80 beats/minute. The patient needs moderate assistance to stand. Flat facial expression, "pill-rolling" bilaterally, and head bobbing noted while in sitting position. Lungs clear throughout the area. Heart without abnormal heart tones. Apical pulses irregular with 60–84 beats/minute.

Highlight the assessment findings in the progress note that would indicate the patient is not progressing as indicated.

21 Drugs for Neuromuscular Disorders and Muscle Spasms

Match the classifications of multiple sclerosis (MS) in Column I with its characteristics in Column II.

Column I

_____ **1.** Relapsing remitting MS

_____ **2.** Primary progressive MS

_____ **3.** Secondary progressive MS

_____ **4.** Progressive relapsing MS

Column II

a. May have relapses, remissions, and plateaus
b. Relapse with full recovery and residual deficit
c. Clear acute relapses with or without full recovery
d. Will have slowly worsening symptoms with no relapses or remissions

Complete the following.

5. Muscle spasms can result from _____ injuries and spasticity from chronic _____ _____.

6. Muscle relaxants suppress the _____ reflex and are prescribed for muscle spasms that do not respond to _____ drugs or other forms of therapy.

7. Baclofen, dantrolene, and tizanidine are some drugs to _____ pain and _____ mobility for hyperexcitable, spastic muscles.

SHORT ANSWER QUESTIONS

Identify the affected neuromuscular site(s) for each of the autoimmune neuromuscular disorders and the drugs to treat the disorders.

8. Myasthenia gravis

9. Multiple sclerosis

Select the best response.

10. The nurse is assessing a patient who is receiving treatment for myasthenia gravis with pyridostigmine. Which clinical manifestations would be noted if the drug's action is therapeutic?
    a. Increased salivation
    b. Maintenance of muscle strength
    c. Miosis
    d. Tachycardia

11. The patient is receiving treatment for myasthenia gravis with an acetylcholinesterase (AChE) inhibitor. The nurse observes that the patient is diaphoretic, drooling, and eyes are tearing. The nurse would be most concerned about the patient exhibiting these clinical manifestations in which medical condition?
    a. Anaphylactic reaction
    b. Cholinergic crisis
    c. Early stages of myasthenic crisis
    d. Vascular spasm

12. Which emergency drug would be administered to a patient exhibiting signs of cholinergic crisis?
    a. Atropine
    b. Diazepam
    c. Neostigmine
    d. Pyridostigmine

13. The patient presents to the health care provider with complaints of double vision, headache, and muscle weakness. The patient states that these symptoms come and go every few weeks, but these "spells" seem to be getting closer together. Which diagnostic test is likely to be obtained if multiple sclerosis is considered?
    a. Angiography
    b. Computerized tomography (CT) scan
    c. Magnetic resonance imaging (MRI)
    d. Myelogram

14. The patient has been receiving pyridostigmine. Which drug when prescribed by the health care provider would the nurse question before administering to the patient?
    a. Histamine$_2$ blocker
    b. Propranolol
    c. Cephalosporin
    d. Tetracycline

15. The patient has been prescribed azathioprine and interferon-β for remissions and exacerbations of multiple sclerosis. The patient inquires, "How will this help me feel better?" Which response would be appropriate by the nurse?
    a. "New neurons and axons will form."
    b. "Your muscle strength will improve."
    c. "Spasticity will decrease and you will have improved muscle movement."
    d. "The disease will not progress."

16. The patient has multiple sclerosis and is experiencing muscle spasms. Centrally acting muscle relaxants improve spasms by which mechanism?
    a. Affect *mu* receptors to decrease pain.
    b. Decrease pain and increase range of motion.
    c. Decrease inflammation of the peripheral nerves.
    d. Speed conduction to improve flexibility.

17. The patient has been involved in a motor vehicle collision and has been prescribed methocarbamol for muscle spasms of the neck and back. Which side effect would the nurse discuss with the patient? **Select all that apply**.
    a. Urine discoloration
    b. Diarrhea
    c. Drowsiness
    d. Increased appetite

18. A nurse is preparing several medications for a patient. Which drug would the nurse seek clarification?
    a. Dantrolene sodium for muscle spasms
    b. Diazepam for narrow-angle glaucoma
    c. Acetylcholine receptor (AChR) antibody for diagnostic testing for myasthenia gravis
    d. Chlorzoxazone for muscle trauma

CLINICAL JUDGMENT STANDALONE CASE STUDY

Read the scenario and answer the following questions on a separate sheet of paper.

SLO: Prioritize care to patients with neuromuscular disorder
NGN Item Type: Drag and Drop
Cognitive Skills: Recognize Cues

A 24-years-old patient is admitted to the medical-surgical unit for a compound fracture to the right tibia and fibula from a parachute jumping accident. The patient is to remain NPO for surgery. Upon history intake, the nurse discovers the patient has a history of myasthenia gravis.

Highlight the findings in the Nurses' Notes and Vital Signs that are of immediate concern that requires immediate action by the nurse.

Health History	Nurses' Notes	Vital Signs	Laboratory Results
Medical History: Asthma and myasthenia gravis **Home Medications:** Pyridostigmine ER 180 mg bid Albuterol MDI PRN Ibuprofen 400 mg q8h			

Health History	Nurses' Notes	Vital Signs	Laboratory Results
1520: Post-op day 1. Splint to right leg dry and intact. 3 × 6 cm pinkish slightly wet area noted to right splint anteriorly mid foreleg. Toes pink with brisk cap refill. C/o "just feeling weak" and "no energy." Lungs clear throughout area. No chest pain. Speech slightly slurred. "My vision seems to be blurry." PERRL.			

Health History	Nurses' Notes	Vital Signs	Laboratory Results
1020: Temp: 100.9°F BP: 92/58 left brachial HR: 54 bpm, regular, left radial RR: 14 bpm SpO_2: 91% RA			

Chapter **21** **Drugs for Neuromuscular Disorders and Muscle Spasms**

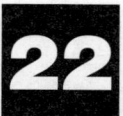

22 Antipsychotics and Anxiolytics

Match the term in Column I to the corresponding statement in Column II.

Column I

_____ **1.** Acute dystonia

_____ **2.** Akathisia

_____ **3.** Anxiolytics

_____ **4.** Neuroleptic

_____ **5.** Psychosis

_____ **6.** Schizophrenia

_____ **7.** Tardive dyskinesia

_____ **8.** Extrapyramidal symptoms

Column II

a. Losing contact with reality

b. Protrusion and rolling of the tongue, sucking and smacking movements of the lips, chewing motion

c. Muscle tremors, rigidity, shuffling gait

d. Restlessness, inability to sit still, foot-tapping

e. Spasms of tongue, face, neck, and back

f. Used to treat anxiety and insomnia

g. Drug that modifies psychotic behavior

h. Chronic psychotic disorder

Complete the following

9. Antipsychotic drugs were developed to improve the _____, _____, and _____ of patients with psychotic symptoms resulting from an imbalance of _____, a neurotransmitter.

10. Typical antipsychotics are subdivided into phenothiazines and nonphenothiazines. Nonphenothiazines are divided into four classes: _____, _____, _____, and _____.

11. The most common side effect of all antipsychotics is _____.

12. Antipsychotics may lead to dermatologic side effects early in drug therapy that include _____ and _____.

13. Phenothiazines (increase/decrease) the seizure threshold; adjustment of anticonvulsants may be required. *(Circle the correct answer.)*

14. Anxiolytics (are/are not) usually given for secondary anxiety. *(Circle the correct answer.)*

15. Long-term use of anxiolytics is not recommended because _____ may develop within weeks or months.

16. The action of anxiolytics resembles that of _____, not antipsychotics.

Match the following drugs in Column I with their drug classification in Column II. Drug classifications in Column II may be used more than once.

Column I

_____ 17. Clozapine

_____ 18. Chlorpromazine

_____ 19. Fluphenazine

_____ 20. Molindone hydrochloride

_____ 21. Haloperidol

_____ 22. Risperidone

Column II

a. Phenothiazine
b. Nonphenothiazine
c. Atypical antipsychotic

REVIEW QUESTIONS

Select the best response.

23. Neuroleptic drugs are useful in the management of which type of medical condition?
    a. Anxiety disorders
    b. Depressive disorders
    c. Psychotic disorders
    d. Psychosomatic disorders

24. A patient who was started on antipsychotic drugs asks the nurse when the drug will take effect. Which response is best by the nurse?
    a. "It may take up to one week to start to feel the full effects."
    b. "Responses vary, but it may be about 6 weeks."
    c. "You will only feel better when you start psychotherapy, too."
    d. "You should start to feel better within 30-60 minutes."

25. The patient has been started on chlorpromazine hydrochloride for treatment of intractable hiccups. Which information would the nurse include in patient education about this class of drug?
    a. "A therapeutic response to this drug will be immediate."
    b. "Change positions slowly from patient sitting to standing to prevent orthostatic hypotension."
    c. "It is all right to have alcohol when taking this drug."
    d. "This drug may be stopped abruptly as soon as your pain stops."

26. Typical antipsychotics may cause extrapyramidal symptoms (EPSs) or pseudoparkinsonism. Which symptom is considered an extrapyramidal symptom?
    a. Downward eye movement
    b. Intentional tremors
    c. Loss of hearing
    d. Shuffling gait

27. Which drug would the nurse expect to administer to decrease extrapyramidal symptoms (EPSs)?
    a. Benztropine
    b. Bethanechol
    c. Buspirone hydrochloride
    d. Doxepin

28. Phenothiazines are grouped into three categories based on their side effects. In which group is fluphenazine?
    a. Aliphatic
    b. Piperazine
    c. Piperidine
    d. Thioxanthene

29. The patient has been prescribed fluphenazine for the treatment of schizophrenia. Which information would the nurse include in the patient teaching for this drug? **Select all that apply.**
    a. "Blood pressure changes are not an indication of an adverse reaction."
    b. "It is all right to take any herbal drugs when taking fluphenazine."
    c. "Notify your health care provider if you have dizziness, headache, or nausea."
    d. "This medication must be taken every day."
    e. "You should not drink alcohol when taking this drug."

30. An 80-year-old patient with diminished renal and hepatic function is prescribed fluphenazine 5 mg every 8 hours for a newly diagnosed schizophrenia. Which statement is correct about the amount of the drug prescribed?
    a. The patient is an adult, and this is in the normal adult range.
    b. The patient's dose should be 10% less than the young and middle - adult dose.
    c. The patient's dose should be 25% to 50% less than the usual young and middle-adult dose.
    d. This drug is contraindicated in patients who are greater than 70 years old.

31. A patient presents to the emergency department with an overdose of chlorpromazine hydrochloride. Which action would be a priority for the nurse to take?
    a. Administer activated charcoal.
    b. Administer anticholinergic drugs.
    c. Establish an intravenous (IV) site.
    d. Maintain the airway.

32. A highly agitated and combative patient presents to the emergency department. The health care provider has ordered haloperidol 5 mg intramuscularly (IM). Which statement is correct about this medication as an antipsychotic?
    a. It has a sedative effect on agitated, combative patients.
    b. It is the drug of choice for older patients with liver disease.
    c. It will not cause extrapyramidal syndrome (EPS).
    d. It can safely be used in patients with narrow-angle glaucoma.

33. Which drug class consists of atypical antipsychotics?
    a. Butyrophenones
    b. Phenothiazines
    c. Serotonin/dopamine antagonists
    d. Thioxanthenes

34. The atypical antipsychotics have a weak affinity for the dopamine subtype 2 (D_2) receptors. Consequently, which outcome to the occurrence of EPS is correct?
    a. An absence of EPS
    b. An increase in EPS
    c. Fewer EPS
    d. No effect on EPS

35. Atypical antipsychotics have a stronger affinity for which type of dopamine subtype receptors that block serotonin receptors?
    a. D_1
    b. D_2
    c. D_3
    d. D_4

36. A young adult patient with bipolar disorder has just been prescribed risperidone. Which side effect would the nurse include in the health teaching about this drug?
    a. Hepatotoxicity
    b. Hyperglycemia
    c. Hearing loss
    d. Urinary frequency

37. The drug alprazolam belongs to which anxiolytic drug group?
    a. Antihistamines
    b. Benzodiazepines
    c. Buspirones
    d. Phenothiazines

38. A patient with which medical condition would fluphenazine be contraindicated? **Select all that apply**.
    a. Narrow-angle glaucoma
    b. Coma
    c. Subcortical brain damage
    d. Continued blood dyscrasias despite lowering dose
    e. Neuromuscular pain

39. Lorazepam is an anxiolytic drug; however, it may be prescribed for other purposes. For which other condition might it be prescribed? **Select all that apply**.
    a. Alcohol withdrawal
    b. Anxiety associated with depression
    c. Muscle spasms
    d. Preoperative induction
    e. Status epilepticus

CASE STUDY: CRITICAL THINKING

Read the scenario, and answer the following questions on a separate sheet of paper.

A young college student who have been cramming for final exams is brought to the emergency department. The patient's friends report that they have been unable to awaken the patient after sleeping for 18 hours. An empty bottle of clonazepam and a bottle of vodka were found at the bedside. Vital signs are temperature 99° F, heart rate 64 beats/minute, respiratory rate 8 breaths/minute, blood pressure 82/40 mm Hg, O_2 saturation 78% on room air. The patient is only responsive to deep pain.

1. Identify the drug class clonazepam belongs.

2. Describe the mechanism of action for clonazepam.

3. Discuss the side effects associated with this category of drug.

4. With the above history, discuss the concerns the nurse would have and the priority actions.

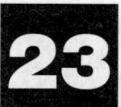# 23 Antidepressants and Mood Stabilizers

STUDY QUESTIONS

Answer the following questions as true or false. If false, make it into a true statement.

1. _____ Herbal supplements, such as St. John's wort, do not interact with selective serotonin reuptake inhibitors (SSRIs).

2. _____ Tyramine-rich foods include aged cheese, yogurt, and soy sauce.

3. _____ Monoamine oxidase inhibitors (MAOIs) are considered first-line therapy for depression.

4. _____ Amitriptyline is considered a serotonin norepinephrine reuptake inhibitor (SNRI).

5. _____ Causes of depression include decreased circulating neurotransmitter levels or the occurrence of major stressors such as the recent death of a family member.

Complete the following.

6. Clinical response of tricyclic antidepressants (TCAs) occurs after _____ of drug therapy.

7. TCAs _____ mood, _____ interest in daily living, and _____ insomnia.

8. Herbal supplements that can be used to treat mild depression include _____.

9. Atypical antidepressants or _____ _____ affect one or two of the three neurotransmitters: _____, _____, and _____.

10. Any drugs that _____ the _____ can cause a hypertensive crisis when taken with an MAOI.

11. _____ was the first drug used to treat _____ _____ disorder.

12. Lithium's therapeutic index has a _____ range from _____.

13. Nonsteroidal antiinflammatory drugs (NSAIDs) can _____ lithium level whereas _____ and _____ diuretics can _____ lithium levels.

14. SNRIs are used for major depression, _____, and _____.

15. Many antidepressants interact with _____ _____ that can lead to _____.

Match the drugs in Column I with the neurotransmitters affected in Column II. The neurotransmitters in Column II may be used more than once.

Column I

_____ **16.** Amitriptyline

_____ **17.** Fluoxetine

_____ **18.** Desvenlafaxine

_____ **19.** Doxepin

_____ **20.** Citalopram

_____ **21.** Duloxetine

_____ **22.** Selegiline

Column II

a. Dopamine
b. Norepinephrine
c. Serotonin

Match the drugs in Column I with their drug classification in Column II. The drug classifications in Column II may be used more than once.

Column I

_____ **23.** Trazodone

_____ **24.** Maprotiline

_____ **25.** Citalopram

_____ **26.** Amitriptyline

_____ **27.** Tranylcypromine

_____ **28.** Paroxetine

Column II

a. Atypical antidepressants
b. SSRIs
c. MAOIs
d. TCAs

REVIEW QUESTIONS

Select the best response.

29. Which drug would the nurse expect to administer to a young patient with enuresis?
    a. Citalopram
    b. Fluvoxamine
    c. Imipramine
    d. Sertraline

30. The patient has been taking phenelzine for several months for depression with minimal improvement. Which dose is the maximum daily dose for this drug?
    a. 15 mg/day
    b. 45 mg/day
    c. 60 mg/day
    d. 90 mg/day

31. The patient has been prescribed amitriptyline as an adjunct to therapy for depression. Which information would the nurse include in the health teaching regarding this drug?
    a. "Check your heart rate daily. It may become very slow."
    b. "Stand up slowly because your blood pressure can drop suddenly."
    c. "You should start to feel less depressed within 12 hours."
    d. "Take your drug in the morning because it will make you alert."

32. Which food or beverage is contraindicated in a patient that is prescribed isocarboxazid? **Select all that apply**.
    a. Bananas
    b. Chocolate
    c. Chicken
    d. Milk
    e. Wine

33. A patient who has been taking fluoxetine and "some herb" for depression is complaining of a severe headache. The patient is diaphoretic and restless. Which herb would the nurse suspect the patient has been taking?
    a. Ephedra
    b. Ginseng
    c. Garlic
    d. St. John's wort

34. Which effect is an advantage of taking SSRIs over TCAs?
    a. Fewer sexual side effects
    b. Increased appetite
    c. Less sedation
    d. Less tachycardia

35. Which nursing intervention is most important for a patient taking lithium?
    a. Advising the patient that the drug can be stopped when not in a manic phase.
    b. Emphasizing the importance of patient-adjusted dosage.
    c. Monitoring for excessive thirst, weight loss, and increased urination.
    d. Teaching the patient to limit fluid intake to prevent weight gain.

36. The patient is currently taking lithium for bipolar disorder, manic phase. Which laboratory value would the nurse monitor?
    a. BUN
    b. Blood glucose
    c. INR
    d. Platelet count

37. The patient has been taking lithium 1800 mg/day in three divided doses for 10 days. The patient remains agitated and hyperactive, with a lithium level of 0.7 mEq/L. Which patient condition would the nurse suspect is occurring?
    a. Lithium toxicity
    b. Subtherapeutic lithium level
    c. Therapeutic lithium level
    d. Allergy to lithium

38. The nurse is teaching the patient about lithium. Which statement by the patient indicates a need for more education?
    a. "I can stop my drug if I have not been manic for 2 weeks."
    b. "I should avoid caffeine products that may aggravate the manic phase."
    c. "I should take my drug with food."
    d. "It is important that I wear or carry ID indicating that I am taking lithium."

39. The patient has been prescribed desvenlafaxine for generalized anxiety disorder. Which statement by the patient indicates the need for further health teaching?
    a. "I need to take my drug even if I am not feeling anxious."
    b. "I need to wear sunscreen when I am outdoors."
    c. "If I have any issues with my sexual performance, I can ask my health care provider."
    d. "It is OK if I keep taking my herbal drugs for my depression and anxiety."

CASE STUDY: CRITICAL THINKING

Read the scenario and answer the following questions on a separate sheet of paper.

A 53-year-old female recently relocated to start a new job after her current position of 20 years was eliminated. The patient was prescribed fluoxetine 20 mg at bedtime for complaints of insomnia, sadness, tearfulness, and inability to concentrate. The patient tells the nurse, "I can't believe I lost my job and have to start over. I feel like such a failure." She is postmenopausal and has a history of hypertension and migraines.

1. Discuss SSRIs and their mechanisms of action.

2. Identify questions the nurse would ask in the initial interview.

3. Discuss the discharge health education regarding fluoxetine the nurse would provide.

24 Antiinflammatories

STUDY QUESTIONS

Match the term in Column I with the definition in Column II.

Column I

_____ 1. Acetylsalicylic acid (ASA)

_____ 2. Indomethacin

_____ 3. Ketorolac

_____ 4. Fenamate

_____ 5. Oxicam

_____ 6. Immunomodulator

_____ 7. Colchicine

_____ 8. Allopurinol

_____ 9. Celecoxib

Column II

a. Disrupts the inflammatory process and delays disease progression

b. Indicated for long-term arthritic conditions

c. One of the first nonsteroidal antiinflammatory drugs (NSAIDs) introduced

d. Oldest antiinflammatory drug

e. The first injectable NSAID

f. The first drug used to treat gout

g. Drug of choice for patients with chronic tophaceous gout

h. Potent class of NSAID used for acute and chronic arthritic conditions

i. Cyclooxygenase inhibitor

Complete the following.

10. Inflammation is a response to tissue _____ and _____.

11. The five cardinal signs of inflammation are _____, _____, _____, _____, and _____.

12. Leukocyte infiltration of the inflamed tissue occurs during the _____ phase of inflammation.

13. The half-life of each NSAID (does/does not) differ greatly. (*Circle correct answer.*)

14. When using NSAIDs for inflammation, the dosage is generally _____ than that for pain relief.

15. Corticosteroids are indicated to control _____ flareups.

REVIEW QUESTIONS

Select the best response.

16. Which body response occurs during the vascular phase of inflammation?
    a. Leukocyte and protein infiltration into inflamed tissue
    b. Vasoconstriction with leukocyte infiltration into inflamed tissue
    c. Vasoconstriction and fluid influx into the interstitial space
    d. Vasodilation with increased capillary permeability

17. A patient who is taking NSAIDs for arthritis complains of persistent heartburn. Which question(s) would the nurse further ask the patient about the heartburn? **Select all that apply**.
    a. "Do you take your drug with food?"
    b. "Have you been drinking an increased amount of water?"
    c. "Have you noticed a change in the color of your bowel movements?"
    d. "What dosage of the NSAID are you taking?"
    e. "Where is the heartburn located?"

18. Which mechanism of action is correct for ibuprofen?
    a. "Ibuprofen is a COX-2 inhibitor, so it blocks prostaglandin synthesis."
    b. "Ibuprofen inhibits prostaglandin synthesis."
    c. "Ibuprofen binds with opiate receptor sites."
    d. "Ibuprofen promotes vasodilation to increase blood flow."

19. A patient with a complicated medical history including hypertension, atrial fibrillation, and arthritis calls the health care provider's office to speak with a nurse about "all of these bruises I have all of a sudden." Which potential drug-to-drug interaction would concern the nurse?
    a. Aspirin and warfarin
    b. Sulfasalazine and acetaminophen
    c. Tolmetin and propranolol
    d. Meloxicam and amlodipine

20. A 4-year-old child was brought to the emergency room for continued fever despite taking aspirin. Which statement is correct about a 4-year-old receiving aspirin?
    a. Aspirin has the potential to cause gastrointestinal (GI) bleeding in children.
    b. Aspirin has the potential to cause ringing in the ears in children.
    c. Aspirin has the potential to cause hyperglycemia in children.
    d. Aspirin has the potential to cause Reye syndrome in children.

21. A patient with a history of asthma has been prescribed sulfasalazine, a salicylate derivative, for arthritis. Which effects can salicylic acid and salicylate derivatives cause that would concern the nurse?
    a. Tachycardia
    b. Increased secretions
    c. Bronchospasm
    d. Fluid retention

22. Which statement is correct about the positive aspect of ibuprofen in relation to other NSAIDs?
    a. It tends to cause less GI irritation.
    b. It may be taken between meals.
    c. It has a long half-life of 20–30 hours.
    d. It has no drug–drug interactions.

23. A patient has been prescribed ibuprofen 400 mg three times a day (tid) for arthritis. Which statement by the patient would indicate a need for further education?
    a. "This drug may cause GI upset."
    b. "Now I won't have to drink so much water."
    c. "I know this drug might cause some diarrhea."
    d. "I will need to stop taking this drug if I get pregnant."

24. Which advantage does piroxicam have over other NSAIDs?
    a. Piroxicam does not cause any GI irritation
    b. Piroxicam has fewer drug-drug interactions
    c. Piroxicam has a long half-life
    d. Piroxicam has a rapid onset

25. By which action does colchicine relieve the symptoms of gout?
    a. Inhibits the migration of leukocytes to the inflamed area.
    b. Blocks reabsorption of uric acid.
    c. Blocks prostaglandin release.
    d. Inhibits uric acid synthesis.

26. Which mechanism of action is primary for probenecid in the treatment of gout?
    a. Probenecid is used for the retention of urate crystals in the body
    b. Probenecid is used for the inhibition of the reabsorption of uric acid
    c. Probenecid is used for the promotion of uric acid removal in the ureters
    d. Probenecid is used for the increasing the release of uric acid

27. Which statement describes the mechanism of action for etanercept for the treatment of severe rheumatoid arthritis?
    a. Etanercept neutralizes tumor necrosis factor, thereby altering the inflammatory response.
    b. Etanercept inhibits IL-1 from binding to interleukin receptor sites in cartilage and bone.
    c. Etanercept blocks COX-2 receptors, which are needed for the biosynthesis of prostaglandins.
    d. Etanercept promotes uric acid reabsorption.

28. When discontinuing steroid therapy, which time frame would the dosage be tapered?
    a. No tapering is necessary
    b. 1 to 4 days
    c. 5 to 10 days
    d. More than 10 days

29. A patient has started taking corticosteroids for an arthritic condition. Which information would the nurse include in a health teaching plan? **Select all that apply**.
    a. Corticosteroids are used to control arthritic flare-ups in severe cases.
    b. Corticosteroids have a short half-life.
    c. Corticosteroids are usually administered once a day.
    d. Corticosteroids are tapered over the course of 5 to 10 days.
    e. Corticosteroids may not be taken with prostaglandin inhibitors.

30. Which information would the nurse include when teaching about antigout drug? **Select all that apply**.
   a. Include large doses of vitamin C supplements.
   b. Increase fluid intake.
   c. Avoid alcoholic beverages.
   d. Avoid foods high in purine.
   e. Take the drug with food.
   f. Avoid direct sunlight.

31. A patient who has been prescribed infliximab for severe rheumatoid arthritis has developed temperature of 101.9° F, chills, nausea, vomiting, and dizziness. Which advise would the nurse provide for the patient to do?
   a. The nurse does not need to advise anything. These are common side effects of infliximab.
   b. Instruct the patient take a cool bath.
   c. The patient should wait 24 hours and, if symptoms continue, call the clinic back.
   d. The patient should contact the health care provider for further evaluation.

CASE STUDY: CRITICAL THINKING

Read the scenario, and answer the following questions on a separate sheet of paper.

A 54-year-old patient comes to the clinic for treatment of an inflammatory condition. The patient reports taking 975 mg of aspirin combined with 65 mg of caffeine every 4 hours for the past week for joint pain without relief. The patient now reports bloody stools. Vital signs include blood pressure 90/62 mm Hg, heart rate 118 beats/min, respiratory rate 24 breaths/min, temperature 100.0°F, and pulse oximetry 98% on room air. Other assessment includes pale and cool skin.

1. Discuss the therapeutic dosage range and maximum dose for aspirin.

2. Describe the common side effects of aspirin.

3. Discuss the signs and symptoms of aspirin overdose.

4. Discuss the possible causes for the patient's abnormal vital signs.

25 Analgesics

Complete the following.

1. The _____ theory proposes tissue injury activates _____ and causes the release of chemical mediators.

2. Opioids such as morphine activate the same receptors as _____ to reduce pain.

3. Nonsteroidal antiinflammatory drugs control pain at the _____ level by blocking pain-sensitizing chemicals and interfering with the production of _____.

4. As a result of unrelieved pain, a patient may develop glucose intolerance and _____ respiratory rate, heart rate, blood pressure, and stress response.

Match the term in Column I to its definition in Column II.

Column I

_____ **5.** Pain threshold

_____ **6.** Pain tolerance

_____ **7.** Neuropathic pain

_____ **8.** Endorphins

_____ **9.** Analgesics

_____ **10.** Nociceptors

Column II

a. Neurohormones that naturally suppress pain conduction
b. Class of drugs that relieve pain
c. Level of stimulus needed to create a painful sensation
d. Sensory receptors for pain
e. Pain due to disease or injury of the peripheral nervous system or central nervous system (CNS)
f. Amount of pain a person can endure without interfering with normal functioning

Complete the following.

11. Opioids act primarily on the _____ and nonopioid analgesics act on the _____ at the pain receptor sites.

12. In addition to suppressing pain impulses, opioids also suppress _____ and _____.

13. In addition to pain relief, many opioids have _____ and _____ effects.

14. Opioids are contraindicated for use in patients with _____ and _____.

15. The patient taking meperidine reports blurred vision. The nurse knows this is a(n) _____ and would report this finding to the _____.

16. Pentazocine, an opioid agonist-antagonist, is classified as a Schedule _____ drug.

Match the term in Column I to its definition in Column II.

Column I

_____ **17.** Acute pain

_____ **18.** Cancer pain

_____ **19.** Somatic pain

_____ **20.** Visceral pain

_____ **21.** Chronic pain

_____ **22.** Superficial pain

_____ **23.** Vascular pain

Column II

a. Originates from smooth muscle and organs
b. Occurs from pressure on nerves and organs
c. Occurs suddenly and is usually less than 3 months in duration
d. Contributes to headaches or migraines
e. Originates in skeletal muscle, ligaments, and joints
f. Persists for more than 3 months and is difficult to treat
g. Originates on surface areas such as skin and mucous membranes

REVIEW QUESTIONS

Select the best response.

24. Which drug effect is considered a major side effect of meperidine?
a. Decreased blood pressure
b. Decreased pulse rate
c. Increased respiration
d. Increased urine output

25. Which assessment finding is an indication of opioid overdose?
a. Dilated pupils
b. Increased urinary output
c. Pinpoint pupils
d. Diarrhea

26. Which nursing assessment would be least important when monitoring a patient who is receiving hydromorphone?
a. Bowel sounds
b. Fluid intake
c. Pain scale
d. Vital signs

27. Which information would the nurse include in a teaching plan for a patient who is being discharged home after knee surgery with a prescription for an opioid? **Select all that apply**.
a. Dietary restrictions while taking hydrocodone.
b. Instructions not to exceed recommended dosage.
c. Instructions not to use alcohol or CNS depressants while taking hydrocodone.
d. Instructions on how to prevent constipation.
e. Side effects to report.

28. Which factor is most relevant to the relief of chronic pain?
a. Administration of drugs at patient's request
b. Use of opioid analgesics
c. Use of injectable drugs
d. Use of drugs with long duration of action

29. The patient is brought to the emergency department with a reported overdose of morphine. Which drug would the nurse anticipate be prescribed?
a. Butorphanol
b. Naloxone
c. Flumazenil
d. Pentazocine

30. Mixed opioid agonist-antagonists were developed in hopes of decreasing which condition?
a. Chronic pain
b. Opioid abuse
c. Renal failure
d. Respiratory depression

31. The patient abruptly stopped taking an opioid after taking it for 8 weeks for a mild back injury sustained at work. Which time frame would the nurse anticipate withdrawal symptoms attributable to physical dependence to begin?
a. 6–12 hours
b. 24–48 hours
c. 48–72 hours
d. 72–96 hours

32. Which time frame is correct on the duration of pain relief for controlled-release morphine?
a. 1–2 hours
b. 4–5 hours
c. 8–12 hours
d. 24–48 hours

33. An 8-year-old child is seen in the emergency room with a broken arm. Which intervention would the nurse perform to be more successful in treating pain in an 8-year-old child? **Select all that apply**.
    a. Assume the child is hurt and administer pain drug.
    b. Discuss the child's typical responses with the caregivers.
    c. Utilize only nonpharmacologic pain control methods.
    d. Use a pain scale appropriate for children.
    e. Utilize developmentally appropriate communication techniques.

34. A patient will be discharged home with a prescription for an opioid-containing acetaminophen. Which drug, when taken with an opioid with acetaminophen, would the nurse question?
    a. Ampicillin
    b. Cholestyramine
    c. Furosemide
    d. Propranolol

35. The nurse is concerned that the patient is experiencing side effects of opioid agonist-antagonists. Which assessment would be a priority for the nurse to monitor?
    a. Constipation
    b. Dysuria
    c. Hypertension
    d. Respiratory depression

36. A patient who is 4 hours postoperative is requesting morphine for the third time for pain rated an 8 on the numeric pain scale. The vital signs include temperature 97.5°F, heart rate 88 beats/min, respiratory rate 12 breaths/min, blood pressure 104/60 mm Hg, and oxygen saturation 98% on room air. Assuming that a dose of the drug is due, which action would be best for the nurse to take?
    a. Administer the dose and contact the health care provider about the respiratory rate.
    b. Administer the dose and contact the health care provider about inadequate pain control.
    c. Hold the dose and contact the health care provider regarding the respiratory rate.
    d. Hold the dose and contact the health care provider about inadequate pain control.

37. An older adult patient has a fentanyl patch 75 mcg for chronic pain. Which statement is correct regarding this drug for the older adult?
    a. This patient should not have a fentanyl patch for chronic pain.
    b. The dose may be too low.
    c. The dose may be too high for this patient.
    d. The dose is appropriate.

38. A patient is taking a combination drug of hydrocodone and ibuprofen after reconstructive knee surgery. Which statement by the patient indicates the need for more teaching?
    a. "I must take only what is prescribed for my pain."
    b. "I may need to take a laxative if I get constipated while I am taking this drug."
    c. "Having a few beers on the weekend will help me relax and ease the pain."
    d. "I should not take anything with ibuprofen in it while I am taking this drug."

39. A patient was prescribed oral ketorolac for postoperative pain. Which time frame indicates the maximum length of time this drug can be taken?
    a. 24 hours
    b. 3 days
    c. 5 days
    d. 2 weeks

40. Which drug would be appropriate for pain management for a patient who sustained multiple abrasions to both knees after falling off a bicycle? **Select all that apply**.
    a. Acetaminophen
    b. Aspirin
    c. Hydrocodone
    d. Ibuprofen
    e. Morphine

CLINICAL JUDGMENT STANDALONE CASE STUDY

Read the scenario and answer the following questions on a separate sheet of paper.
SLO: Apply clinical judgment on a patient requiring analgesic therapy
NGN Item Type: Drop-Down Cloze
Cognitive Skills: Recognize Cues

A 25-year-old presents to the emergency department with a severe left-sided headache. The patient states the headaches have been present for 24 hours and "it just won't go away" and that the "lights hurt my eyes and everything is just loud." The patient is also nauseated and has been vomiting. Assessment findings include:

Temporal temperature 98.2°F
Heart rate 120 beats per minute
Respiratory rate 22 breaths per minute
Blood pressure 142/76 mm Hg
Oxygen saturation 100% on room air
Pain is rated at a 13 on a numerical scale of 1–10
Lying supine in bed with lights off, head of the bed at a 30 degrees
Alert and oriented to person, place, time, and situation
Physical examination unremarkable

Choose the *most likely* options for the information missing from the statements in the following by selecting from the list of options provided.

The nurse anticipates the patient is suffering from a migraine in which cerebral neurons are ___1___.

Unrelieved pain can cause ___2___ blood pressure, heart rate, and respiratory rate. After administering sumatriptan, the nurse would monitor for side effects and/or adverse drug reactions, such as ___3___, dizziness, and hypotension.

Options for 1	Options for 2	Options for 3
Hypoexcited	Decreased	Increased oral secretions
Hyperexcited	Normal	Altered taste
Normal	Elevated	Anxiety
		Orange urine

26 Penicillins, Other Beta-lactams, and Cephalosporins

STUDY QUESTIONS

Match the antibiotic in Column I to its category in Column II.

Column I

_____ **1.** Penicillin G

_____ **2.** Cefaclor

_____ **3.** Oxacillin

_____ **4.** Ceftolozane/tazobactam

_____ **5.** Cefazolin

_____ **6.** Amoxicillin

_____ **7.** Cefdinir

_____ **8.** Cefepime

_____ **9.** Piperacillin/tazobactam

Column II

a.   First-generation cephalosporin
b.   Second-generation cephalosporin
c.   Third-generation cephalosporin
d.   Fourth-generation cephalosporin
e.   Fifth-generation cephalosporin
f.   Basic penicillin
g.   Penicillinase-resistant penicillins
h.   Broad-spectrum penicillin
i.   Extended-spectrum penicillins

REVIEW QUESTIONS

Select the best response.

10. A patient, who recently completed five days of antibiotics, presents to the clinic with complaints of severe vaginal itching and discharge. Which mechanism would the nurse recognize as a possible cause of vaginal itching and discharge?
a. Poor hygiene
b. Hypersensitivity
c. Kidney infection
d. Superinfection

11. A patient is scheduled to receive ceftriaxone for an infection due to *Klebsiella*. Which patient teaching would the nurse provide?
a. It is given intramuscularly (IM) or intravenously (IV).
b. There is no cross-reaction to penicillins.
c. Ceftriaxone is safe to take with anticoagulants.
d. There is no effect on lab values.

12. A patient with renal dysfunction and *Staphylococcus aureus* skin infection is prescribed cefprozil monohydrate. Which dose indicates the maximum amount the nurse would anticipate?
a. 250 mg/d
b. 500 mg/d
c. 750 mg/d
d. 1 g/d

13. A young patient is admitted to the intensive care unit with a severe lower respiratory tract infection and is started on aztreonam. Which dose of aztreonam would the nurse anticipate administering?
a. 500 mg q8h
b. 500 mg q6h
c. 1500 mg q8h
d. 2000 mg daily

14. Which class of drug would increase the risk of nephrotoxicity in a patient taking ceftriaxone?
a. Angiotensin-converting enzyme inhibitor
b. Antidysrhythmic
c. Loop diuretic
d. A pain medication that is not a nonsteroidal anti-inflammatory drug

15. A patient is concerned about some nausea and weight loss while on ceftriaxone. Which information would the nurse tell the patient regarding the side effects of ceftriaxone?
a. Nausea and loss of appetite are common side effects.
b. Gastrointestinal bleeding may occur frequently.
c. Ceftriaxone causes nutrient absorption problems.
d. The patient will eat more when the infection is cured.

127

16. Which statement by a parent indicates more discharge teaching is necessary for the care of a 5-year-old child who has been prescribed dicloxacillin for otitis media?
    a. "Abdominal pain can be a side effect."
    b. "She needs to drink plenty of orange juice with this medication."
    c. "My child must take all of the drug until it is gone."
    d. "If my child develops a rash, I should bring her back to the doctor."

17. Which category of drugs is known to increase the serum levels of cefotetan?
    a. Antacids
    b. Laxatives
    c. Opioids
    d. Uricosurics

18. Which mechanism of action is correct about penicillin V potassium?
    a. Alteration in membrane permeability
    b. Inhibition of cell-wall synthesis
    c. Inhibition of protein synthesis
    d. Interference with cellular metabolism

19. A patient, who is allergic to dextromethorphan, is diagnosed with strep throat and is prescribed amoxicillin/clavulanate potassium. The patient takes oral contraceptives, vitamin C, and fexofenadine. Which instruction would the nurse include in the discharge teaching regarding amoxicillin/clavulanate potassium?
    a. "Increase calcium intake."
    b. "Wear sunscreen at all times."
    c. "Use an alternate method of birth control."
    d. "Stop the fexofenadine."

20. A patient is started on ceftazidime. Which nursing intervention would the nurse perform? **Select all that apply**.
    a. Obtain a culture.
    b. Administer IV dose over 20 minutes every day.
    c. Assess for allergic reaction.
    d. Monitor urine output.
    e. Restrict oral fluid intake.

21. A nurse is administering morning medications to several patients. Which patient would the nurse be concerned about in administering amoxicillin?
    a. A child with skin infection
    b. A pregnant patient
    c. A patient with asthma
    d. A patient with diabetes

22. An adult patient has been prescribed cefaclor for otitis media. Which order would the nurse seek further clarification?
    a. Immediate release (IR), 250 mg q8h
    b. Immediate release (IR), 500 mg q8h
    c. Immediate release (IR), 750 mg q8h
    d. Extended release (ER), 500 mg q12h

CASE STUDY: CRITICAL THINKING

A 54-year-old patient is seen in the clinic with complaints of burning and pain during urination and fever. The initial urinalysis was positive for protein and white blood cells and a culture and sensitivity was ordered. The patient has no known drug allergies and was prescribed amoxicillin 500 mg every 12 hours.

1. Identify if amoxicillin has a narrow spectrum or broad spectrum of activity and against which organisms it is effective.

2. Describe the purpose of using an antibiotic with a broad spectrum of activity.

3. After two days of being on amoxicillin, the symptoms continued. The antibiotic was switched to cefadroxil 1 gram every 12 hours.

4. Discuss the class of antibacterials for cefadroxil and the differences among the different generations of this class.

5. Discuss what the nurse would include when teaching the patient about cefadroxil.

27 Macrolides, Oxazolidinones, Lincosamides, Glycopeptides, and Lipopeptides

STUDY QUESTIONS

Match the drug in Column I with the category in Column II. Categories in Column II may be used more than once.

Column I

_____ 1. Clindamycin

_____ 2. Linezolid

_____ 3. Erythromycin

_____ 4. Azithromycin

_____ 5. Daptomycin

_____ 6. Clarithromycin

Column II

a. Macrolides
b. Lincosamides
c. Lipopeptides
d. Oxazolidinones

REVIEW QUESTIONS

Select the best response.

8. A trough level is obtained in a patient receiving daptomycin. Which trough level would the nurse know is appropriate?
   a. 5 mcg/mL by the second dose
   b. 5.9 mcg/mL by the third dose
   c. 6 mg/mL by the third dose
   d. 6.5 mg/L by the fourth dose

9. For which reason is acid-resistant salt added to macrolides, such as erythromycin?
   a. Acid-resistant salts decrease gastric acid from destroying the antibacterial.
   b. The salts decrease the absorption of the antibacterial in the small intestine.
   c. The risk of superinfection is minimized.
   d. The salts assist in dissolving the drug in the stomach.

10. Which teaching would the nurse include for a patient who is taking clindamycin for skin infection? **Select all that apply**.
    a. Clindamycin may cause diarrhea.
    b. Observe for superinfection like vaginitis.
    c. Take the medicine with a full glass of water.
    d. Anticipate urinary urgency.
    e. Complete the antibiotic.

11. A patient is diagnosed with Legionnaires' disease. Which macrolide would the nurse anticipate in being prescribed?
    a. Azithromycin
    b. Clarithromycin
    c. Vancomycin
    d. Erythromycin

12. A patient with bronchitis has been taking azithromycin. The patient tells the nurse they have been taking acetaminophen for headaches. The nurse reviews the patient's laboratory results knowing that which condition can occur?
    a. Leukocytosis
    b. Hepatotoxicity
    c. Elevated platelets
    d. Decreased bilirubin

13. A patient who has been on antibacterials for pneumonia developed profuse watery diarrhea. Stool culture revealed the patient has pseudomembranous colitis due to *Clostridium difficile*. Which antibacterial would the nurse anticipate in being prescribed?
    a. Telavancin intravenously
    b. Daptomycin intravenously
    c. Vancomycin orally
    d. Clarithromycin orally

14. The nurse is noting the urine output has decreased to 500 mL/day in an older adult patient receiving vancomycin intravenously. Which action would be best by the nurse?
    a. Increase the patient's oral fluid intake.
    b. Increase the rate on patient's intravenous fluid.
    c. Contact the health care provider.
    d. Document this in the patient's chart.

15. The patient has been prescribed azithromycin for an upper respiratory tract infection. Which statement by the patient indicates understanding of drug's side effects?
    a. "I need to stay out of the sun or wear sunscreen."
    b. "I have to take it on an empty stomach to prevent nausea."
    c. "If my eyes get red and itchy, I shouldn't wear my contacts."
    d. "I cannot take anything for pain if I get a headache."

CASE STUDY: CRITICAL THINKING

A 38-year-old is seen in the clinic with complaints of pharyngitis and fever. The patient was prescribed azithromycin 500 mg for "strep throat."

1. Describe the class of antibacterials that includes azithromycin and its mechanism of action.

2. Discuss the potential side effects and/or adverse drug reactions the nurse would teach the patient who is on azithromycin.

After three days of taking azithromycin, the patient develops severe, watery stool.

3. Discuss the concerns the nurse may have.

The patient was started on vancomycin 125 mg po q6hr for *C. difficile*.

4. Discuss the difference between oral and intravenous vancomycin.

28 Tetracyclines, Glycylcyclines, Aminoglycosides, and Fluoroquinolones

Complete the following.

1. Streptomycin sulfate was the first _____ available against the bacterium *Streptomyces griseus*.

2. Aminoglycosides cross the blood-brain barrier in (adults/children) but not in (adults/children). (*Circle the correct answers.*)

3. An increased risk for ototoxicity can occur when taking aminoglycosides concurrently with _____.

4. Fluoroquinolones interfere with the enzyme _____ _____, which is needed to synthesize bacterial _____.

5. Patients taking fluoroquinolones should (increase/decrease) fluid intake. (*Circle the correct answer.*)

Match the drug in Column I with its category in Column II. Categories in Column II may be used more than once.

Column I

_____ **6.** Amikacin

_____ **7.** Doxycycline

_____ **8.** Gentamicin

_____ **9.** Ciprofloxacin

_____ **10.** Tigecycline

_____ **11.** Tobramycin

Column II

a. Aminoglycosides
b. Fluoroquinolones
c. Glycylcyclines
d. Tetracycline

REVIEW QUESTIONS

Select the best response.

12. Which fluoroquinolone prescription would the nurse seek clarification?
    a. Levofloxacin 750 mg IV q12h
    b. Ofloxacin 200 mg PO q12h
    c. Moxifloxacin 400 mg PO q day
    d. Ciprofloxacin 250 mg PO bid

13. The nurse assesses a patient who is taking gentamicin. Which assessment finding would be cause for concern? **Select all that apply**.
    a. Nausea
    b. Ototoxicity
    c. Headache
    d. Photosensitivity
    e. Elevated renal function tests

14. A patient is taking gentamicin intravenously for a postsurgical infection at 9:00 am and 9:00 pm. Which time is most correct for the nurse to check drug peak level?
    a. 9:15 am
    b. 10:00 am
    c. 9:15 pm
    d. 10:30 pm

15. The trough level that the nurse drew for a patient taking gentamicin is 3.5 mcg/mL. Which action would be taken by the nurse?
    a. Administer the medication at the correct time.
    b. Hold the drug and contact the health care provider.
    c. Repeat the trough level after the next dose of medication.
    d. Give the patient diphenhydramine to decrease the risk of a reaction.

131

16. The patient has developed vaginal discharge since beginning gentamicin. Which cause would the nurse suspect may have occurred?
    a. The patient has been exposed to other infectious agents.
    b. The patient is experiencing an allergic reaction.
    c. A superinfection has developed.
    d. A drug-drug interaction is taking place.

17. Which assessment would the nurse routinely monitor in a patient receiving gentamicin? **Select all that apply**.
    a. Changes in hearing
    b. Color and clarity of urine
    c. AST/ALT laboratory values
    d. Blood glucose values
    e. Changes in visual acuity

18. A patient has been prescribed doxycycline. Which statement made by the patient indicate(s) that the nurse needs to provide more discharge teaching? **Select all that apply**.
    a. "It is best if I take this with food."
    b. "I should drink milk."
    c. "I have to take this drug on an empty stomach."
    d. "I should wait a half-hour after meals to take the medication."
    e. "I cannot eat eggs when I take this drug."

19. Which teaching would the nurse include to a patient taking tetracycline for a respiratory tract infection? **Select all that apply**.
    a. Outdated tetracycline breaks down into toxic by-products and must be discarded.
    b. Observe for superinfection like vaginitis.
    c. Avoid tetracycline during the first and third trimesters of pregnancy.
    d. Anticipate urinary urgency.
    e. Wear sunscreen and limit outdoor exposure during peak daylight hours.

20. Which drug, if prescribed for a patient taking oral doxycycline, would the nurse seek clarification? **Select all that apply**.
    a. Prenatal vitamins
    b. Antacids
    c. Warfarin
    d. Morphine
    e. Omeprazole

21. Which nursing intervention would the nurse implement for a patient taking doxycycline for chlamydia? **Select all that apply**.
    a. Restricting fluids
    b. Storing the drug away from light
    c. Ordering renal and liver profiles
    d. Obtaining a specimen for culture and sensitivity
    e. Advising the patient to use additional contraceptives when taking this drug

22. The nurse is performing a morning assessment on a patient receiving gentamicin. The patient reports tinnitus all night. The nurse prepares to educate the patient based on which information?
    a. Only low-pitched sounds are affected by gentamicin.
    b. Tinnitus is a sign of gentamicin allergy.
    c. Ototoxicity from gentamicin is caused by damage to cranial nerve VIII.
    d. Only female patients have ringing in their ears from gentimicin.

23. Which laboratory test is most likely influenced by doxycycline?
    a. Serum potassium
    b. Serum calcium
    c. Platelets
    d. Hemoglobin and hematocrit

CLINICAL JUDGMENT STANDALONE CASE STUDY

SLO: Plan nursing actions for a patient receiving antibacterials for abdominal discomfort
NGN Item Type: Matrix Multiple Choice
Cognitive Skills: Generate Solutions

A 48-year-old male patient recently underwent an esophagogastroduodenoscopy (EGD) because of complaints of continued abdominal distention and pain. He was diagnosed with acute gastritis and was discharged on oral famotidine. Two weeks later, the patient presents to the emergency department with continued abdominal pain and distention and states the medication did not help. Patient's history includes type 2 diabetes, gastritis, and chronic pain syndrome. Home medications include metformin/sitagliptin daily, ibuprofen twice daily for chronic pain, bismuth subsalicylate twice daily, and famotidine twice daily. The nurse observes the patient to be mildly distressed, moaning slightly and gently rubbing the abdominal area. Other assessments include the following:

Blood pressure 142/83 mm Hg
Heart rate 98 and regular rhythm
Respiratory rate 22 and regular
Oxygen saturation 98% on room air
Skin warm and dry, with pink undertone
Mucous membranes moist and pink
Respirations even and regular, lungs clear with diminished bases
Heart sounds without murmurs, rubs, or gallops
No edema noted to extremities.

Abdomen slightly distended with active bowel sounds in all quadrants, hyperresonance to percussion and tender to upper quadrants with mild palpation.

The patient underwent a second EGD and was found to have gastric ulcer which was positive for *Helicobacter pylori* (*H. pylori*). He is being discharged home on tetracycline, bismuth subsalicylate, and metronidazole to treat *H. pylori*. **Place an X for the nursing actions listed below that are Indicated (appropriate or necessary) or** **Contraindicated (could be harmful) for tetracycline to optimize patient care.**

Nursing Action	Indicated	Contraindicated
Advise the patient to stop taking the medications once the pain is relieved		
Tell the patient to not take over-the-counter antacids		
Inform the patient that tetracycline can be kept in the car		
Teach patient proper oral care to avoid mouth ulcers		
Instruct the patient to take the medication with food or glass of milk		
Teach patient to use sun block and wear protective clothing during sun exposure		

29 Sulfonamides and Nitroimidazoles Antibiotics

Complete the following.

1. Sulfonamides inhibit bacterial synthesis of _____.

2. Clinical use of sulfonamides has decreased because of the availability and effectiveness of _____.

3. The antibacterial drug that has a synergistic effect with sulfonamides is _____.

4. Sulfonamides (are/are not) effective against viruses and fungi. (*Circle the correct answer.*)

5. Anaphylaxis (is/is not) common with the use of sulfonamides. (*Circle the correct answer.*)

6. Sulfonamide drugs are metabolized in the _____ and excreted by the _____.

7. Sulfonamides are (bacteriostatic/bactericidal). (*Circle the correct answer.*)

8. The use of warfarin with sulfonamides (increases/decreases) the anticoagulant effect. (*Circle the correct answer.*)

Match the drug in Column I with its duration of action in Column II. Duration of action in Column II may be used more than once.

Column I

_____ 9. Trimethoprim-sulfamethoxazole

_____ 10. Sulfasalazine

_____ 11. Sulfadiazine

Column II

a. Short-acting
b. Intermediate-acting

REVIEW QUESTIONS

Select the best response.

12. A patient has sustained partial-thickness and full-thickness burns over 20% of the body. Which drug would be useful for this patient?
    a. Sulfadiazine
    b. Sulfasalazine
    c. Sulfacetamide sodium
    d. Silver sulfadiazine

13. A recent postpartum patient was prescribed TMP-SMZ for urinary tract infection (UTI). Which important question would the nurse ask? **Select all that apply**.
    a. "What kind of juice do you like to drink?"
    b. "Are you breastfeeding?"
    c. "Are you allergic to any medications?"
    d. "Do you have a history of kidney stones?"
    e. "What drugs do you take regularly?"

14. Which intervention would the nurse implement in a patient with bronchitis who is receiving TMP-SMZ and lisinopril? **Select all that apply**.
    a. Encourage fluids.
    b. Monitor urinary output.
    c. Observe for undesired side effects.
    d. Assess lung sounds.
    e. Administer laxatives.

15. Which dose is the usual adult dose of TMP-SMZ?
    a. 160 mg TMP/800 mg SMZ q6h
    b. 160 mg TMP/800 mg SMZ q12h
    c. 40 mg TMP/60 mg SMZ q6h
    d. 40 mg TMP/60 mg SMZ q12h

16. For which reason are sulfonamides not classified as antibiotics?
    a. They do not inhibit cell-wall growth.
    b. They are only bacteriostatic, not bactericidal.
    c. They were not obtained from biological sources.
    d. They are only effective against viruses and fungi.

17. A patient has been started on TMP-SMZ for otitis. The nurse will advise the patient about which side effect?
    a. Confusion
    b. Constipation
    c. Fever
    d. Insomnia

18. Which amount is the maintenance dose for sulfasalazine in the treatment of an inflammatory bowel disease, such as ulcerative colitis?
    a. 500 mg q6h
    b. 1000 mg q6h
    c. 1250 mg per day
    d. 1500 mg per day

19. For which bacteria is quinupristin-dalfopristin appropriate for life-threatening infection?
    a. Vancomycin-resistant *Enterococcus faecium*
    b. *Escherichia coli*
    c. *Proteus mirabilis*
    d. *Klebsiella pneumoniae*

Read the scenario and answer the following questions on a separate sheet of paper.

A 72-year-old presents to the emergency department from a long-term acute care facility with complaints of fever, shaking chills, flank pain, and burning on urination. Vital signs include temperature 100.3°F, heart rate 94 beats/min, respiratory rate 16 breaths/min, and blood pressure 102/70 mm Hg. The patient's medical history includes type 2 diabetes mellitus and cerebrovascular accident with residual left-sided weakness. Current drugs include glyburide, warfarin, and a daily multivitamin. The patient is allergic to all cephalosporins. The patient was diagnosed with an *E. coli* urinary tract infection and was prescribed oral trimethoprim-sulfamethoxazole (TMP-SMZ).

1. Describe the mechanism of action and standard dosage for oral TMP-SMZ.

2. Discuss the plan of care as it relates to TMP-SMZ.

3. Determine the adverse reactions the nurse would monitor.

30 Antituberculars, Antifungals, and Antivirals

Complete the following.

1. *Mycobacterium* species is a/an _____ bacillus that can cause _____.

2. Multidrug-resistant tuberculosis (TB) continues to be a problem because people (do/do not) complete the drug regimen. (*Circle the correct answer.*)

3. TB is transmitted by droplets when people _____, _____, or _____ and people in close contact _____ the particles.

4. A person who had _____ _____ _____ can develop TB disease.

5. Since isoniazid is metabolized through the liver and excreted by the kidneys, isoniazid is contraindicated in persons with severe _____ and _____ disease. List the other contraindications for receiving isoniazid.

6. Psychotic behavior (is/is not) a side effect of isoniazid. (*Circle the correct answer.*)

7. (Single/Combination) therapy against TB disease is more effective in eradicating infection. (*Circle the correct answer.*)

8. A common adverse effect with isoniazid is peripheral neuropathy. A supplement with _____ is usually taken concomitantly to prevent neuropathy.

9. Children who have latent TB infection should be treated with _____ for _____ months.

Match the drug in Column I with its type in Column II. The type in Column II may be used more than once.

Column I

_____ **10.** Ethambutol

_____ **11.** Rifapentine

_____ **12.** Pyrazinamide

_____ **13.** Capreomycin

_____ **14.** Isoniazid

_____ **15.** Aminosalicylate

_____ **16.** Ethionamide

_____ **17.** Streptomycin

_____ **18.** Rifampin

Column II

a. First-line drug
b. Drug-resistant TB medication

Complete the following.

19. Overgrowth of fungus usually occurs in persons who are immunocompromised and is classified as an _____ infection.

20. Rapid intravenous infusion of echinocandins can cause _____ reactions.

21. Herpes virus type 1 (HSV-1) is usually associated with _____, and herpes virus type 2 (HSV-2) is associated with _____.

22. Varicella-zoster virus that has lain dormant in nerve root ganglia can be reactivated as _____. Painful vesicular rash occurs along the _____.

23. Currently, hepatitis _____ and hepatitis _____ are vaccine preventable.

24. Specific therapy (does/does not) exist to cure persons with acute hepatitis B. (*Circle correct answer.*)

25. Hepatitis _____ and hepatitis _____ can develop into chronic hepatitis.

REVIEW QUESTIONS

Select the best response.

26. Which outcome is a life-threatening adverse effect of isoniazid?
    a. Crystalluria
    b. Hepatotoxicity
    c. Ototoxicity
    d. Palpitations

27. Which person should not receive prophylactic treatment for TB with isoniazid?
    a. 29-year-old concurrently taking theophylline
    b. 46-year-old with alcoholism
    c. 57-year-old taking warfarin
    d. 65-year-old with parkinsonism

28. The patient has just started taking rifapentine as part of the combination therapy for active TB. The nurse knows that rifapentine would be taken how often?
    a. Twice per day
    b. Daily
    c. Twice per week
    d. Every other day

29. An immunocompromised patient has recently been diagnosed with histoplasmosis. The patient has been started on amphotericin B. The nurse would anticipate administering which drug to alleviate side effects? **Select all that apply**.
    a. Diphenhydramine
    b. Acetaminophen
    c. Diazepam
    d. Hydrocortisone

30. Which drug would be ordered for a patient with hepatitis C viral infection?

a.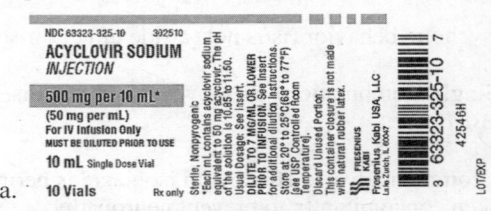

b.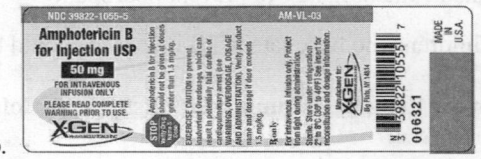

c.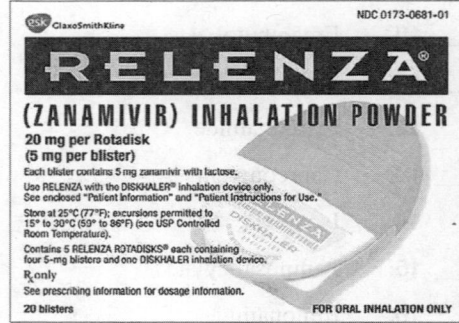

d.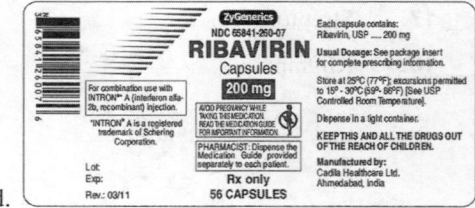

31. During the admission interview, which information would the nurse seek to obtain from a patient taking isoniazid? **Select all that apply**.
    a. Blood glucose level
    b. Drug allergies
    c. History of TB exposure
    d. Date of last purified protein derivative and chest x-ray

32. The 28-year-old patient has been diagnosed with TB disease. The patient weighs 80 kg. Which dose of isoniazid (INH) would the nurse anticipate administering *initially*?
    a. 160 mg/day
    b. 400 mg/day
    c. 600 mg/day
    d. 800 mg/day

33. A patient with active TB is prescribed isoniazid (INH). The nurse would teach the patient that frequent laboratory test to monitor liver function is needed for which reason?
    a. INH is excreted by the liver.
    b. INH causes liver cancer.
    c. INH can be hepatotoxic.
    d. INH cannot be metabolized by patients who have liver disease.

34. The patient has just been prescribed isoniazid (INH) for active TB. Which drug taken by the patient would be of concern to the nurse?
    a. Cetirizine
    b. Lisinopril
    c. Aluminum hydroxide/magnesium hydroxide
    d. Metformin

35. Which priority health teaching would the nurse include for the patient who has just started a course of isoniazid (INH)? **Select all that apply**.
    a. The patient may need to take vitamin B_6 supplements.
    b. Alcohol should be avoided.
    c. Fluid intake should be restricted.
    d. Body fluids including urine and tears may turn a brownish-orange color.
    e. Daily weights should be monitored.

36. Which instruction would rifampin be taken to decrease the incidence of resistance?
    a. Take rifampin on a daily basis
    b. Rifampin is taken in conjunction with other antitubercular drug
    c. Take rifampin once a week
    d. Rifampin is given only if patient is symptomatic

37. An immunocompromised patient has aspergillosis and has been prescribed amphotericin B. Which route would the nurse administer this drug?
    a. Intramuscularly
    b. Intravenously
    c. Orally
    d. Rectally

38. A patient with coccidioidomycosis is in the intensive care unit and has been prescribed amphotericin B. Which administration instruction would the nurse anticipate?
    a. Dilute and infuse over 30 minutes while monitoring vital signs every 5 minutes.
    b. Dilute, protect from light, and infuse slowly using an in-line filter.
    c. Prepare to administer undiluted by intravenous push slowly over 15 minutes.
    d. Prepare the drug in a solution and have the patient drink it slowly.

39. A patient is being treated with amphotericin B for histoplasmosis. Which statement by the patient would be concerning to the nurse?
    a. "I know I can only get this drug by having an intravenous site."
    b. "This drug may make me feel flushed."
    c. "I should not eat for 12 hours before receiving the drug."
    d. "I should let my health care provider know if I am not urinating as much."

40. A patient has been prescribed acyclovir. Which information would be part of the teaching plan for this patient? **Select all that apply**.
    a. Be sure to drink plenty of water to maintain hydration.
    b. Be sure to use spermicide to prevent infecting others.
    c. Drug can be taken at mealtime.
    d. Arise slowly because of the risk for orthostatic hypotension.
    e. Report any decreased urinary output, dizziness, or confusion.

41. A patient has been prescribed peginterferon. Which symptom would the nurse advise the patient to report to the health care provider? **Select all that apply**.
    a. Mood changes
    b. Fever
    c. Vision changes
    d. Photophobia
    e. Urinary urgency

42. Available:

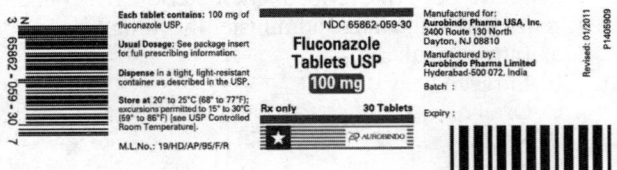

The patient's prescription is for a maintenance dose of fluconazole, 150 mg/day. How many tablets should the patient take per dose?
   a. 1 tablet
   b. 1.5 tablets
   c. 2 tablets
   d. 2.5 tablets

43. Which laboratory value must be frequently monitored in the patient taking fluconazole? **Select all that apply**.
   a. AST
   b. ALT
   c. BUN
   d. Glucose
   e. Potassium
   f. PT

SLO: Determine appropriate nursing actions for patients with TB
NGN Item Type: Matrix Multiple Choice
Cognitive Skills: Take Action

A 22-year-old male was directly admitted to the hospital from the clinic for complaints of nighttime diaphoresis, loss of appetite, and weight loss for 2 weeks for possible infection with *Mycobacterium tuberculosis*. The patient has a long history of intravenous drug use and was recently diagnosed with acquired immunodeficiency syndrome (AIDS). **For each nursing actions, use an X to indicate whether the nursing actions are Appropriate (correct) or Inappropriate (not correct) in caring for a patient suspected of TB.**

Nursing Actions	Appropriate	Inappropriate
Hold rifampin if body fluids, such as urine, sweat, and saliva, turns red-orange color		
Administer isoniazid on empty stomach		
Obtain initial follow-up appointment with a medical provider prior to patient being discharged		
Explain that his partner does not need to be treated		
Obtain sputum samples to test for acid-fast bacilli		
Anticipate in administering pyridoxine with isoniazid		
Place patient in reverse isolation		
Assess for numbness, tingling, or burning sensations		
Assist the patient in developing a plan to remain adherent to the drug regimen		

31 Antimalarials, Anthelmintics, and Peptides

STUDY QUESTIONS

Match the term in Column I with the appropriate definition in Column II.

Column I

_____ **1.** Tissue phase

_____ **2.** Erythrocyte phase

_____ **3.** Prophylaxis

_____ **4.** Helminthiasis

_____ **5.** Trichinosis

_____ **6.** Drug-resistant infection

_____ **7.** Peptides

Column II

a. Prevention
b. Worm infection
c. Invasion of the body tissue
d. Infection caused by eating raw or undercooked pork
e. Invasion of the blood cells
f. Provides the ability to kill a range of parasites and viruses
g. When microbes are not sensitive to antimicrobials

REVIEW QUESTIONS

Select the best response.

8. Which site is common for helminthiasis?
   a. Blood
   b. Intestines
   c. Liver
   d. Urinary tract

9. Which pathogen is the causative species for malaria?
   a. Bacterium
   b. Fungus
   c. Protozoan
   d. Virus

10. A patient who recently returned from an archeology dig overseas presents to the emergency department with complaints of fever, chills, and body aches. Which drug would the nurse anticipate in giving for a patient diagnosed with malaria?
    a. Acyclovir
    b. Chloroquine
    c. Delavirdine
    d. Tobramycin

11. Which laboratory value is affected by chloroquine usage? **Select all that apply**.
    a. Creatinine
    b. Glucose
    c. Hemoglobin
    d. Hematocrit
    e. Red blood cell count
    f. Aspartate aminotransferase (AST)

12. The patient is planning an overseas mission trip to a mosquito-infested area and was prescribed chloroquine as prophylaxis for malaria. Which statement by the patient indicates the need for more health education by the nurse?
    a. "I may have some abdominal cramping and nausea."
    b. "I only need to take my medication before my trip."
    c. "If my ears start ringing, I should contact my health care provider."
    d. "I should avoid taking any antacid while I am taking this drug."

13. A patient returns to the clinic complaining of not getting better after completing treatment with chloroquine for malaria. Vital signs are temperature 104.5°F, heart rate 120 beats/min, respiratory rate 22 breaths/min, blood pressure 138/82 mm Hg, and oxygen saturation 99% on room air. Which treatment would the nurse anticipate next?
    a. Continue 5 more days of chloroquine.
    b. Change medication to artemether/lumefantrine.
    c. Start thiabendazole.
    d. Start zidovudine.

14. Which instruction would be included in the teaching for anthelmintics? **Select all that apply**.
   a. Bathing in hot water instead of showering.
   b. Changing clothing, linen, and towels daily.
   c. Taking the drug on an empty stomach to aid in absorption.
   d. Understanding the importance of hand hygiene.
   e. Thoroughly cooking all foods containing pork.

15. The patient diagnosed with taeniasis (tapeworms) is being treated with praziquantel. Which possible side effect would the nurse include in patient teaching? **Select all that apply**.
   a. Blurred vision
   b. Difficulty hearing
   c. Dizziness
   d. Headache
   e. Weakness

16. Which statement by a patient who is being treated with colistimethate would concern the nurse about a potential risk for antibiotic resistance? **Select all that apply**.
   a. "If I run out of my antibiotic, I can use my leftovers from a previous infection."
   b. "I will take the antibiotics as prescribed."
   c. "Sometimes my friends ask me if I have any antibiotics. If I feel better, I will give my friends my leftovers."
   d. "When I stop having a fever I can stop taking the drug."

CASE STUDY: CRITICAL THINKING

Read the scenario and answer the following questions on a separate sheet of paper.

A 28-year-old patient started having abdominal pain and anal itching after working on a farm and ranch. The patient was diagnosed with helminths.

1. Describe helminths.

2. Identify the common helminths causing infection in humans and how they infect humans.

3. Discuss how helminths are treated.

32 HIV- and AIDS-Related Drugs

Match the drug in Column I to its drug classification of antiretroviral therapy in Column II. The drug class in Column II may be used more than once.

Column I

_____ **1.** Didanosine

_____ **2.** Enfuvirtide

_____ **3.** Raltegravir

_____ **4.** Maraviroc

_____ **5.** Indinavir

_____ **6.** Ritonavir

_____ **7.** Efavirenz

_____ **8.** Tenofovir

_____ **9.** Nevirapine

_____ **10.** Zidovudine

Column II

a. Nucleoside/nucleotide reverse transcriptase inhibitors

b. Protease inhibitors

c. Integrase strand transfer inhibitors

d. Fusion inhibitors

e. Nonnucleoside reverse transcriptase inhibitors

f. CCR5 antagonists

Complete the following.

11. The phases of the human immunodeficiency virus (HIV) life cycle include _____, _____, reverse transcription, integration, _____, _____, and budding.

12. Individuals who fail antiretroviral therapy (ART) (*should/should not*) be tested for drug resistance. (*Circle the correct answer.*)

13. Patients on medication for HIV should strive for _____ percent adherence.

14. Drug-drug interactions can occur when drugs are metabolized by the _____ system.

15. _____ is the only NNRTI that penetrates cerebrospinal fluid.

16. Selection of a protease inhibitor-based regimen should consider _____. (*List at least three considerations.*)

17. _____ is a syndrome that is related to a disease- or pathogen-specific inflammatory response in patients on ART.

Select the best response.

18. A nurse is teaching a patient who is positive for HIV. Which statement by the patient indicates a need for further teaching on HIV transmission? **Select all that apply**.
    a. "It is okay to share my razor."
    b. "I need to wear a condom with any type of sexual intercourse."
    c. "I can spread HIV by sharing my toothbrush."
    d. "I can donate my sperm."

19. Which laboratory test is used to monitor the efficacy of HIV drug therapy?
    a. White blood cell count
    b. CD4+ T-cell count
    c. Plasma B-cells
    d. Complete blood count

20. Which statement is correct on the goal of combination ART?
    a. Decrease the viral load and decrease the CD4+ count.
    b. Decrease the CD4+ count and increase the viral load.
    c. Increase the CD4+ count and decrease the viral load.
    d. Replace the memory cells within the immune system.

21. If therapy is to be initiated, the selection of ART would be based on which patient status? **Select all that apply**.
    a. Comorbid conditions
    b. Age and support system
    c. Willingness to accept therapy
    d. Probability of adherence to therapy
    e. Pregnancy status

22. Drug adherence has improved since the advent of ART. Which advancements to ART helped in increasing adherence?
    a. More pill burden
    b. Increased potency of newer ART
    c. Improved side effect profile
    d. Decreased potency of newer ART to reduce side effects

23. An adult patient is scheduled to begin taking zidovudine 300 mg by mouth. Which time frame is zidovudine usually prescribed?
    a. Daily
    b. Every 12 hours
    c. Every 6 hours
    d. Every 8 hours

24. An 8-week-old neonate has been diagnosed with HIV and will be receiving zidovudine orally. The child weighs 4.5 kg. Which dose would the nurse anticipate for this child?
    a. 9 mg/kg/dose bid
    b. 12 mg/kg/dose bid
    c. 120 mg/kg/dose bid
    d. 300 mg/kg/dose bid

25. During the time that a patient is taking zidovudine, frequent monitoring of which laboratory value is required? **Select all that apply**.
    a. Liver enzymes ALT/AST
    b. Complete blood count (CBC) with differential
    c. Creatinine
    d. Serum sodium
    e. Urine sedimentation rate

26. The nurse is assessing a patient taking zidovudine. Which common side effects would the nurse assess for? **Select all that apply**.
    a. Constipation
    b. Headache
    c. Myalgia
    d. Rash
    e. Seizures

27. Which nonnucleoside reverse transcriptase inhibitor (NNRTI) penetrates the blood-brain barrier?
    a. Rilpivirine
    b. Delavirdine
    c. Efavirenz
    d. Nevirapine

28. Efavirenz is initially scheduled to be taken at which intervals?
    a. 600 mg q6h
    b. 600 mg q8h
    c. 600 mg q12h
    d. 600 mg daily

29. During the time that a patient is taking efavirenz, periodic monitoring of which laboratory value is required?
    a. BUN/creatinine
    b. CBC
    c. Electrolytes
    d. Liver panel

30. Which side effect would be common in a patient taking efavirenz? **Select all that apply**.
    a. Diarrhea
    b. Difficulty swallowing
    c. Dizziness
    d. Rash
    e. Seizures

31. A patient is being discharged on efavirenz. Which teaching point would be important for the nurse to provide? **Select all that apply**.
    a. "Avoid alcohol while taking this drug."
    b. "Be sure to drink 2500 mL of fluid a day."
    c. "Don't take St. John's wort with this drug, as it will decrease its effectiveness."
    d. "This drug can cause convulsions and possibly liver failure."
    e. "Vomiting is a serious adverse reaction to efavirenz."

32. Which laboratory value would the nurse to monitor in a patient taking tenofovir? **Select all that apply**.
    a. Blood glucose
    b. Cholesterol
    c. Liver enzymes
    d. Triglycerides
    e. Potassium

33. A patient is being discharged on tenofovir. Which teaching would this patient receive? **Select all that apply**.
    a. "You cannot take St. John's wort while taking this drug."
    b. "You can take this drug with or without food."
    c. "You will need to learn to measure your blood glucose level."
    d. "Side effects may include nausea, vomiting, and diarrhea."
    e. "You will not be able to drive until you stop taking this drug."

34. Which treatment is the standard of care for prophylactic therapy of a pregnant patient who is positive for HIV and is asymptomatic?
    a. Combination drug therapy
    b. No therapy since all ART is contraindicated during pregnancy
    c. Single drug therapy with zidovudine only
    d. No therapy since the patient is asymptomatic

35. Which side effect would the nurse expect to see in a patient taking atazanavir? **Select all that apply**.
    a. Diarrhea
    b. Nausea
    c. Rash
    d. Urinary retention
    e. Vomiting

36. Which modalities can help increase HIV drug adherence? **Select all that apply**.
    a. Pill organizers
    b. Drug charts
    c. Scheduled pill holidays
    d. Alarms on cell phone or watch
    e. Taking drugs at the same time each day, such as after brushing teeth.

CLINICAL JUDGMENT STANDALONE CASE STUDY

SLO: Utilize knowledge of occupational exposure and postexposure prophylaxis treatment for HIV.
NGN Item Type: Cloze
Cognitive Skills: Analyze Cues
Post-exposure case

A nurse, following all the appropriate safety protocols, was inserting an intravenous (IV) needle into a patient who tested positive for HIV. Just when the needle was inserted, the patient jerked causing the IV needle to prick the nurse's gloved hand to the left index finger. Upon immediate inspection, the nurse did not observe any evidence of a needle stick. After regloving and obtaining a new IV needle, the nurse successfully started an IV line. Upon removing the gloves, the nurse noticed some bleeding on the left index finger. **Choose the most likely options for the missing information from the statements below by highlighting the correct response from the lists of options provided**.

After washing their hands with soap and water, the nurse was seen in the emergency room. After the nurse's blood sample was sent to the laboratory, the nurse was prescribed medications for HIV, also known as _____**1**_____. The nurse will anticipate completing _____**2**_____ of treatment. Periodic laboratory testing will be conducted to assess the levels of _____**3**_____ and _____**4**_____.

Options for 1	Options for 2	Options for 3	Options for 4
Preexposure prophylaxis (PrEP) treatment	72 hours	White blood cell (WBC)	HIV RNA
Postexposure prophylaxis (PEP) treatment	1 week	Hemoglobin	HIV DNA
Non-HIV antiviral treatment	4 weeks	Neutrophils	HIV mRNA
	6 months	CD4+ T-cell	

33 Transplant Drugs

Complete the following.

1. Transplantation of a healthy organ at the time of the donor's death is called _____.

2. A critical component of the cellular immune response is the activation of _____.

3. Patients on belatacept are at increased risk for _____ _____ _____ if they do not have immunity to _____ _____.

4. Sirolimus is in the class of _____ drugs that block _____ and _____ activation.

5. Combining corticosteroids with potassium-wasting diuretics increases the risk of _____.

6. Patients taking trimethoprim-sulfamethoxazole should protect their _____ from the _____.

Make the following false statements into true statements.

7. Induction therapy includes transplant drugs that provide improved immunity.

8. An example of a living-donor transplantation is when a kidney donated by a living person is transplanted into the body with severe kidney disease.

9. Transplant recipients receiving immunosuppressive drugs can receive live vaccines.

10. Sirolimus is primarily excreted by the kidneys.

11. Antithymocyte globulin alters B-cell function and prolongs T-cell addition.

Match the drug in Column I to the correct drug classes in Column II. Drug classes in Column II may be used more than once.

Column I

_____ 12. Tacrolimus

_____ 13. Everolimus

_____ 14. Basiliximab

_____ 15. Cyclosporine

_____ 16. Belatacept

_____ 17. Sirolimus

_____ 18. Azathioprine

_____ 19. Mycophenolate mofetil

_____ 20. Prednisone

Column II

a. Purine antimetabolites
b. Corticosteroids
c. Calcineurin inhibitors
d. Inosine monophosphate dehydrogenase inhibitors
e. Mammalian target of rapamycin inhibitors
f. T-cell co-stimulation blocker
g. Monoclonal antibody

Select the best response.

21. A nurse believes cytokine release syndrome is occurring in a patient receiving basiliximab before renal transplant surgery. Which clinical manifestations are related to cytokine release syndrome? **Select all that apply**.
    a. Hypotension
    b. Bradycardia
    c. Dyspnea
    d. Hypothermia
    e. Headache

22. A nurse would anticipate administering which drug to reduce the symptoms from cytokine release syndrome?
    a. Corticosteroid
    b. Diltiazem
    c. Furosemide
    d. Naloxone

23. Cyclosporine oral solution should not be mixed in which type of fluid?
    a. Apple juice
    b. Orange juice
    c. Grape juice
    d. Grapefruit juice

24. Which statement by the patient demonstrates an understanding of cyclosporine?
    a. "If I get an infection, I can take any antibiotics."
    b. "I can take cimetidine if I get an upset stomach."
    c. "If I have a fever, I need to call my doctor."
    d. "If I get mild muscle aches, I can take ibuprofen."

25. A patient is scheduled to receive a maintenance dose of belatacept postrenal transplant. The provider prescribed belatacept 10 mg/kg IV starting at week 10. Which action would be correct by the nurse?
    a. Call the provider who ordered the drug.
    b. Give the drug since the order is correct.
    c. Give the drug; the provider wanted the lower dose.
    d. Give the drug but at the correct recommended dose.

26. A patient with which organ transplant is appropriate to treat with mammalian target of rapamycin (mTOR) inhibitors?
    a. Lung
    b. Heart
    c. Liver
    d. Kidney

27. Which organ transplant is appropriate for mycophenolate mofetil? **Select all that apply**.
    a. Heart transplant
    b. Pancreas transplant
    c. Liver transplant
    d. Kidney transplant
    e. Corneal transplant

28. A patient is taking high doses of corticosteroids for acute transplant rejection. For which reason would a nurse teach the patient to avoid abrupt discontinuation of corticosteroids?
    a. Corticosteroids prevent infections by promoting leukocytes.
    b. Corticosteroids promote the inflammatory response that suppresses the immune system.
    c. Corticosteroids suppress adrenal function.
    d. Corticosteroids promote leukocyte activation.

29. Before receiving antithymocyte globulin, the patient would receive which drugs to decrease the incidence and severity of adverse reactions?
    a. Corticosteroid and antibiotic
    b. Antihistamine and antibiotic
    c. Antibiotic and diuretic
    d. Corticosteroid and antihistamine

30. A patient who had a heart transplant is to receive immunosuppressive drugs to prevent rejection. Which nursing action would be a priority?
    a. Advise the patient to avoid anyone with an active infection.
    b. Instruct the patient to take blood pressure and temperature measurements each day.
    c. Instruct the patient that exercising places undue stress on the body, further suppressing the immune system.
    d. Promote proper nutrition by cooking all foods, including fruits, and vegetables.

CASE STUDY: CRITICAL THINKING

Read the scenario and answer the following questions on a separate sheet of paper.

A middle-aged adult patient is scheduled to receive a liver transplant. Several hours before the surgery, the patient is to receive cyclosporine and methylprednisolone sodium succinate.

1. Describe the types of drugs cyclosporine and methylprednisolone sodium succinate are, and their general mechanisms of action.

2. Discuss some of the common side effects and adverse effects of cyclosporine and methylprednisolone sodium succinate.

3. Explain why patients receiving immunosuppressive drugs should not receive live vaccines.

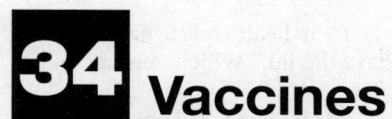 **Vaccines**

STUDY QUESTIONS

Match the term in Column I to its definition in Column II.

Column I

_____ **1.** Seroconversion

_____ **2.** Pathogen

_____ **3.** Vaccine

_____ **4.** Antibody

_____ **5.** Attenuated viruses

_____ **6.** Passive immunity

_____ **7.** Toxoids

Column II

a. Immediate and short-lived
b. Weakened microorganisms
c. Another term for immunoglobulins
d. Acquisition of detectable levels of antibodies
e. A small amount of antigen that is administered to stimulate the immune response
f. Microorganisms, such as bacteria, viruses, and fungi that invade the body
g. Inactivated toxins to stimulate antitoxins

Complete the following.

8. In the United States, there are more than _____ infectious diseases that may be prevented with vaccination.

9. The Advisory Committee on Immunizations identifies recommended _____, _____ to vaccinate, _____, and _____.

10. Yellow fever is transmitted by _____.

11. Adverse effects of vaccines must be reported through a surveillance system called _____.

12. _____ zoster is the reactivation of _____ zoster, usually settling in a dorsal root ganglion and causing severe pain.

REVIEW QUESTIONS

Select the best response.

13. Which term is used for vaccines made from the inactivated toxic substances produced by some microorganisms?
a. Attenuated vaccines
b. Conjugate vaccines
c. Recombinant subunit vaccines
d. Toxoids

14. In which situation would persons receive immuno-globulin for acquired passive immunity? **Select all that apply**.
a. Fetuses in utero.
b. When time does not permit active vaccination alone.
c. When the exposed individual is at high risk for complications of the disease.
d. During pregnancy.
e. Someone who is immunosuppressed.

15. By which process are antibodies received by an individual, used for protection against a particular pathogen, and acquired from another source?
a. Active immunity
b. Childhood immunity
c. Passive immunity
d. Toxoids

16. Which action occurs when there is an acquisition of detectable levels of antibodies in the bloodstream after receiving vaccines?
a. Passive immunity
b. Acquired natural immunity
c. Immunization
d. Seroconversion

149

17. When a parent asks about vaccine's action, which response by the nurse is correct?
    a. "Vaccines are perceived by the body as antibodies."
    b. "Vaccines cause an allergic reaction."
    c. "Vaccines produce a mild form of the disease."
    d. "Vaccines stimulate an immune response."

18. Which type of immunity develops that usually persists for the remainder of the individual's life after being infected with a disease?
    a. Natural acquired
    b. Humoral
    c. Active acquired artificial
    d. Passive natural

19. Which age is a child's first vaccine usually administered?
    a. At birth
    b. 2 months of age
    c. 4 months of age
    d. 6 months of age

20. Which condition is rubella commonly known as?
    a. German measles
    b. Hard measles
    c. Herpes zoster
    d. Smallpox

21. Susceptible individuals age 13 years or older receive two doses of varicella vaccine spaced how far apart?
    a. At least 4 weeks
    b. 3 months
    c. 6 months
    d. 1 year

22. Which organization would a health care provider report the details of an adverse reaction to a vaccine?
    a. Centers for Disease Control and Prevention (CDC)
    b. National Vaccine Injury Compensation Program (NVICP)
    c. Vaccine Adverse Events Reporting System (VAERS)
    d. Vaccine manufacturer

23. Which type of immunity is conferred by the Td vaccine?
    a. Active
    b. Inactive
    c. Natural
    d. Passive

24. Which immunizations are examples of live, attenuated vaccines?
    a. Influenza and hepatitis B
    b. Measles-mumps-rubella (MMR) and poliomyelitis
    c. MMR and varicella
    d. Varicella and Td

25. A patient presents to a health care provider and states, "I think I have the flu." Which cues are indicative of influenza?
    a. Abdominal pain, cough, and nasal congestion
    b. Fever, diarrhea, and dizziness
    c. Fever, myalgia, and cough
    d. Vomiting, diarrhea, and headache

26. When the MMR vaccine is not given the same day as the varicella vaccine, which time frame should be the minimum interval between administrations?
    a. 1 week
    b. 2 weeks
    c. 3 weeks
    d. 4 weeks

27. A parent reports their child developed some redness and tenderness at the injection site after the first dost of DTaP. Which action would the nurse take?
    a. Administer DTaP again, because these are common side effects, not contraindications.
    b. Provide DT in the right thigh.
    c. Give DTaP subcutaneously instead of intramuscularly to prevent muscle soreness.
    d. Inject half the usual dose of DTaP to reduce the likelihood of a reaction.

28. Which information would the nurse provide the parent of a 4-month-old child who just received immunizations? **Select all that apply**.
    a. Appointment card for the next immunization clinic visit
    b. Immunization record
    c. List of side effects to observe
    d. Report of adverse reaction form
    e. Vaccine Information Statements (VIS) for all vaccines administered

29. Which source would be a good resource for health and immunization information before international travel?
    a. Centers for Disease Control and Prevention.
    b. No source is necessary because there are no special immunization needs for travelers.
    c. The patient's travel agent.
    d. U.S. embassy in the destination country.

30. In the case of an anaphylactic reaction to a vaccine, which drug would the nurse have readily available?
    a. Acetaminophen
    b. Diphenhydramine
    c. Epinephrine
    d. Ranitidine

CLINICAL JUDGMENT STANDALONE CASE STUDY

Read the scenario and answer the following questions on a separate sheet of paper.

SLO: Apply knowledge of recommended immunization schedule for adults.

NGN Item Type: Multiple Response Select All That Apply

Cognitive Skills: Analyze Cue

A 74-year-old sustained a deep puncture wound to the right foot from a gardening tool. The nurse observes localized redness and swelling on the injured foot. The patient has no known drug allergy and takes "only aspirin for my arthritis because I don't really like coming to the doctor much." Prior immunizations include annual influenza and vaccine for COVID-19 at a local pharmacy store but has not received other vaccinations in more than 20 years. The patient reported having usual childhood illnesses, such as chicken pox, measles, and mumps. Labs are unremarkable except for mildly decreased hemoglobin, hematocrit, and total white blood cells. Which immunizations would be appropriate for this patient? **Select all that apply**.

_____**A.** Influenza, live attenuated

_____**B.** Varicella

_____**C.** Zoster recombinant

_____**D.** Tetanus, diphtheria, and pertussis

_____**E.** Meningococcal B

_____**F.** Pneumococcal

35 Anticancer Drugs

Match the chemotherapy drugs/terms in Column I with the most appropriate description in Column II. Each description is used only once.

Column I

_____ 1. Alkylating drugs

_____ 2. Aromatase inhibitors

_____ 3. Cyclophosphamide

_____ 4. Doxorubicin

_____ 5. Palliative chemotherapy

_____ 6. Fluorouracil

_____ 7. Hormonal agents

_____ 8. Methotrexate

_____ 9. Personal protective equipment

_____ 10. Vincristine

Column II

a. Associated with hemorrhagic cystitis
b. Leucovorin rescue
c. Stomatitis is early sign of toxicity
d. Associated with cardiotoxicity
e. Associated with neurotoxicity
f. Powder-free gloves, mask, impermeable gown
g. Mask cancer cells and prevent them from using hormones
h. Cause cross-linking of DNA strands, abnormal base pairing, or DNA strand breaks
i. Used to relieve symptoms associated with advanced disease
j. Block conversion of androgens to estrogen

For the following environmental factors, identify the type of cancers that are promoted.

11. _____ Benzene

12. _____ Ultraviolet rays

13. _____ Epstein-Barr virus

14. _____ Animal fat

15. _____ Alcohol

REVIEW QUESTIONS

Select the best response.

16. The nurse is caring for a patient receiving combination chemotherapy. The patient asks why more than one drug is prescribed. Which response by the nurse would be correct?
    a. "It has better response rates than single-drug chemotherapy."
    b. "It has fewer side effects than when given alone."
    c. "It is always more effective than surgery or radiation."
    d. "Survival rates are always better."

17. The nurse is teaching a community group about factors that influence the development of cancer. Which information would the nurse include?
    a. Aflatoxin is associated with cancer of the lung.
    b. Benzene is associated with cancer of the tongue.
    c. Epstein-Barr virus is associated with cancer of the stomach.
    d. Human papillomavirus is associated with cancer of the cervix.

18. Which information is correct concerning the side effects of chemotherapy?
   a. They are minimal because chemotherapy drugs are highly selective.
   b. Side effects usually occur during the first cycle of treatment.
   c. Toxicities to normal cells cause the side effects.
   d. Side effects of chemotherapy are usually permanent.

19. An older adult patient is diagnosed with advanced metastatic cancer and is scheduled to receive palliative chemotherapy. Which response by the nurse would be appropriate when the patient questions the benefits of palliative chemotherapy?
   a. "Quality of life is improved."
   b. "Limits further growth of the cancer."
   c. "Growth of cancer will be slower."
   d. "Tumors will shrink throughout your body."

20. The patient will be receiving chemotherapy that will lower white blood cell count. Monitoring for which finding would be a nursing priority?
   a. Change in temperature
   b. Evidence of petechiae
   c. Increase in diarrhea
   d. Taste changes

21. The patient has thrombocytopenia secondary to chemotherapy. Which nursing action would be most appropriate?
   a. Apply pressure to the injection site and assess for bleeding.
   b. Help the patient conserve energy by scheduling care.
   c. Monitor breath sounds and vital signs.
   d. Provide small, frequent meals, and monitor loss of fluids from diarrhea.

22. The patient has diarrhea secondary to chemotherapy. Which information would be included in patient teaching about chemotherapy-related diarrhea?
   a. Eat only very hot or very cold foods.
   b. Increase intake of fresh fruits and vegetables.
   c. Increase intake of high-fiber foods.
   d. Limit caffeine intake.

23. An older adult patient is to receive cyclophosphamide for treatment of lymphoma. Medical history includes atrial fibrillation, arthritis, and cataracts. Digoxin 0.125 mg daily and naproxen 500 mg at bedtime are the current drugs the patient is on. For which drug-drug interaction would the nurse need to be aware?
   a. Cyclophosphamide increases digoxin levels.
   b. Cyclophosphamide decreases digoxin levels.
   c. Digoxin increases cyclophosphamide levels.
   d. These drugs cannot be given together.

24. The patient is in the outpatient oncology clinic for treatment with fluorouracil (5-FU) for colon cancer. The patient has recently been started on metronidazole for treatment of trichomoniasis. Which drug-drug interactions would concern the nurse?
   a. 5-FU may decrease the effectiveness of metronidazole.
   b. 5-FU cannot be given with metronidazole.
   c. Metronidazole may increase the side effects of 5-FU.
   d. Metronidazole may increase 5-FU toxicity.

25. An older adult patient is receiving acetaminophen, cyclophosphamide, doxorubicin, and methotrexate (CAM) for the treatment of prostate cancer. During morning rounds, the patient complains of feeling short of breath. Physical assessment reveals crackles in both lungs. Which drug most likely caused this clinical manifestation?
   a. Acetaminophen
   b. Cyclophosphamide
   c. Doxorubicin
   d. Methotrexate

26. A patient is to receive an antiemetic and fluorouracil (5-FU) intravenously as part of a treatment protocol for colon cancer. Which time frame would the nurse administer the antiemetic?
   a. 1 day after administering 5-FU
   b. 1 day before administering 5-FU
   c. 30-60 minutes before administering 5-FU
   d. 4 hours before administering 5-FU

27. Which outcome would be most appropriate when generating solutions for a patient scheduled to receive cyclophosphamide?
   a. Patient will be free from symptoms of stomatitis.
   b. Patient will maintain cardiac output.
   c. Patient will show no signs of hemorrhagic cystitis.
   d. Patient will show no signs of syndrome of inappropriate antidiuretic hormone secretion.

28. The patient is to receive cyclophosphamide as part of cancer treatment. Which nursing action would the nurse expect to complete?
   a. Assess for signs of hematuria, urinary frequency, or dysuria.
   b. Decrease fluids to reduce the risk of calculus formation.
   c. Hydrate the patient with intravenous (IV) fluids only after administration of cyclophosphamide.
   d. Medicate with an antiemetic only after the patient complains of nausea.

29. The nurse is administering doxorubicin to a patient diagnosed with cancer. Which time frame would the nurse assess for tissue necrosis due to doxorubicin?
   a. 3–4 weeks after administration.
   b. Immediately after administration.
   c. 2–4 days after administration.
   d. Tissue necrosis rarely occurs with this drug.

30. The nurse is preparing to administer intravenous (IV) vinblastine, bleomycin, and cisplatin (VBP). Which precaution would the nurse take when administering these drugs?
    a. Wear a clean cotton gown.
    b. Wear shoe covers.
    c. Wear a hair net.
    d. Wear two pairs of gloves.

31. A patient is being discharged after receiving intravenous (IV) chemotherapy. Which statement made by the patient indicates a need for additional teaching?
    a. "Chemotherapy is excreted in my bodily fluids."
    b. "I will not need to know how to check my temperature."
    c. "My spouse should wear gloves when emptying my urinal."
    d. "The chemotherapy will remain in my body for 2–3 days."

32. A patient with breast cancer is scheduled to receive anastrozole, an aromatase inhibitor. Which information would the nurse include in the teaching?
    a. Peripheral conversion of androgens to estrogens is blocked.
    b. Tumors that are not hormonally sensitive are treated with aromatase inhibitors.
    c. Premenopausal women with breast cancer are treated with aromatase inhibitors.
    d. Postmenopausal women with breast cancer are treated with aromatase inhibitors.

33. A patient is scheduled to receive vincristine as part of a treatment for cancer. The medication record for the patient indicates that phenytoin is taken to control a seizure disorder. Which medical condition would the nurse monitor in this patient?
    a. Headaches
    b. Increased blood pressure
    c. Renal failure
    d. Seizures

34. A patient in the outpatient oncology clinic has developed stomatitis secondary to cancer therapy. Which statement made by the patient would indicate that additional teaching about stomatitis is needed?
    a. "I will rinse my mouth out frequently with normal saline."
    b. "I will try using ice pops or ice chips to help relieve mouth pain."
    c. "I will use a mouthwash that is alcohol base."
    d. "I will use a soft toothbrush."

CASE STUDY: CRITICAL THINKING

Read the scenario and answer the following questions on a separate sheet of paper.

An adult patient is being treated for multiple myeloma with cyclophosphamide.

1. Which class does cyclophosphamide belong to, and what is its mechanism of action?

2. Discuss the major side effects of cyclophosphamide.

3. What are the key factors in the nursing assessment for patients receiving cyclophosphamide?

4. Discuss the priority teaching points for the patient about the drug regimen.

36 Targeted Therapies to Treat Cancer

Complete the following.

1. _____ normally prompt cells to divide through the signal transduction pathways.

2. _____ are multienzyme complexes that degrade proteins intracellularly.

3. Targeted therapies block the _____ and _____ of cancer cells.

4. The largest class of targeted therapy drugs that attack one particular molecular target is _____ inhibitor.

5. _____ are enzymes that activate other proteins, including signal transduction pathways.

Match the class of targeted therapy drug in Column I to the mechanism of action in Column II.

Column I

_____ **6.** mTOR kinase inhibitor

_____ **7.** EGFR inhibitor

_____ **8.** Angiogenesis inhibitor

_____ **9.** Monoclonal antibody

_____ **10.** Tyrosine kinase inhibitor

Column II

a. Prevents formation of new blood vessels
b. Binds to different areas of EGFR, blocking its activity
c. Primarily affects BCR-ABL kinase enzyme
d. Leads to G_1 arrest and cell death
e. Targets cell-membrane surface antigens

REVIEW QUESTIONS

Select the best response.

11. During the first dose of trastuzumab, the patient complains of shortness of breath and pruritus. Which action would be the best by the nurse?
    a. Decrease the infusion rate by 50% and notify the health care provider.
    b. Disconnect the IV and attach a 0.22-micron filter.
    c. Review the pretreatment multigated acquisition scan.
    d. Stop the infusion and manage the reaction.

12. Which rationale for administering bevacizumab in a patient with metastatic colon cancer is correct?
    a. The patient's immune response is enhanced.
    b. Apoptosis is increased.
    c. Tumor's microvascular growth is inhibited.
    d. An inflammatory response is modulated.

13. Gefitinib most frequently causes which side/adverse effect?
    a. Hypocalcemia
    b. Diarrhea
    c. Myelosuppression
    d. Seizures

14. Which antibodies are types of monoclonal antibodies? **Select all that apply**.
    a. Fully human antibodies
    b. Chimeric antibodies
    c. Equine antibodies
    d. Porcine antibodies
    e. Murine antibodies

15. A patient with nonsmall-cell lung cancer (NSCLC) is to begin treatment with gefitinib. The nurse notes on the medical record that the patient is also taking warfarin daily for atrial fibrillation. Which statement indicates the nurse is aware of gefitinib's mechanism of action?
    a. Increases the effects of warfarin.
    b. May require a dose increase when taken with warfarin.
    c. Gefitinib should not be given to a patient taking anticoagulants.
    d. Gefitinib may reach toxic levels when given concurrently with warfarin.

16. A patient in the outpatient oncology clinic is receiving sunitinib as part of the treatment for gastrointestinal stromal tumors. The health care provider prescribes ketoconazole to treat a fungal infection. Which drug-drug interaction would concern the nurse if these drugs are taken concurrently?
    a. Ketoconazole may decrease the effectiveness of sunitinib.
    b. Ketoconazole may potentiate sunitinib toxicity.
    c. Sunitinib may decrease the effectiveness of ketoconazole.
    d. Sunitinib may lead to toxic levels of ketoconazole.

17. A patient is beginning therapy with an epidermal growth factor/receptor inhibitor erlotinib for NSCLC. Which status would be important for the nurse to assess before beginning therapy?
    a. Cardiac status
    b. Hearing function
    c. Lung sounds
    d. Mental status

18. A patient is admitted to the hospital 1 week after receiving imatinib. On physical assessment, the nurse notes the presence of petechiae, ecchymoses, and bleeding gums. Which hypothesis (problem) would be most appropriate?
    a. Bleeding
    b. Falls
    c. Fatigue
    d. Altered nutrition

19. A patient is to start ziv-aflibercept, in addition to the already prescribed 5-fluorouracil, leucovorin, and irinotecan. Which statement made by the patient indicates a lack of understanding for receiving ziv-aflibercept?
    a. "The new drug is going to starve cancer cells."
    b. "I will need to stay indoors because medicine will make my skin more sensitive to the sun."
    c. "The drug will allow my good cells to grow new vessels."
    d. "The drug will prevent the cells from dividing."

20. A patient who is to receive rituximab has a blood pressure of 90/52 mm Hg and a heart rate of 82 beats/min. Upon reviewing the patient's routine drugs, the nurse notes antihypertensives. Which action would be best for the nurse to take?
    a. Start the infusion. The blood pressure and heart rate are within the parameters.
    b. Notify the health care provider.
    c. Infuse 250 mL of 0.9% sodium chloride over 2 hours before infusing rituximab.
    d. Retake the blood pressure in the other arm.

CASE STUDY: CRITICAL THINKING

Read the scenario and answer the following questions on a separate sheet of paper.

An adult patient has been diagnosed with ovarian cancer and presents to the outpatient oncology clinic for treatment. The patient is being treated with bevacizumab for metastatic disease.

1. Describe how the nurse would administer bevacizumab.

2. Describe the mechanism of action for bevacizumab.

3. Discuss the potential side effects and adverse effects of bevacizumab.

4. What teaching would the nurse provide in relation to bevacizumab therapy?

37 Biologic Response Modifiers

Complete the following.

1. Immunomodulators, also called _____ _____ _____, enhance, direct, or _____ the body's immune system.

2. Two advances in biologic therapies include _____ _____ and _____ _____.

3. Biologic response modifiers assist the immune system through _____ and prevent cancer cells from _____.

4. Macrophages are considered mature _____.

5. Erythropoietin stimulates the production of _____ _____ _____ in the bone marrow.

6. Granulocyte colony-stimulating factor is produced by macrophages, _____, and other immune cells and stimulates the synthesis of _____.

7. Many adverse effects of exogenous interleukins are due to _____ _____ _____.

Match the appropriate term in Column I with the description in Column II.

Column I

_____ 8. Colony-stimulating factors (CSFs)

_____ 9. Erythropoietin

_____ 10. Granulocyte colony-stimulating factor (G-CSF)

_____ 11. Granulocyte-macrophage colony-stimulating factor (GM-CSF)

Column II

a. Glycoprotein that stimulates the production of neutrophils

b. Proteins that stimulate growth and maturation of bone marrow stem cells

c. Glycoprotein produced by the kidneys in response to low oxygen (hypoxia)

d. Supports survival, proliferation, and differentiation of hematopoietic progenitor cells

REVIEW QUESTIONS

Select the best response.

12. Which mechanism of action is correct for biologic response modifiers (BRMs)? **Select all that apply**.
    a. Slow spread of tumor cells
    b. Enhance host's normal immunologic function
    c. Improve liver functioning
    d. Change cancers cells to behave more like healthy cells
    e. Replicate red blood cells

13. A patient is receiving GM-CSF infusion therapy. Which system would the nurse focus attention on both during and after these infusions?
    a. Cardiac system
    b. Central nervous system
    c. Musculoskeletal system
    d. Respiratory system

14. Before administering erythropoietin, which assessment would the nurse conduct?
    a. Renal function
    b. Hemoglobin level
    c. Liver function
    d. Chest X-ray

15. A patient is being treated with interferon for chronic myelogenous leukemia. For which adverse drug effect would the nurse monitor that may require the treatment to be stopped? **Select all that apply**.
    a. Severe depression
    b. Hepatic decompensation
    c. Absolute neutrophil count <500/mm³
    d. Platelets >140,000/mm³

16. A patient with hairy cell leukemia is being treated with interferon. Which information would the nurse educate the patient about the neurological side effects?
    a. "These side effects are common and will subside after the drug is stopped."
    b. "These side effects rarely occur."
    c. "These side effects will diminish as treatment goes on."
    d. "The worst effect is mild confusion."

17. For which dermatologic effect would the nurse assess in a patient taking interferon? **Select all that apply**.
    a. Alopecia
    b. Bruising
    c. Xerostomia
    d. Rash

18. Which health teaching is appropriate for a patient who is being treated with interferon alpha for hairy cell leukemia? **Select all that apply**.
    a. Report any unusual weight loss.
    b. Teach information on the effect of BRM-related fatigue on activities of daily living
    c. Side effects from a BRM disappear within 12-24 hours after discontinuation of therapy.
    d. Persistent headache or blurred vision should be reported to the health care provider.

19. For which condition may GM-CSF be administered? **Select all that apply**.
    a. Absolute neutrophil count >1500/mm³
    b. Autologous bone marrow transplant (BMT) recipient
    c. Allogeneic BMT recipient
    d. 12 hours after high-dose chemotherapy administration
    e. Kaposi sarcoma

20. A patient is to start aldesleukin for metastatic renal cell cancer. Which potential drug effect would the nurse monitor to determine if dose interruption or discontinuation is warranted? **Select all that apply**.
    a. New irregular cardiac rhythm
    b. Oxygen saturation less than 95%
    c. Stool positive for blood
    d. Existing skin rash that was present before starting aldesleukin
    e. Hypoglycemia

CASE STUDY: CRITICAL THINKING

Read the scenario, and answer the following questions on a separate sheet of paper.

An adult patient has been diagnosed with acute myelogenous leukemia and will be undergoing treatment. The patient is scheduled to receive G-CSF and wants to know what this drug will do to cure the cancer. The prescribed dose of G-CSF is 75 mcg/kg/day intravenously.

1. Describe the type of medication G-CSF is and how it works.

2. Discuss the potential side effects the patient may experience from G-CSF.

3. Which priority teaching will the nurse provide to the patient and patient's significant others?

38 Upper Respiratory Disorders

STUDY QUESTIONS

Match the drug class in Column I to the description in Column II.

Column I

_____ **1.** Antihistamines

_____ **2.** Antitussives

_____ **3.** Decongestants

_____ **4.** Expectorants

Column II

a. Act on the cough-control center in the medulla

b. Loosen bronchial secretions so they can be removed by coughing

c. H_1 blockers or H_1 antagonists

d. Stimulate the alpha-adrenergic receptors, producing vascular constriction in the nasal capillaries

Complete the following.

5. Antihistamines are _____ antagonists that have effects on the _____ muscles.

6. Many over-the-counter (OTC) cold remedies contain a _____ _____ antihistamine that can cause side effects such as _____ _____ and _____.

7. Second-generation antihistamines are considered _____ and have fewer _____ side effects.

8. Frequent use of nasal decongestants can result in _____ and _____ _____ _____, which can occur in as little as _____ _____.

9. Nasal decongestants stimulate the _____ receptors that cause _____, which can also cause _____.

Match the antihistamine in Column I to the correct generation in Column II. The generation in Column II may be used more than once.

Column I

_____ **10.** Diphenhydramine

_____ **11.** Cetirizine

_____ **12.** Loratadine

_____ **13.** Chlorpheniramine

_____ **14.** Azelastine

_____ **15.** Clemastine fumarate

Column II

a. First generation

b. Second generation

Select the best response.

16. Antihistamines are another group of drugs used for the relief of cold symptoms. Which property of these drugs result in decreased secretions?
    a. Analgesic
    b. Anticholinergic
    c. Antitussive
    d. Cholinergic

17. Compared to first-generation antihistamines, second-generation antihistamines have a lower incidence of which side effect?
    a. Drowsiness
    b. Headache
    c. Tinnitus
    d. Vomiting

18. The U.S. Food and Drug Administration has ordered removal of all cold remedies containing which drug?
    a. Dextromethorphan
    b. Guaifenesin
    c. Histamine
    d. Phenylpropanolamine

19. The patient has seasonal allergies and asks the student health nurse about the appropriate dose of diphenhydramine. Which amount is the recommended dosage of diphenhydramine?
    a. 25–50 mg q4-6h
    b. 25–50 mg daily
    c. 50–100 mg q4-6h
    d. 100 mg daily

20. Diphenhydramine has which therapeutic effect?
    a. Anticoagulant
    b. Anticonvulsant
    c. Antihypertensive
    d. Antitussive

21. Which advice would the nurse provide to a breastfeeding patient who is also taking diphenhydramine?
    a. Breastfeeding provides allergy relief to the infant.
    b. Large amounts of the drug pass into breast milk; breastfeeding is not recommended.
    c. Small amounts of the drug pass into breast milk; breastfeeding is contraindicated.
    d. The drug does not affect breastfeeding.

22. Which statement indicates an advantage of systemic decongestants over nasal sprays and drops?
    a. Fewer side effects
    b. Less costly
    c. Preferred by older patients
    d. Provide longer relief

23. Which expectorant is frequently an ingredient in cold remedies?
    a. Dextromethorphan
    b. Ephedrine
    c. Guaifenesin
    d. Promethazine

24. Which group of drugs is used to treat cold symptoms? **Select all that apply**.
    a. Antihistamines
    b. Antitussives
    c. Decongestants
    d. Expectorants
    e. Xanthines

25. Decongestants are contraindicated or to be used with extreme caution for patients with which condition? **Select all that apply**.
    a. Cardiac disease
    b. Diabetes mellitus
    c. Hypertension
    d. Hyperthyroidism
    e. Obesity

26. A patient with a history of atrial fibrillation and depression has been taking medications for a "common cold." Which teaching would the nurse provide? **Select all that apply**.
    a. Administer 4 puffs of nasal spray for a full 10 days.
    b. Antibiotics are also needed to fight a common cold virus.
    c. Do not drive during initial use of a cold remedy containing an antihistamine.
    d. Read labels of OTC drugs for any interactions with current drugs.
    e. Take cold remedies with a decongestant for a better night's sleep.

CASE STUDY: CRITICAL THINKING

Read the scenario and answer the following questions on a separate sheet of paper.

A patient is preparing to fly across the country for a conference and presents to the health care provider with nasal stuffiness. The patient tells the provider "I hate to fly when my nose is this way. It just makes the trip all that much longer." A decongestant, oxymetazoline, is ordered.

1. What is the purpose of oxymetazoline, and how does it work?

2. What is the standard dosage for this drug?

3. Describe rebound congestion.

4. What other side effects might be expected, and how can they be prevented?

5. Are there any other options for a decongestant?

39 Lower Respiratory Disorders

STUDY QUESTIONS

Match the drug in Column I with its class in Column II. Drugs may belong to more than one class.

Column I

_____ **1.** Acetylcysteine

_____ **2.** Zafirlukast

_____ **3.** Albuterol

_____ **4.** Ipratropium bromide

_____ **5.** Dexamethasone

_____ **6.** Epinephrine

_____ **7.** Arformoterol tartrate

_____ **8.** Tiotropium

Column II

a. Alpha-adrenergic agonist
b. Beta-adrenergic agonist
c. Glucocorticoid
d. Mucolytic
e. Leukotriene receptor antagonist
f. Anticholinergic

Complete the following.

9. The natural substance in the cytoplasm of bronchial cells responsible for maintaining bronchodilation is _____ _____ _____.

10. In an acute bronchospasm caused by anaphylaxis, the nonselective sympathomimetic drug administered subcutaneously to promote bronchodilation and elevate the blood pressure is _____.

11. The class of drugs that are considered the first line of defense in an acute asthmatic attack are categorized as _____ _____.

12. Sympathomimetics cause dilation of the bronchioles by increasing _____.

13. Theophylline (increases/decreases) the risk of digitalis toxicity. (*Circle the correct answer.*)

14. When theophylline and beta$_2$-adrenergic agonists are given together, a(n) _____ effect can occur.

15. The half-life of theophylline is (shorter/longer) for smokers than for nonsmokers. (*Circle the correct answer.*)

16. Aminophylline, theophylline, and caffeine are _____ derivatives used to treat _____.

17. The drugs commonly prescribed to treat unresponsive asthma are _____.

18. Cromolyn is used as a _____ treatment for bronchial asthma. It acts by inhibiting the release of _____.

19. A serious side effect of cromolyn is _____ _____.

20. The newer drugs for asthma are more selective for _____ receptors.

21. The leukotriene receptor antagonist (is/is not) considered safe for use in children 6 years and older. (*Circle the correct answer.*)

22. The preferred time of day for the administration of leukotriene receptor antagonists is _____.

23. The usual dose of montelukast for an adult is _____.

24. A group of drugs used to liquefy and loosen thick mucous secretions is _____.

25. With infection resulting from retained mucous secretions, a(n) _____ may be prescribed.

REVIEW QUESTIONS

Select the best response.

26. A patient is being treated for chronic obstructive pulmonary disease (COPD) with a drug that is delivered via a metered-dose inhaler. Related health teaching would include which priority information?
   a. Hold the inhaler upside down.
   b. Refrigerate the inhaler.
   c. Shake the inhaler well just before use.
   d. Test the inhaler each time to see if the spray works.

27. When compared to oral drugs for asthma, which information of a metered-dose inhaler would the nurse be aware? **Select all that apply**.
   a. Inhaled dose will deliver more of the drug directly to the lungs.
   b. There are fewer side effects with an inhaled drug.
   c. Inhaled drug is longer-lasting.
   d. Inhaled drug has a more rapid onset.
   e. Some oral and inhaled drugs can be taken together.

28. A patient expresses not having the time to wait between taking an inhaled beta agonist and an inhaled steroid for asthma. Which response would be appropriate by the nurse?
   a. "The inhaled beta agonist allows the bronchioles to dilate so the steroid works better."
   b. "This is done so you remember which one comes first."
   c. "The inhaled beta agonist will make your heart circulate the steroid faster."
   d. "The steroid may make your nose stuffy, so you take the inhaled beta agonist first."

29. Which condition is a side effect of long-term use of glucocorticoids? **Select all that apply**.
   a. Impaired immune response
   b. Insomnia
   c. Hyperglycemia
   d. Vomiting
   e. Weight loss

30. Which anticholinergic drug has few systemic effects and is administered by aerosol?
   a. Albuterol
   b. Ipratropium
   c. Isoproterenol
   d. Tiotropium

31. A patient who has been taking theophylline for asthma has also been taking ephedra to stay alert while finishing a project at work. Heart rate is 124 beats/min, respiratory rate 18 breaths/min, blood pressure 170/90 mm Hg, and oxygen saturation 99% on room air. Fingerstick blood glucose is 210 mg/dL and the theophylline level is 26 mcg/mL. Which side effect or reaction would the nurse suspect may be occurring in this patient?
   a. Acute allergic reaction
   b. Asthma attack
   c. Stevens-Johnson syndrome
   d. Theophylline toxicity

32. The patient has exercise-induced bronchospasm and is being treated with a short-acting $beta_2$ agonist. Which priority information would the nurse include? **Select all that apply**.
   a. "Cleanse all washable parts of inhaler equipment daily."
   b. "Hold your breath for a few seconds, remove mouthpiece, and exhale slowly."
   c. "Keep your lips secure around the mouthpiece and inhale while pushing the top of the canister once."
   d. "Monitor your heart rate while taking this medication."
   e. "Wait 5 minutes and repeat the procedure if a second inhalation is needed."

33. Which medication when prescribed with theophylline would concern the nurse? **Select all that apply**.
   a. Beta blockers
   b. Digitalis
   c. Lithium
   d. Stool softeners
   e. Phenytoin

34. Which statement by a patient who is prescribed cromolyn indicates the need for more education?
    a. "I must take this drug every day."
    b. "It will stop an asthma attack when taken immediately."
    c. "I can rinse my mouth out with water to get rid of the taste."
    d. "It is important for me to take this exactly as directed."

35. Which level of theophylline would fall in the therapeutic range?
    a. 2 mcg/mL
    b. 8 mcg/mL
    c. 14 mcg/mL
    d. 23 mcg/mL

CASE STUDY: CRITICAL THINKING

Read the scenario, and answer the following questions on a separate sheet of paper.

An adult patient has recently been diagnosed with asthma and has been prescribed albuterol, montelukast sodium, and fluticasone propionate/salmeterol 100/50 mcg.

1. Identify the classifications for each of the drugs.

2. Describe the mechanisms of action for each drug.

3. Identify the priority teaching points for this patient with a new diagnosis of asthma.

40 Cardiac Glycosides, Antianginals, and Antidysrhythmics

STUDY QUESTIONS

Match the electrocardiogram waveform in Column I to its definition in Column II.

Column I

_____ **1.** P wave

_____ **2.** QRS complex

_____ **3.** T wave

_____ **4.** PR interval

_____ **5.** QT interval

Column II

a. Ventricular action potential duration
b. Atrial activation (depolarization)
c. Ventricular repolarization
d. Atrioventricular conduction time
e. Ventricular depolarization

Complete the following.

6. Heart failure occurs when the myocardium (strengthens/weakens) and (shrinks/enlarges), which causes the heart to lose its ability to pump blood through the heart and circulatory system. (*Circle the correct answers.*)

7. With heart failure there is a(n) (increase/decrease) in preload and afterload. (*Circle the correct answer.*)

8. Cardiac glycosides are also called _____ _____ which _____ the sodium-potassium pump.

9. The action of antianginal drugs is to increase blood flow and to (increase/decrease) oxygen supply or to (increase/decrease) oxygen demand by the myocardium. (*Circle the correct answers.*)

10. Name three of the four effects digitalis preparations have on the heart muscle (myocardium): _____, _____, and _____.

11. Beta blockers and calcium channel blockers (decrease/increase) the workload of the heart. (*Circle the correct answer.*)

12. To prevent thromboembolus in patients with atrial dysrhythmias, _____ is prescribed concurrently with antidysrhythmics.

13. Electrolyte imbalances such as _____, _____, and _____ can increase digitalis toxicity.

14. Angiotensin converting enzyme inhibitors help patients with heart failure by _____ venules and _____, which improves _____ blood flow and _____ blood fluid volume.

15. Short-acting nitroglycerin (NTG) is not swallowed because it undergoes _____, thereby decreasing its effectiveness.

16. NTG acts directly on the _____, causing relaxation and dilation.

17. NTG sublingually acts within _____ minutes. Administration may be repeated _____ times.

18. The most common side effect of NTG is _____.

19. The two drug groups that may be used as an antianginal, antidysrhythmic, and antihypertensive are _____ _____ and _____ _____ _____.

20. Calcium channel blockers that are effective in the long-term treatment of angina, dysrhythmia, and hypertension and have the side effect of bradycardia are _____ and _____.

21. Beta blockers and calcium channel blockers should not be discontinued without health care provider approval. Withdrawal symptoms may include _____ _____ and _____.

22. Classic angina occurs when the patient is _____.

23. Unstable angina (preinfarction) has the following pattern of occurrence: Occurs _____, is _____, and manifests with _____ severity.

24. Variant angina (Prinzmetal's angina) occurs when the patient is _____.

25. Prinzmetal's angina is due to _____ of the vessels.

26. The major systemic effect of nitrates is _____.

27. Cardiac dysrhythmias can result from (hypoxia/hyperoxia) and (hypocapnia/hypercapnia). (*Circle correct answers.*)

28. Examples of antidysrhythmics include _____, _____, and _____.

29. Patients with heart failure should avoid _____ and _____.

Match the herbs in Column I with their effects on digoxin in Column II. Effects in Column II may be used more than once.

Column I

_____ 30. St. John's wort

_____ 31. Ephedra

_____ 32. Aloe

_____ 33. Goldenseal

_____ 34. Ginseng

Column II

a. Increased risk of digitalis toxicity
b. Decreased digoxin absorption
c. Decreased effects of digoxin
d. Falsely elevated digoxin levels

REVIEW QUESTIONS

Select the best response.

35. Phosphodiesterase inhibitors promote which actions in treating heart failure?
    a. Increase serum sodium and potassium levels
    b. Promote negative inotropic action
    c. Promote positive inotropic action
    d. Promote vasoconstriction

36. A patient with a history of atrial flutter is prescribed quinidine. Which response by the nurse is most appropriate when answering a patient who asks how the drug helps the heart?
    a. "It will help your heart pump stronger."
    b. "It will prevent you from having chest pain."
    c. "It will decrease myocardial oxygen consumption."
    d. "It will slow down the speed of your heart so that it will work more effectively."

37. Which drug is more effective when other drugs are ineffective in treating ventricular fibrillation?
    a. Amiodarone
    b. Atropine
    c. Acebutolol HCl
    d. Propafenone HCl

38. Which cardiac disorder is lidocaine primarily used to treat?
    a. Atrial fibrillation
    b. Bradycardia
    c. Complete heart block
    d. Ventricular dysrhythmias

39. A patient with angina has been prescribed verapamil. Which priority teaching point would the nurse include? **Select all that apply**.
   a. "Eat lots of fiber to avoid constipation."
   b. "High blood pressure can be caused by verapamil."
   c. "This drug is taken three times per day."
   d. "Wear sunscreen due to photosensitivity."
   e. "You should not take this drug if you are diabetic."

40. A patient has been prescribed amlodipine to help control hypertension. Which laboratory values must be monitored carefully?
   a. Arterial blood gasses
   b. Blood glucose
   c. Complete blood count
   d. Liver enzymes

41. Elevated levels of atrial natriuretic peptide and brain natriuretic peptide (BNP) indicate which disease process?
   a. Aneurysm
   b. Cerebrovascular accident
   c. Heart failure
   d. Myocardial infarction

42. An older adult patient taking digoxin daily along with several other drugs has a BNP level of 630 pg/mL. Which statement is correct about the BNP level?
   a. It is below the normal/reference range for the patient's age.
   b. It is within the normal range.
   c. It is slightly elevated.
   d. It is markedly elevated.

43. The nurse knows that digitalis is usually prescribed for which dysrhythmia?
   a. Atrial fibrillation
   b. Paroxysmal atrial tachycardia
   c. Second-degree heart block
   d. Ventricular tachycardia

44. Which dose of digoxin is the usual maintenance dose?
   a. 0.125–5 mg/d
   b. 0.025–1 mg/d
   c. 0.05–1.75 mg/d
   d. 6–10 mg/d

45. A patient who has been on digoxin presents to the clinic complaining of nausea, malaise, and "just not feeling well." The nurse suspects digoxin toxicity. Which value represents therapeutic digitalis level?
   a. 0.15–0.5 ng/mL
   b. 0.8–2 ng/mL
   c. 2–3.5 ng/mL
   d. 3.5–4 ng/mL

46. Which product is the antidote for digitalis toxicity?
   a. Cardizem
   b. Digoxin immune fab
   c. Gamma globulin
   d. Protamine

47. The nurse is reviewing the patient's medication administration record (MAR). Which drug on the MAR would concern the nurse, given that the patient is taking digitalis? **Select all that apply**.
   a. Cortisone
   b. Furosemide
   c. Hydrochlorothiazide
   d. NTG
   e. Potassium supplement

48. The nurse is providing health teaching to a patient prescribed digoxin for heart failure. Which food would the nurse inform the patient to avoid? **Select all that apply**.
   a. Apples
   b. Celery
   c. Hot dogs
   d. Lettuce
   e. Potatoes

49. Which priority health teaching would be given to a patient taking sublingual (SL) NTG? **Select all that apply**.
   a. Sips of water may be taken before placing NTG SL to aid in absorption.
   b. NTG should be stored in its original container and away from light.
   c. The tablet is to be chewed and swallowed.
   d. Call your health care provider if chest pain is not relieved after three tablets.
   e. Patients should not take vitamin C supplements while taking NTG.

50. Which duration of action of a NTG transdermal patch is correct?
   a. 6–8 hours
   b. 10–12 hours
   c. 18–24 hours
   d. 36–48 hours

51. Which priority teaching would the nurse provide to a patient who is prescribed acebutolol?
   a. "Do not abruptly stop this drug, or you risk your heart rate beating very fast or irregularly."
   b. "Drowsiness is a common side effect."
   c. "No laboratory work will be required while taking this drug."
   d. "Fluid intake should be increased to prevent dehydration."

52. Which herbal product must be avoided when taking digitalis preparations? **Select all that apply**.
   a. Aloe
   b. Feverfew
   c. Ginkgo biloba
   d. Ginseng
   e. Ma-huang

53. Which condition can directly lead to cardiac dysrhythmias? **Select all that apply**.
  a. Electrolyte imbalances
  b. Excess catecholamines
  c. Hepatitis
  d. Hypocapnia
  e. Hypoxia

CASE STUDY: CRITICAL THINKING

Read the scenario and answer the following questions on a separate sheet of paper.

An adult patient with a history of hypertension, diet-controlled diabetes, and vasospastic angina presents to the emergency department with severe left-sided chest pain, nausea, shortness of breath, and diaphoresis. Vital signs include the following: temperature 97.7° F, heart rate 102 beats/min, respiratory rate 20 breaths/min, blood pressure 164/100 mm Hg, and oxygen saturation on room air of 99%. Five minutes after administering one sublingual NTG tablet, repeat vital signs include heart rate 120 beats/min, respiratory rate 22 breaths/min, and blood pressure 110/60 mm Hg. The patient now feels lightheaded and nauseated, but the chest pain persists. A NTG drip is started, and the patient is admitted to critical care.

1. Describe the three different types of angina.

2. Describe nonpharmacologic and pharmacologic treatments for vasospastic angina.

3. Which drugs other than NTG can be used to treat angina?

4. Discuss the reason the patient's blood pressure decreased.

41 Diuretics

Chapter **41** Diuretics

STUDY QUESTIONS

Labeling Diagram

Label the different segments of the renal tubules, the major class of diuretics for each, and the primary electrolytes influenced by the diuretic.

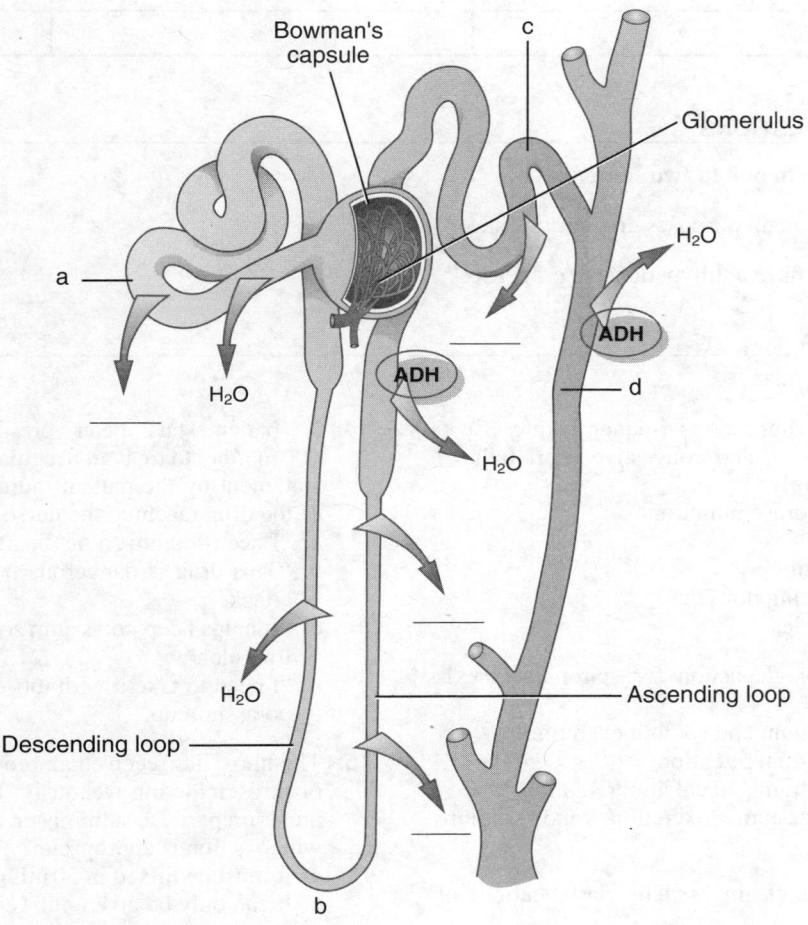

a. _____
_____

b. _____
_____

c. _____
_____

d. _____
_____

Identify the normal levels of the chemistry panel, and list the possible abnormal results (hypo- or hyper-) associated with thiazide diuretics.

Laboratory Test	Normal Levels	Abnormal Results
1. Potassium		
2. Magnesium		
3. Ionized calcium		
4. Chloride		
5. Bicarbonate		
6. Uric acid		
7. Blood sugar		
8. Blood lipids		

SHORT ANSWER QUESTIONS

Answer the following in one to two sentences.

9. Which of the two main purposes do diuretics have?

10. How do diuretics have antihypertensive properties?

REVIEW QUESTIONS

Select the best response.

11. Which group of diuretics is frequently prescribed to treat hypertension and congestive heart failure? Select all that apply.
    a. Carbonic anhydrase inhibitors
    b. Loop diuretics
    c. Osmotic diuretics
    d. Potassium-sparing diuretics
    e. Thiazide diuretics

12. Which pharmacologic action for spironolactone is correct?
    a. Increase potassium and sodium excretion
    b. Promote potassium retention
    c. Promote potassium and calcium retention
    d. Promote potassium excretion and sodium retention

13. Furosemide belongs in which classification of diuretics?
    a. Loop diuretic
    b. Osmotic diuretic
    c. Potassium-sparing diuretic
    d. Thiazide diuretic

14. A patient has been prescribed spironolactone 100 mg/day to treat an irregular heart rhythm. Which statement by the patient indicates an understanding of the drug teaching the nurse provided?
    a. "I need sodium so my heart beats regularly."
    b. "This drug is dangerous if you have had a heart attack."
    c. "It helps keep potassium so my heart does not get irregular."
    d. "I need to take it with lots of bananas to keep my potassium up."

15. The nurse has received an order to administer 40 mg of furosemide intravenously (IV) to the patient. The nurse prepares to administer the drug knowing that which action is appropriate?
    a. It must be mixed in 50 mL of normal saline.
    b. It can only be given in a central line.
    c. The patient must be on a cardiac monitor.
    d. It should be given over 1-2 minutes.

16. Which lab value would a nurse monitor in a patient receiving chlorothiazide? Select all that apply.
    a. Potassium
    b. Sodium
    c. Bicarbonate
    d. Calcium
    e. AST/ALT

17. A patient who has had an acute myocardial infarction has been started on spironolactone 50 mg/day. When evaluating routine laboratory work, the nurse discovers the patient has a potassium level of 5.8 mEq/L. Which intervention would be a priority by the nurse?
    a. The spironolactone dose should be held and the intake of foods rich in potassium should be restricted.
    b. The spironolactone dose should be continued and the patient should be encouraged to eat fruits and vegetables.
    c. The spironolactone dose should be increased and the patient instructed to decrease foods rich in potassium.
    d. Instruct the patient to continue with the current dose of spironolactone and report any signs or symptoms of hypokalemia.

18. Which type of acid-base imbalance could occur if a patient is taking high doses of acetazolamide or uses the drug constantly?
    a. Metabolic acidosis
    b. Metabolic alkalosis
    c. Respiratory acidosis
    d. Respiratory alkalosis

19. The patient with heart failure has been prescribed hydrochlorothiazide. Which statement by the patient indicates understanding of the dosing regimen?
    a. "I need to take it on an empty stomach for it to work."
    b. "I really only need to take my medicine when I am having a hard time breathing."
    c. "It may take several weeks before it starts to work."
    d. "I should take it in the morning so I don't have to go to the bathroom at night."

20. The patient with a complicated medical history including heart failure, cardiac arrhythmias, arthritis, and depression was started on furosemide for heart failure. Which drug if taken with furosemide would be of major concern to the nurse?
    a. Amiodarone
    b. Acetaminophen
    c. Amitriptyline
    d. Zolpidem

21. A patient taking furosemide reports being weak, having severe leg cramps, and unable to ambulate. Knowing the mechanism of action of furosemide, the nurse would be concerned about which electrolyte imbalance?
    a. Hyponatremia
    b. Hypermagnesemia
    c. Hypokalemia
    d. Hyperchloremia

22. A patient with which condition would loop diuretics be contraindicated?
    a. Anuria
    b. Asthma
    c. Ceftriaxone allergy
    d. Gastric ulcers

23. A patient diagnosed with hypertension and diabetes was started on hydrochlorothiazide. Which statement by the patient indicates an understanding of the drug teaching the nurse provided?
    a. "It will start working within minutes."
    b. "I don't need to monitor my blood sugar."
    c. "I should take my drug on an empty stomach so it works better."
    d. "I need to keep track of my weight and blood pressure at home."

CASE STUDY: CRITICAL THINKING

Read the scenario, and answer the following questions on a separate sheet of paper.

An adult patient was involved in a motorcycle collision suffering a severe traumatic brain injury. While preparing to take the patient to surgery, the neurosurgeon orders mannitol to be administered. The patient weighs 80 kg. Vital signs include temperature 97.9° F, heart rate 62 beats/min, respiratory rate controlled on a ventilator at 18 breaths/min, and blood pressure 194/132 mm Hg. The patient has an increased intracranial pressure (ICP) of 36 mm Hg.

1. Describe the class of diuretic mannitol is and its mechanism of action.

2. What is the standard dosage range for mannitol? How is mannitol administered?

3. Calculate the correct dose for this patient?

42 Antihypertensives

STUDY QUESTIONS

Complete the following.

1. When hypertension cannot be controlled with lifestyle and diet changes, antihypertensive drugs may be prescribed. Three of the five sympatholytic groups are _____, _____, and _____.

2. Two categories of antihypertensives in addition to the sympatholytics are _____ and _____.

3. Thiazide diuretics may be combined with other antihypertensive drugs. Examples of other antihypertensives include _____ and _____.

4. Many antihypertensive drugs can cause fluid retention. To decrease body fluid, the drug group often administered with antihypertensive drugs is _____.

5. Beta-adrenergic blockers reduce cardiac output by diminishing the sympathetic nervous system response. With continued use of beta blockers, vascular resistance is (increased/diminished) and blood pressure is (lowered/increased). *(Circle the correct answers.)*

6. Atenolol and metoprolol are examples of (cardioselective/noncardioselective) antihypertensive drugs. *(Circle the correct answer.)*

7. The alpha blockers are useful in treating hypertensive patients with lipid abnormalities. The effects they have on lipoproteins include (decreased/increased) VLDL and LDL; and (decreased/increased) HDL. *(Circle the correct answers.)*

Match the drug name in Column I with the class of antihypertensive in Column II.

Column I

_____ **8.** Captopril

_____ **9.** Verapamil

_____ **10.** Prazosin

_____ **11.** Atenolol

_____ **12.** Methyldopa

_____ **13.** Hydralazine

_____ **14.** Candesartan

_____ **15.** Carvedilol

Column II

a. Cardioselective beta blocker
b. Selective alpha blocker
c. Angiotensin-converting enzyme (ACE) inhibitor
d. Calcium channel blocker
e. Centrally acting alpha$_2$ agonist
f. Direct-acting vasodilator
g. Angiotensin II-receptor antagonist (A-II blocker)
h. Nonselective beta$_1$ and beta$_2$ blocker

16. Which patient would be most suited for treatment with a nonselective alpha-adrenergic blocker?
    a. A patient with mild to moderate renal failure
    b. A patient with hypertension associated with pheochromocytoma
    c. A patient with hyperlipidemia
    d. A patient with type 2 diabetes

17. Which area of the body do direct-acting vasodilators act to decrease blood pressure?
    a. Cardiac valves
    b. Dopaminergic receptors in kidneys
    c. Renal tubules
    d. Smooth muscles of the blood vessels

18. Which class of drugs would be given to avoid fluid retention?
    a. Anticoagulants
    b. Antidysrhythmics
    c. Cardiac glycosides
    d. Diuretics

19. Which mechanism of action is correct for angiotensin II-receptor blockers (ARBs)? **Select all that apply**.
    a. Block angiotensin II
    b. Cause vasodilation
    c. Decrease peripheral resistance
    d. Increase sodium retention
    e. Slow heart rate

20. For which purpose are ARBs combined with the thiazide diuretic?
    a. To decrease rapid blood pressure drop.
    b. To enhance the antihypertensive effect by promoting sodium and water loss.
    c. To increase sodium and water retention for controlling blood pressure.
    d. To promote potassium retention.

21. Valsartan may be prescribed for patients with hypertension instead of captopril. Which factor is the most limiting in the use of captopril?
    a. Coughing
    b. Dizziness
    c. Constipation
    d. Sneezing

22. A nurse is preparing to administer cardiac drugs to several patients. The nurse would be concerned about administering lisinopril as a monotherapy to which patient?
    a. A Hispanic
    b. An Asian
    c. A Caucasian
    d. An African American

23. An African American patient presents to a health care provider for continued high blood pressure. Which group of drugs would be more effective for this patient?
    a. Angiotensin II blockers
    b. Beta blockers
    c. Calcium blockers
    d. Direct renin inhibitor

24. Which drug-herb interaction can occur when ma-huang (ephedra) is taken concomitantly with an antihypertensive drug?
    a. A decrease or counteraction of the effects of the antihypertensive drug.
    b. A decrease in the hypertensive state.
    c. An increase in the hypotensive effects of the antihypertensive drug.
    d. No effect on the action of the antihypertensive drug.

25. If a patient takes captopril with nitrates, diuretics, or adrenergic blockers, which side effect would the nurse assess in this patient?
    a. Hypoglycemic reaction
    b. Hypotensive reaction
    c. Hyperkalemic reaction
    d. Hypertensive reaction

26. Which electrolyte imbalance might occur if a patient takes captopril with a potassium-sparing diuretic?
    a. Hypokalemia
    b. Hyperkalemia
    c. Hypocalcemia
    d. Hypercalcemia

27. A patient wishes to stop taking captopril for the treatment of hypertension. Which response is most appropriate by the nurse?
    a. "Blood pressure can be controlled by diet and exercise, so you don't have to take drug."
    b. "It is important to keep taking your drug as directed until you speak with your health care provider."
    c. "Once your blood pressure is normal for one month, you can stop taking your drug."
    d. "Wean yourself off of the drug over a 10-day period."

28. Amlodipine has which protein-binding power?
    a. Highly protein-bound
    b. Moderately to highly protein-bound
    c. Moderately protein-bound
    d. Low protein-bound

29. Which assessment finding would the nurse assess in a patient who is experiencing side effects from metoprolol? **Select all that apply**.
   a. Dizziness
   b. Headache
   c. Increased blood pressure
   d. Nausea
   e. Paranoia

30. A patient taking amlodipine complains of swelling in the ankles. Which response by the nurse is correct?
   a. "Swelling is common when taking amlodipine. You should cut the tablet in half to reduce your dosage."
   b. "Swelling may occur with amlodipine. I will contact your health care provider to determine if the drug should be changed."
   c. "You should not be taking that drug because of your age. I will see what other antihypertensive drug you can take."
   d. "You should stop taking the drug for several days and check that the swelling has decreased."

31. Which statement is true about the advantage of using cardioselective beta-adrenergic blockers as an antihypertensive? **Select all that apply**.
   a. They can be abruptly discontinued without causing rebound symptoms.
   b. They help prevent bronchodilation.
   c. They increase serum electrolyte levels.
   d. They maintain renal blood flow.
   e. They minimize the hypoglycemic effect.

32. Which statement best describes the direct renin inhibitor aliskiren?
   a. It is effective for treating severe hypertension.
   b. It can be combined with another antihypertensive drug.
   c. It can cause hypokalemia when taken as a monotherapy drug.
   d. It is more effective than calcium channel blockers in treating hypertension in Black patients.

CLINICAL JUDGMENT UNFOLDING CASE STUDY

Read the scenario and answer the following questions on a separate sheet of paper.

Question 1:
SLO: Apply knowledge of antihypertensives to determine which assessment data require immediate follow-up by the nurse.
NGN Item Type: Highlight Text
Cognitive Skills: Recognize Cues

A 70-year-old female patient, who has a history of hypertension, presents to the clinic with complaints of dizziness. Home medications include clonidine/chlorthalidone 0.2 mg/15 mg daily. The patient reports that at times she "forgets to take a dose here and there."

Assessment findings include:
   Reports dizziness
   Reports "feels like a band around my head"
   Serum sodium 149 mEq/L
   Reports occasional epistaxis
   Blood pressure 232/136 mm Hg
   Serum potassium 4.8 mEq/L
   Heart rate 92 beats/minute
   Respiratory rate 16 breaths/minute
   Temperature 98.3°F
   Hgb 12.5 g/dL
   Blood urea nitrogen (BUN) 23 mg/dL
   Creatinine 1.9 mg/dL

Electrocardiogram (ECG)

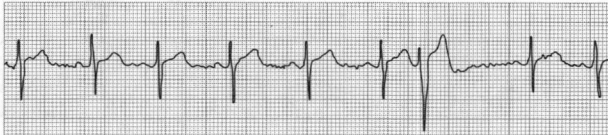

(Aehlert, B. 2018. ECGs Made Easy, 6th ed. p. 167, fig 6.4)

Highlight the assessment findings that require immediate follow up by the nurse.

Question 2:
SLO: Analyze patient's data on antihypertensives to determine potential health risk
NGN Item Type: Drop-Down Table
Cognitive Skills: Analyze Cues

A 70-year-old female patient who has a history of hypertension, presents to the clinic with complaints of dizziness. Home medications include clonidine/chlorthalidone 0.2 mg/15 mg daily. The patient reports that at times "forgets to take a dose here and there."

Assessment findings include:
   Reports dizziness
   Reports "feels like a band around my head"
   Serum sodium 149 mEq/L
   Reports occasional epistaxis
   Blood pressure 232/136 mm Hg
   Serum potassium 4.8 mEq/L
   Heart rate 92 beats/minute
   Respiratory rate 16 breaths/minute
   Temperature 98.3°F
   Hgb 12.5 g/dL
   Blood urea nitrogen (BUN) 23 mg/dL
   Creatinine 1.9 mg/dL

Electrocardiogram (ECG)

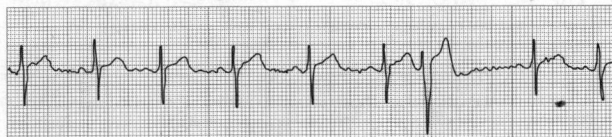

(Aehlert, B. 2018. ECGs Made Easy, 6th ed. p. 167, fig 6.4)

Drag each potential issue that this patient is at risk for to the second column.

Potential Issues	Risk to the Patient
Low-renin hypertension	
Orthostatic hypotension	
Fluid retention	
Renal insufficiency	
Hyperkalemia	
Rebound hypertension	
Hypernatremia	

Phase 2
Question 3:
SLO: Prioritize nursing care for patients receiving antihypertensives.

NGN Item Type: Drop-Down Cloze
Cognitive Skills: Prioritize Hypotheses

A 70-year-old female patient who has a history of hypertension, presented to the clinic with complaints of dizziness. Home medications include clonidine/chlorthalidone 0.2 mg/15 mg daily. She was directly admitted to the cardiac unit for hypertensive emergency. The patient has been receiving nitroprusside 0.6 mcg/kg/min intravenously for 3 hours. The patient's current weight is 178 pounds. In the last 8 hours, total fluid intake was 850 mL and total fluid output was 436 mL.

Choose the most likely options for the missing information from the statements below by selecting from the lists of options provided.

The patient received a total of __1__ mcg in 3 hours. The nurse would assess the patient for signs and symptoms of cyanide toxicity, such as __2__, profound __3__, dyspnea, dizziness, and vomiting. Nitroprusside can also cause reflex __4__ and palpitations.

Options for 1	Options for 2	Options for 3	Options for 4
44	Metabolic acidosis	Bradycardia	Bradycardia
243	Metabolic alkalosis	Tachypnea	Tachycardia
2410	Respiratory acidosis	Diarrhea	Drowsiness
8739	Respiratory alkalosis	Hypotension	Bleeding

Questions 4:
SLO: Generate nursing actions for patients receiving antihypertensives.
NGN Item Type: Drop-Down Table
Cognitive Skills: Generate Solutions

A 70-year-old female patient who has a history of hypertension, presented to the clinic with complaints of dizziness. Home medications include clonidine/chlorthalidone 0.2 mg/15 mg daily. She was directly admitted to the cardiac unit for hypertensive emergency. Her blood pressure normalized with nitroprusside without any unwanted side effects. The patient was started on oral metoprolol with hydrochlorothiazide. The patient voices frustration and asks the nurse several questions about the antihypertensives.

Indicate in the third column the appropriate nursing response listed in the first column in response for each patient's question in the second column. Note that not all nursing responses will be used.

Nurse's Responses	Patient Questions	Appropriate Nurse's Response for Each Patient Question
"That is the only way you can take the metoprolol and hydrochlorothiazide."	"Why do I need to take two pills when I used to take only one?"	
"Metoprolol has lower tendency to cause rebound high blood pressure."	"Couldn't I just continue with my other blood pressure medicine?"	
"The metoprolol and hydrochlorothiazide come as a single pill."	"How do I know if the medicine is working?"	
"If you start feeling dizzy when you stand from a sitting position, then it is working."	"Hopefully this medicine will not cause my blood pressure to skyrocket."	

Nurse's Responses	Patient Questions	Appropriate Nurse's Response for Each Patient Question
"As long as you do not stop taking the medicine, you will not have problems with high blood pressure."		
"The other pill caused a significant rebound high blood pressure. This new pill has less tendency."		
"Let me show you how to take your blood pressure and heart rate. If your blood pressure is really low or you feel dizzy or your heart rate is less than 60, call your doctor."		

Phase 3
Question 5:
SLO: Determine appropriate nursing actions for patients taking antihypertensives
NGN Item Type: Matrix Multiple Choice
Cognitive Skills: Take Action

A 70-year-old female patient who has a history of hypertension, presented to the clinic with complaints of dizziness. Her blood pressure normalized on nitroprusside and was started on oral metoprolol 25 mg with hydrochlorothiazide 12.5 mg daily. While preparing to administer the medication, the nurse assesses the patient. **Use an X for the nursing action below that is Indicated (appropriate or necessary) or Contraindicated (could be harmful).**

Nursing Actions	Indicated	Contraindicated
Administer with heart rate 54		
Hold for blood pressure 90/68		
Administer when patient complains of fatigue		
Hold for urine output of 90 mL in 4 hours		
Check blood pressure in sitting and standing		

Question 6:
SLO: Evaluate the action of antihypertensives.
NGN Item Type: Highlight Text
Cognitive Skills: Evaluate Outcomes

A 70-year-old female patient who has a history of hypertension, presented to the clinic with complaints of dizziness. Her blood pressure normalized on nitroprusside and was started on oral metoprolol 25 mg with hydrochlorothiazide 12.5 mg daily. While preparing to administer the medication, the nurse assesses the patient.

Highlight the assessment findings in the progress note that would indicate potential complications from metoprolol and hydrochlorothiazide.

Progress Notes:
Awake, alert, and oriented in all fields. States "feel weaker than usual. I don't seem to have a lot of oomph." Vital signs include blood pressure 98/64, apical pulse 86, and radial pulse 72 beats/minute; respiratory rate 18 regular and even; temp 97.9° F. Skin warm with pink undertone. Cardiac without extra heart sounds. Lung sounds with few crackles to bases bilaterally. Denies cough. Abdomen soft, mild tenderness to lower quadrants. Reports no bowel movements for 3 days. Trace edema to ankles bilaterally. Labs: sodium 132 mEq/L, potassium 3.4 mEq/L, calcium 11.3 mg/dL, glucose 84 mg/dL. Cardiac monitor showing sinus rhythm with 1st-degree atrioventricular (AV) block and occasional premature ventricular beats at 70–92 beats/minute.

43 Anticoagulants, Antiplatelets, and Thrombolytics

STUDY QUESTIONS

Complete the following.

1. A thrombus can form in a(n) _____ or in a(n) _____.

2. Anticoagulants are used to inhibit _____ _____. They (do/do not) dissolve clots. (*Circle the correct answer.*)

3. Anticoagulants and thrombolytics (have/do not have) the same action. (*Circle the correct answer.*)

4. The most frequent use of heparin is to prevent _____ _____ that may lead to _____ _____.

5. Heparin can be given (orally/subcutaneously/intravenously). (*Circle all the correct answers.*)

6. The low-molecular-weight heparins (LMWHs) are derivatives of _____ heparin. The advantage of LMWHs is that they lower the risk of _____.

7. The international normalized ratio (INR) is a laboratory test to monitor the therapeutic effect of (warfarin/heparin). (*Circle the correct answer.*)

8. Heparin can (decrease/increase) the platelet count, causing thrombocytopenia. (*Circle the correct answer.*)

9. A thrombus disintegrates when a thrombolytic drug is administered. Ideally, the drug should be administered within _____ hours following an acute MI.

10. The action of the thrombolytic drugs streptokinase and urokinase is the conversion of _____ to _____.

11. The major complication with the use of thrombolytic drugs is _____.

12. A synthetic anticoagulant, _____, indirectly inhibits thrombin production and is closely related in structure to heparin and LMWH.

13. **Number the following steps of heparin activity in the correct order.**

    _____a.   Inhibits conversion of fibrinogen to fibrin.

    _____b.   Inactivates antithrombin III to prevent the formation of thrombin.

    _____c.   Clot prevented.

    _____d.   Heparin binds with antithrombin III.

Match the drug in Column I with its drug group in Column II. The drug group in Column II may be used more than once.

Column I

_____	14.	Warfarin
_____	15.	Aspirin
_____	16.	Enoxaparin
_____	17.	Dalteparin
_____	18.	Protamine sulfate
_____	19.	Clopidogrel
_____	20.	Streptokinase
_____	21.	Bivalirudin
_____	22.	Alteplase (tissue plasminogen activator [tPA])

Column II

a. Anticoagulant: LMWH
b. Direct thrombin inhibitor (parenteral)
c. Oral anticoagulant
d. Antiplatelet
e. Anticoagulant antagonist
f. Thrombolytic

REVIEW QUESTIONS

Select the best response.

23. A patient on warfarin for a DVT asks the nurse how warfarin works. Which response by the nurse would be the best?
    a. "Warfarin will help dissolve the blood clots."
    b. "Warfarin is given with thrombolytics to help break up clots."
    c. "Warfarin prevents new clots from forming."
    d. "Warfarin dilates the veins to improve blood flow."

24. The nurse has several patients receiving warfarin. Which INR would concern the nurse? **Select all that apply**.
    a. 1.2
    b. 1.4
    c. 1.8
    d. 2.0
    e. 2.4

25. Which drug is not considered an LMWH? **Select all that apply**.
    a. Enoxaparin sodium
    b. Clopidogrel
    c. Dalteparin
    d. Apixaban

26. A patient with unstable angina is having an emergent percutaneous transluminal coronary angioplasty (PTCA). The nurse is completing preprocedural teaching and explains a drug will be given right before the procedure and then for the next 12 hours by an intravenous (IV) drip to prevent ischemia. Which drug is the nurse teaching the patient about?
    a. Abciximab
    b. Aminocaproic acid
    c. Protamine sulfate
    d. Warfarin

27. A patient weighs 168 pounds and is going to receive abciximab for unstable angina. Which dosage is correct for a continuous infusion?
    a. 9.5 mcg/min
    b. 19 mcg/min
    c. 25 mg/min
    d. 42 mg/min

28. Which statement best describes clopidogrel?
    a. It is the most effective anticoagulant when used with ibuprofen.
    b. It is most effective when prescribed as a single drug to prevent stroke.
    c. It is an inexpensive alternative to warfarin.
    d. It can be used together with aspirin after myocardial infarction (MI) or cerebrovascular accident (CVA) to prevent platelet aggregation.

29. A patient with a history of atrial fibrillation is being discharged from the hospital on warfarin. Which teaching intervention would be a priority?
    a. "INR will be monitored closely."
    b. "Periodic evaluation of your electrolytes is very important."
    c. "Your blood must be monitored for BUN/creatinine values to evaluate for new renal failure."
    d. "You will not need any further lab work while taking this medication."

30. A patient on warfarin has an INR of 10.3 seconds. Physical assessment reveals the patient with multiple petechiae to the body. Which drug would the nurse prepare to administer?
    a. Anagrelide
    b. Protamine sulfate
    c. Ticagrelor
    d. Vitamin K (phytonadione)

31. The patient is given heparin for early treatment of DVT. Later, warfarin is prescribed. If the patient is also taking fluoxetine, which is highly protein-bound, which drug-drug interaction can occur?
    a. Drug displacement of the highly protein-bound drug but not displacement of warfarin.
    b. Drug displacement of warfarin.
    c. Drug displacement varies from patient to patient.
    d. No drug displacement of either drug.

32. A patient, who has been on fondaparinux at home, presents to the emergency department with complaints of gastrointestinal bleeding. Which condition would the nurse anticipate is occurring?
    a. Adverse reaction
    b. Allergic reaction
    c. Insufficient dose of fondaparinux
    d. Stevens-Johnson syndrome

33. A patient who received alteplase for treatment of CVA begins to hemorrhage. Which drug would the nurse anticipate administering?
    a. Reteplase
    b. Aminocaproic acid
    c. Calcium gluconate
    d. Protamine sulfate

34. Which action would the nurse perform when caring for a patient who is receiving tenecteplase? **Select all that apply**.
    a. Assess for reperfusion arrhythmias.
    b. Monitor liver panel.
    c. Observe for signs and symptoms of bleeding.
    d. Obtain a type and crossmatch.
    e. Record vital signs and report changes.

35. Which patient would be a candidate for anticoagulant? **Select all that apply**.
    a. A patient with deep vein thrombosis (DVT)
    b. A patient with an artificial heart valve
    c. A patient with migraines
    d. A patient who has had a knee replacement
    e. A patient with a CVA

CLINICAL JUDGMENT STANDALONE STUDY

Read the scenario, and answer the following questions on a separate sheet of paper.

SLO: Determine treatment priority for patients with pulmonary embolus.
NGN Item Type: Drop-Down Cloze
Cognitive Skills: Prioritize Hypotheses

A 28-year-old patient who is diagnosed with a large pulmonary embolus and is admitted to the intensive care unit for further diagnostic studies and treatment. A nurse starts performing an assessment and finds the patient to be restless. The patient reports the inability to "catch my breath" and having "sharp" chest pain. After completing a quick focused assessment, the nurse reviews the patient's medication administration record and current laboratory values. **Choose the *most likely* options for the information missing from the statements by selecting from the lists of options provided**.

The patient with a pulmonary embolus will most likely be started on oral and/or parenteral _____1_____, such as oral _____2_____ and parenteral _____3_____. In addition to monitoring the patient's hemoglobin, hematocrit, and any evidence of active bleeding, the INR would be maintained at _____4_____ if the patient is receiving oral warfarin.

Option 1	Option 2	Option 3	Option 4
Anxiolytics	Aspirin	Rivaroxaban	1–2 seconds
Thrombolytics	Warfarin	Apixaban	2–3 seconds
Anticoagulants	Argatroban	Phytonadione	20–30 seconds
Antihypertensives	Phytonadione	Dabigatran	2–3 minutes
Antiplatelets	Fondaparinux	Enoxaparin	1–2 hours

44 Antihyperlipidemics and Drugs to Improve Peripheral Blood Flow

STUDY QUESTIONS

Complete the following.

1. The four major categories of lipoprotein are _____, _____, _____, and _____.

2. High-density lipoproteins (HDLs) are the densest lipoproteins and contain more _____ and less _____ than the other lipoproteins.

3. Persons with elevated low-density lipoproteins (LDLs) have the risk of developing _____ _____ and _____ _____.

4. In addition to LDL, _____ (a lipoprotein) is a better indicator of risk for coronary artery disease (CAD).

5. Statin drugs inhibit _____ _____ in cholesterol biosynthesis and are called _____ _____ _____.

6. B vitamins and folic acid can lower serum _____ levels.

7. Primary causes of peripheral arterial disease include _____ and _____.

Match the drug in Column I with its drug group in Column II. Drug group in Column II may be used more than once.

Column I

_____ 8. Colestipol hydrochloride

_____ 9. Gemfibrozil

_____ 10. Atorvastatin

_____ 11. Simvastatin

_____ 12. Cholestyramine resin

_____ 13. Niacin

_____ 14. Ezetimibe

Column II

a. Statins
b. Bile-acid sequestrants
c. Fibrates
d. Cholesterol absorption inhibitors
e. Nicotinic acid

REVIEW QUESTIONS

Select the best response.

15. Which elevated apolipoprotein can be an indication of risk for CAD?
    a. apoA-1
    b. apoA-2
    c. apoB-100
    d. apoC-4

16. A patient who was prescribed atorvastatin 80 mg/day presented to the emergency department feeling weak and complaining of muscle pain. Which severe side effect of statins would the nurse suspect?
    a. Stevens-Johnson syndrome
    b. Pseudomembranous colitis
    c. Gastric ulcers
    d. Rhabdomyolysis

17. Homocysteine is a protein in the blood that has been linked to cardiovascular disease and stroke. Which other negative action can it also promote?
    a. Flushing of skin
    b. Loss of blood vessel flexibility
    c. Photosensitivity and sunburn
    d. Lowering of LDL levels

18. A patient who has intermittent claudication and leg pain tells the nurse, "I don't believe in taking all of that medicine stuff. I prefer to use only natural things." Which herb would the nurse recognize as being used by some patients with intermittent claudication?
    a. Ginger
    b. Ginseng
    c. Ginkgo
    d. Goldenseal

19. LDLs are the so-called "bad" lipoproteins. Which statement best reflects why high levels of LDL are considered unhealthy?
    a. There is an increased risk of hyperthyroidism.
    b. There is the possibility of digestive problems.
    c. There is an increased risk of rhabdomyolysis.
    d. There is an increased risk of heart disease.

20. The patient with hyperlipidemia has an HDL of 22 mg/dL. Which conclusion by the nurse would be correct?
    a. An HDL level of 22 mg/dL puts the patient in a high-risk category.
    b. An HDL level of 22 mg/dL places the patient in a moderate-risk category.
    c. The HDL level must be compared with all other levels before a decision can be made.
    d. An HDL level of 22 mg/dL is within the standard preferred range.

21. A patient with a total cholesterol level of 228 mg/dL has been on a low-fat, low-cholesterol diet for 2 months. A follow-up total cholesterol level is 212 mg/dL. Which response by the nurse would be most appropriate for the reason why the level is not lower?
    a. The patient most likely did not adhere to the diet.
    b. Diet modification usually decreases cholesterol levels by only 10-30%.
    c. The patient lost less than 10 pounds on the diet.
    d. The patient's exercise program was not rigorous enough.

22. A patient who is prescribed simvastatin asks if dietary modification is still needed. Which response by the nurse would be most appropriate?
    a. "Yes, you may eat whatever you want as long as you are taking simvastatin."
    b. "Diet is not an important factor if you are compliant with your drugs."
    c. "You should maintain a low-fat, low-cholesterol diet and exercise as well."
    d. "With simvastatin, you must lose weight as well as exercise."

23. Which priority information would the nurse include in the health teaching for a patient taking cilostazol? **Select all that apply**.
    a. Take medications with meals.
    b. Avoid drinking grapefruit juice.
    c. Do not take acetaminophen.
    d. Monitor for side effects such as headache and abdominal pain.
    e. Monitor blood pressure.

CASE STUDY: CRITICAL THINKING

Read the scenario and answer the following questions on a separate sheet of paper.

A young adult female patient has a family history of CAD and has recently been having intermittent chest pain. The patient's cholesterol level is 267 mg/dL; LDL level is 146 mg/dL; and HDL level is 44 mg/dL. Atorvastatin 10 mg/day was initially prescribed. The dosage has now been increased to 20 mg/day. The patient's medical history is positive for type 2 diabetes and has no allergies. The patient states there are plans on "getting pregnant."

1. Discuss the mode of action for atorvastatin and the purpose of this drug.

2. Discuss the implications of atorvastatin and pregnancy.

3. Discuss the nursing actions on what would be monitored during drug therapy, and how long the drug therapy will last.

4. Which teaching points would be included in patient education?

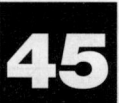 **Gastrointestinal Tract Disorders**

STUDY QUESTIONS

Match the substance in Column I with the description commonly associated with in Column II.

Column I

_____ **1.** Adsorbents

_____ **2.** Cannabinoids

_____ **3.** Chemoreceptor trigger zone (CTZ)

_____ **4.** Emetics

_____ **5.** Opiates

_____ **6.** Osmotics

_____ **7.** Purgatives

Column II

a. Harsh cathartics that cause a watery stool with abdominal cramping

b. Induce vomiting (used after poisoning)

c. Hyperosmolar laxatives

d. Relieve chemotherapy-induced nausea/vomiting

e. Lies near the medulla

f. Adsorb bacteria or toxins that cause diarrhea

g. Decrease intestinal motility, thereby decreasing peristalsis

Complete the following.

8. The _____ lies near the medulla, and the vomiting center is in the _____.

9. Nonprescription drugs for emesis include _____, _____, and _____ solutions.

10. Antihistamine antiemetics have similar side effects to those of _____.

11. Antiemetic drugs in the classes of anticholinergics and antihistamines should not be used in patients with _____ because of their side effects.

12. Phenothiazines and benzodiazepines are classified as _____ that suppress emesis by blocking the _____ trigger zone.

13. Serotonin receptor antagonists suppress _____ and _____ by blocking the _____ receptors.

14. A drug to alleviate nausea and vomiting, such as a _____, can also be used as an appetite stimulant.

15. _____ promotes a soft stool, whereas _____ results in a soft to watery stool.

16. Saline osmotic laxative products consist of _____ or _____.

17. Laxative abuse can cause fluid volume _____ and _____ losses.

SHORT ANSWER

18. List the eight classes of prescription antiemetics.

19. List at least five common causes of constipation.

20. Which instructions would be given to a patient who is prescribed psyllium, a bulk-forming laxative?

_____21. Prescription or nonprescription antiemetics are safe for pregnant women to take.

_____22. A person should have one bowel movement per day to be "normal."

_____23. Chronic use of laxatives can cause laxative dependence.

_____24. Because castor oil is a natural substance, it is safe for women in early pregnancy to use for occasional constipation.

REVIEW QUESTIONS

Select the best response.

25. Which class of drugs can be used as antiemetics? **Select all that apply**.
    a. Anticholinergics
    b. Antihistamines
    c. Cannabinoids
    d. Opioids
    e. Phenothiazines

26. A patient with severe nausea and vomiting asks how promethazine works. Which response by the nurse would be correct?
    a. "It stimulates the dopamine receptors in the brain associated with vomiting."
    b. "It blocks the histamine receptor sites and inhibits the CTZ."
    c. "It blocks the acetylcholine receptors associated with vomiting."
    d. "It prohibits the muscle contraction in the abdominal wall, preventing vomiting."

27. Which nonpharmacologic method would the nurse suggest to a patient who has been vomiting for 18 hours to decrease nausea and vomiting? **Select all that apply**.
    a. "Drink weak tea."
    b. "Takes sips of flat soda."
    c. "Eat small amounts of gelatin if tolerated."
    d. "Crackers may be helpful."
    e. "Eat toast with butter on it."

28. A patient who overdosed on prescription drugs is given activated charcoal orally. Which therapeutic action is a goal behind giving activated charcoal?
    a. Absorb poison
    b. Cause diarrhea
    c. Promote vomiting
    d. Stop nausea

29. The patient is receiving diphenoxylate with atropine for diarrhea. Which side effect would the nurse expect to see during treatment? **Select all that apply**.
    a. Headache
    b. Drowsiness
    c. Hypertension
    d. Hypoglycemia
    e. Urinary retention

30. Which substance is a type of laxative/cathartic? **Select all that apply**.
    a. Adsorbents
    b. Bulk-forming
    c. Emetics
    d. Emollients
    e. Stimulants

31. The patient who is scheduled for a barium enema is prescribed bisacodyl the day before the procedure. Which response by the nurse would be appropriate when the patient asks how bisacodyl works?
    a. "Bisacodyl increases peristalsis by irritating the lining of the intestines."
    b. "By stimulating more smooth muscle contraction, bisacodyl will cause your bowel to empty."
    c. "Bisacodyl increases water in the gut."
    d. "Bisacodyl is an emetic, so you will vomit, and your stomach will be empty for the test."

32. The patient who is on several vitamins is taking mineral oil as a laxative. Which side effect would the nurse inform the patient could occur?
    a. Abdominal bloating and flatulence.
    b. Decreased absorption of fat-soluble vitamins A, D, E, and K.
    c. Dependence on the drug.
    d. Excessive fluid loss attributable to diarrhea.

33. Which patient would laxative/cathartic be contraindicated?
    a. A patient with cirrhosis
    b. A patient with Parkinsonism
    c. A patient with stable angina
    d. A patient with bowel obstruction

34. The patient with migraines has been prescribed promethazine 25 mg PO for nausea. Which side effect would be included in the teaching? **Select all that apply**.
    a. Blurred vision
    b. Diarrhea
    c. Drowsiness
    d. Dry mouth
    e. Hypotension

35. The patient is experiencing diarrhea. Which food would the nurse advise the patient to avoid? **Select all that apply**.
   a. Bottled water
   b. Clear liquids
   c. Fried foods
   d. Milk products
   e. Gelatin

CASE STUDY: CRITICAL THINKING

Read the scenario and answer the following questions on a separate sheet of paper.

An older adult patient, who lives independently at a senior living center, presents to the clinic with complaints of constipation. Approximately 2 months ago, the patient fell and broke the left hip. The patient had surgery to fix the left hip, received physical therapy, and has returned home. Current drugs the patient is taking include digoxin, a calcium supplement, omeprazole, and hydrocodone as needed (PRN) for pain. The patient is prescribed bisacodyl 5 mg orally (PO) for the constipation.

1. Discuss the potential causes of constipation for this patient.

2. Describe the mechanism of action of bisacodyl to treat constipation.

3. Are there any contraindications with any of the patient's other drugs? If so, what?

4. Discuss the priority teaching instructions that are important for the patient regarding bisacodyl.

46 Antiulcer Drugs

Match the descriptor in Column I with the drug/factor in Column II. Drug/factor in Column II may be used more than once.

Column I

_____ 1. Risk factor for the development of peptic ulcer disease (PUD)

_____ 2. Two drugs/factors that neutralizes gastric acid

_____ 3. The first proton pump inhibitor marketed

_____ 4. Associated with the development of PUD

_____ 5. Prostaglandin analogue for prevention of NSAID-induced ulcer

_____ 6. Binds with protein to form a protective viscous coat covering the ulcer

_____ 7. Eradication of *H. pylori* requires addition of this antimicrobial

_____ 8. An antacid that can have a diarrheal effect

_____ 9. Over-the-counter (OTC) proton pump inhibitor used in combination to eradicate *H. pylori*

_____ 10. H_2 antagonist with multiple drug interactions

Column II

a. Magnesium hydroxide
b. Helicobacter pylori
c. Sucralfate
d. Cimetidine
e. Omeprazole
f. Misoprostol
g. Smoking
h. Antacids
i. Metronidazole

Match the drug in Column I with the class to which it belongs in Column II. Class in Column II may be used more than once.

Column I

_____ 11. Rabeprazole

_____ 12. Ranitidine

_____ 13. Glycopyrrolate

_____ 14. Nizatidine

_____ 15. Esomeprazole magnesium

_____ 16. Sucralfate

_____ 17. Calcium carbonate

_____ 18. Famotidine

_____ 19. Sodium bicarbonate

Column II

a. Anticholinergics
b. Antacid
c. Proton pump inhibitor
d. Histamine$_2$ blocker
e. Pepsin inhibitors

Select the best response.

20. A patient asks the nurse when the best time would be to take an over-the-counter (OTC) antacid for "heartburn." Which time frame would the nurse provide?
a. 1 hour before meals
b. 1-3 hours after meals and at bedtime
c. With meals and at bedtime
d. With meals and 1 hour after

21. Which drug class may be used to prevent ulcers? **Select all that apply**.
a. Antibiotics
b. Anticholinergics
c. Antacids
d. Histamine$_2$ blockers
e. Opiates
f. Proton pump inhibitors

22. Which drug class is most used to treat gastroesophageal reflux disease (GERD)? **Select all that apply**.
a. Antacids
b. Anticholinergics
c. Histamine$_2$ blockers
d. Pepsin inhibitors
e. Proton pump inhibitors

23. A patient with peptic ulcer disease has been on propantheline bromide 15 mg 30 minutes before meals and 30 mg at bedtime. Which action describes propantheline bromide?
a. It blocks H$_2$ receptors.
b. It coats the lining of the stomach.
c. It increases gastric motility.
d. It inhibits gastric secretions.

24. A patient diagnosed with an ulcer was prescribed nizatidine. Which information would the nurse include in the teaching plan? **Select all that apply**.
a. "Antacids should not be taken within 1 hour of taking your nizatidine."
b. "Avoid alcoholic beverages and caffeine."
c. "Eating small, frequent meals may be helpful."
d. "This drug should be taken with meals and at bedtime."
e. "You will need to take this for the rest of your life."

25. A patient is taking famotidine for GERD. Which side effect of famotidine would the nurse monitor in this patient? **Select all that apply**.
a. Dizziness
b. Headache
c. Hypertension
d. Erectile dysfunction
e. Nausea

26. Which drug would concern the nurse if prescribed to a patient who is taking esomeprazole? **Select all that apply**.
a. Ampicillin
b. Digoxin
c. Ketoconazole
d. Lisinopril
e. Propranolol

27. A patient who is taking a high-dose nonsteroidal anti-inflammatory drug (NSAID) for arthritis is also taking sucralfate. Which laboratory value would concern the nurse?
a. Hgb 14.1 gm/dL
b. Potassium 4.2 mEq/L
c. Blood glucose 185 mg/dL
d. INR 1.1

CLINICAL JUDGMENT STANDALONE CASE STUDY

Read the scenario and answer the following questions on a separate sheet of paper.

SLO: Demonstrate an understanding of antiulcer drugs
NGN Item Type: Drop-Down Cloze
Cognitive Skills: Recognize Cues

A 54-year-old patient with a high-stress job as a county judge is seen in a medical clinic complaining of abdominal distress after meals. The patient reports drinking liquid antacids containing aluminum hydroxide before every meal and at bedtime for an "aggravating ulcer" which helped at the beginning but is increasing in its intensity and frequency. The patient also complains of some "bloating" and difficulty "in passing stool."

Choose the *most likely* options for the information missing from the statements below by selecting from the list of options provided.

The nurse recognizes that the patient is experiencing a(an) ___1___ effect to the antacid. Failure to reverse these effects can lead to ___2___, hypophosphatemia, nephrolithiasis, and gastrointestinal obstruction. The usual dosage for aluminum hydroxide is ___3___ mL every 3–6 hours or 1–3 hours after meals and at bedtime.

Options for 1	Options for 2	Options for 3
Therapeutic	Hypercalcemia	10–15
Side	Hypermagnesemia	20–40
Adverse	Hyperphosphatemia	40–60
Toxic	Diarrhea	

47 Eye and Ear Disorders

Complete the following.

1. Topical anesthetics (locally/systemically) block the pain signals during selected or ophthalmologic procedures. (*Circle the correct answer.*)

2. Lubricants can be used to moisten contact lenses and _____ _____.

3. Classes of ophthalmic antiinflammatories include immunomodulators, _____, and _____.

4. Ophthalmic cyclosporine, an antiinflammatory, allows _____ production.

5. Miotics are used to lower _____ pressure by widening the _____ network to improve the drainage of aqueous humor.

6. Ocular decongestants are contraindicated in patients with _____ _____.

7. Carbonic anhydrase inhibitors were developed as _____. They are effective in treating _____.

8. The drug group used to paralyze the muscles of accommodation is _____.

9. Instruct patients with glaucoma to avoid anticholinergic drugs because they (decrease/increase) intraocular pressure. (*Circle the correct answer.*)

10. Antiinfectives are used to treat infections of the eye, including inflammation of the membrane covering the eyeball and inner eyelid known as _____.

11. Drugs that interfere with the production of carbonic acid, leading to decreased aqueous humor formation and decreased intraocular pressure, belong to the group _____ _____ _____.

12. Cholinesterase inhibitors can produce systemic _____ effects that include cardiac dysrhythmias, diarrhea, and respiratory depression.

Match the term in Column I with its definition in Column II.

Column I

_____ 13. Otalgia

_____ 14. Optic

_____ 15. Cerumen

_____ 16. Lacrimal duct

_____ 17. Cerumenolytics

_____ 18. Otic

_____ 19. Chalazion

_____ 20. Keratitis

_____ 21. Hordeolum

_____ 22. Acute otitis externa

Column II

a. Also known as tear ducts
b. Drugs that soften or break up earwax
c. Infection of the meibomian glands of the eyelids
d. Ear
e. Swimmer's ear
f. Eye
g. Also known as stye
h. Ear pain
i. Earwax
j. Corneal infection and inflammation

REVIEW QUESTIONS

Select the best response.

23. The patient presents to an ophthalmologist for a routine eye examination. Before the exam, eyedrops are used to dilate the eyes. Such drug belongs to which class of drugs?
    a. Carbonic anhydrase inhibitors
    b. Cerumenolytics
    c. Mydriatics
    d. Osmotics

24. A patient is taking acetazolamide for acute angle-closure glaucoma. The nurse would assess for which side effect associated with this drug class?
    a. Agitation
    b. Constipation
    c. Electrolyte imbalances
    d. Urinary retention

25. The patient has frequent cerumen buildup. Which drug would the nurse anticipate in administering?
    a. Bimatoprost
    b. Carbamide peroxide
    c. Echothiophate
    d. Proparacaine

26. The patient is receiving pilocarpine eyedrops for treatment of glaucoma. Which side effect would the nurse teach the patient to monitor? **Select all that apply**.
    a. Blurred vision
    b. Cardiac dysrhythmias
    c. Eye pain
    d. Headache
    e. Respiratory depression
    f. Vomiting

27. A patient has been diagnosed with dry age-related macular degeneration (AMD). Which drug is available for treatment? **Select all that apply**.
    a. Aflibercept
    b. Bevacizumab
    c. Pegaptanib
    d. Ranibizumab
    e. There is no treatment for dry AMD.

28. A patient, who works as a landscaper, presents to an ophthalmologist with complaints of dry, itching eyes. Which treatment option would be prescribed? **Select all that apply**.
    a. Azelastine
    b. Olopatadine
    c. Epinastine
    d. Ketotifen
    e. Tetracaine HCl

29. A patient with a painful and swollen ear is prescribed ofloxacin otic solution. Before discharge, the nurse inserts a cotton wick into the right external canal. Which statement describes the purpose of the wick?
    a. To keep the external auditory canal dry.
    b. To allow the drug to reach the external auditory canal.
    c. To protect the tympanic membrane from infection.
    d. To keep the external auditory canal free of cerumen.

CASE STUDY: CRITICAL THINKING

Read the scenario and answer the following questions on a separate sheet of paper.

An older adult patient who has chronic open-angle glaucoma and ocular hypertension, presents to the health care provider for a follow-up appointment. Current drug for the glaucoma is timolol solution 2 drops every 8 hours. The patient's medical history includes hypertension, depression, arthritis, and atrial fibrillation. The patient denies any specific complaints except for blurred vision.

1. Describe open-angle glaucoma.

2. Discuss the type of drug timolol is and how its mechanism of action.

3. Discuss the proper procedures to instill eyedrops.

4. Is this the appropriate dose for this patient? Why or why not?

48 Dermatologic Disorders

Match the term in Column I with the correct description in Column II.

Column I

_____ **1.** Macule

_____ **2.** Vesicle

_____ **3.** Plaque

_____ **4.** Papule

Column II

a. Raised, palpable lesion 10 mm in diameter

b. Hard, rough, raised lesion; flat on top, usually >10 mm in diameter

c. Flat, nonpalpable lesion with varying color

d. Raised lesion filled with clear fluid and <1 cm in diameter

Match the condition in Column I to the drug that treats it in Column II. More than one drug in Column II may be used for a condition in Column I.

Column I

_____ **5.** Psoriasis

_____ **6.** Burns

_____ **7.** Acne vulgsaris

_____ **8.** Verruca vulgaris

_____ **9.** Rosacea

Column II

a. Cantharidin

b. Tetracycline

c. Isotretinoin

d. Azelaic acid

e. Adapalene

f. Methotrexate

g. Silver sulfadiazine

h. Calcineurin inhibitors

COMPLETE THE FOLLOWING

10. Tinea pedis is also called _____ _____, and tinea capitis is called _____.

11. _____ are noninflammatory acne lesions that may be _____ (closed) or _____ (open).

12. Isotretinoin is a known _____ and should not be used during pregnancy. Any person started on isotretinoin must be enrolled in a risk-management program called _____.

13. Psoriasis is a _____ disease affecting predominantly the _____ and _____.

14. Worsening psoriasis with the use of topical corticosteroids is called a/an _____ effect.

15. Cyclosporine inhibits _____ activation.

16. Salicylic acid promotes _____ when used for verruca vulgaris.

17. Prolonged use of topical corticosteroids is discouraged because it can cause _____ of the skin and _____ of the dermis and epidermis.

Select the best response.

18. Which class of drug is used to treat acne vulgaris? **Select all that apply**.
    a. Antibiotics
    b. Antifungals
    c. Glucocorticoids
    d. Keratolytics
    e. Nonsteroidal antiinflammatories
    f. T-cell antagonists

19. The health care provider prescribes calcipotriene to treat psoriasis. When the patient asks how this drug will work, which statement would be the nurse's best answer?
    a. "This medication will help stop the proliferation of cells."
    b. "It will be very effective against the itching that goes with psoriasis."
    c. "Calcipotriene will cure psoriasis."
    d. "It can be used like makeup to cover up the scales."

20. The patient with psoriasis is started on a course of infliximab. Which response would the nurse inform the patient about the dosing regimen?
    a. "Infliximab is a gel that you will use after bathing."
    b. "Infliximab is a drug that is administered by IV at prescribed intervals."
    c. "You will be able to give yourself an injection once per week."
    d. "This is an oral drug that you will be on for the rest of your life."

21. Which substance is a common cause of contact dermatitis? **Select all that apply**.
    a. Anesthetics
    b. Cosmetics
    c. Dyes
    d. Peanuts
    e. Sumac

22. A patient with acne vulgaris has been prescribed tetracycline. Which dose would be used as the initial standard dose?
    a. 125 mg q12h
    b. 250 mg bid
    c. 500 mg q12h
    d. 1000 mg bid

23. Which priority information would be provided to the patient taking tetracycline for acne? **Select all that apply**.
    a. Alert the health care provider if pregnant or possibly pregnant.
    b. Avoid the use of harsh cleansers.
    c. Eat a high-fiber diet.
    d. It should not be used with isotretinoin.
    e. Use a sunscreen with SPF 20.

24. Which drug can be utilized to treat male pattern baldness?
    a. Acitretin
    b. Methotrexate
    c. Minoxidil
    d. Tretinoin

25. A patient has been diagnosed with contact dermatitis from poison ivy. Which antipruritic drug can be utilized? **Select all that apply**.
    a. Triamcinolone
    b. Dexamethasone
    c. Diphenhydramine
    d. Fluconazole
    e. Salicylic acid

CASE STUDY: CRITICAL THINKING

Read the scenario and answer the following questions on a separate sheet of paper.

An 18-year-old patient sustained full-thickness burns over the anterior chest and partial-thickness burns over the forearms bilaterally. Mafenide acetate is prescribed to be applied to the burns.

1. Discuss the difference between full- and partial-thickness burns.

2. Discuss the type of drug mafenide acetate.

3. Determine other options that are available for a topical burn preparation.

4. Discuss the priority nursing interventions for this patient.

49 Pituitary, Thyroid, Parathyroid, and Adrenal Disorders

Match the information in Column I with the correct term in Column II.

Column I

_____ **1.** Growth hormone hypersecretion causes excessive growth after puberty

_____ **2.** Another name for the anterior pituitary gland

_____ **3.** Adrenocorticotropic hormone released by the anterior pituitary gland

_____ **4.** A hormone secreted by the posterior pituitary gland to resorb water

_____ **5.** Severe hypothyroidism in children causes delayed physical and mental growth

_____ **6.** Growth hormone hypersecretion causes excessive growth during childhood

_____ **7.** Cortisol hormone secreted from the adrenal cortex affects inflammatory response

_____ **8.** Another name for the pituitary gland

_____ **9.** Aldosterone hormone secreted from the adrenal cortex that regulates sodium, potassium, and hydrogen ions

_____ **10.** Severe hypothyroidism in adults causes physical, emotional, and mental changes

_____ **11.** Another name for the posterior pituitary gland

_____ **12.** Also called Graves' disease; caused by hyperfunction of the thyroid gland

_____ **13.** T_4 hormone secreted by the thyroid gland

_____ **14.** T_3 hormone secreted by the thyroid gland

Column II

a.   ADH
b.   Gigantism
c.   Mineralocorticoid
d.   Neurohypophysis
e.   Triiodothyronine
f.   Acromegaly
g.   Myxedema
h.   Adenohypophysis
i.   ACTH
j.   Thyrotoxicosis
k.   Thyroxine
l.   Glucocorticoid
m.   Cretinism
n.   Hypophysis

15. Place the signs and symptoms under the appropriate endocrine disorder.

SIGNS AND SYMPTOMS		
Hypernatremia	Anemia	Edema
Hypoglycemia	Weight loss	Delayed wound healing
Weight gain	Hyperlipidemia	Hyperglycemia
Fatigue	Hirsutism	Hyperpigmentation
Tachycardia	Hypotension	Hypokalemia
Diarrhea	Peptic ulcers	Hypertension
Buffalo hump	Hyponatremia	Hyperkalemia

ENDOCRINE DISORDERS	
Addison Disease: Adrenal Hyposecretion	Cushing Syndrome: Adrenal Hypersecretion

Match the nursing intervention in Column I with the correct rationale related to glucocorticoid drug administration in Column II.

Column I

_____ **16.** Monitor vital signs.

_____ **17.** Monitor weight after taking a cortisone preparation for more than 10 days.

_____ **18.** Monitor laboratory values, especially blood glucose and electrolytes.

_____ **19.** Instruct patients to take the cortisone with food.

_____ **20.** Advise patients to eat foods rich in potassium.

_____ **21.** Instruct patients not to abruptly discontinue the cortisone preparation.

_____ **22.** Teach patients to report signs and symptoms of drug toxicity.

Column II

a. Corticosteroids increase sodium and water retention and increase blood pressure.

b. Adrenal crisis may occur if cortisone is abruptly stopped.

c. Glucocorticoid drugs promote loss of potassium.

d. Weight gain occurs with cortisone use as a result of water retention.

e. Glucocorticoid drugs promote sodium retention, potassium loss, and increased blood glucose.

f. Glucocorticoid drugs may cause moon face, puffy eyelids, edema in the feet, dizziness, and menstrual irregularity at high doses.

g. Glucocorticoid drugs can irritate the gastric mucosa and may cause peptic ulcers.

REVIEW QUESTIONS

Select the best response.

23. A patient with hypothyroidism is taking levothyroxine 100 mcg/day. Which concern by the nurse would be appropriate about the patient's dose of levothyroxine?
   a. The dose is too low.
   b. The dose is too high.
   c. Nothing; it is within the normal maintenance dosage range.
   d. Nothing; dose should start at a low dose.

24. Which time frame after starting levothyroxine would the patient most likely report feeling its therapeutic effects?
   a. 3-4 days
   b. 4-7 days
   c. 1-2 weeks
   d. 2-4 weeks

25. The nurse assesses the patient for clinical manifestations of hyperthyroidism. Which symptom can indicate hyperthyroidism? **Select all that apply**.
   a. Palpitations
   b. Constipation
   c. Excessive sweating
   d. Tachycardia
   e. Tinnitus

26. Which time frame for dosing would the nurse instruct the patient to take levothyroxine?
   a. Before breakfast
   b. With breakfast
   c. After breakfast
   d. With lunch

27. Which patient teaching would be a priority for hypothyroidism? **Select all that apply**.
   a. Avoid over-the-counter (OTC) drugs.
   b. Report numbness and tingling of the hands to the health care provider.
   c. Increase food and fluid intake.
   d. Take the drug with food.
   e. Wear a medical alert identification information device.

28. While a patient is taking prednisone, which laboratory value would be closely monitored?
   a. Hematocrit
   b. Hemoglobin
   c. Magnesium
   d. Sodium

29. The patient has been started on prednisone for bronchitis to decrease inflammation. Which time frame would be best to take prednisone?
   a. Before meals
   b. With meals
   c. 1 hour after meals
   d. At bedtime

30. Which drug would be used with caution when taking a glucocorticoid? **Select all that apply**.
   a. Acetaminophen
   b. Nonsteroidal antiinflammatory drugs (NSAIDs), including aspirin
   c. Digitalis preparations
   d. Phenytoin
   e. Potassium-wasting diuretics

31. Which nursing intervention would be a priority for a patient taking prednisone? **Select all that apply**.
   a. Follow the physical therapy regimen.
   b. Monitor for signs and symptoms of hyponatremia.
   c. Monitor vital signs.
   d. Obtain a complete medication history.
   e. Record daily weight.

32. Which statement by a patient taking prednisone indicates a need for more teaching?
   a. "I should wear a medical alert identification device or carry a card."
   b. "I will make sure I force fluids daily."
   c. "I will not abruptly stop taking my drug."
   d. "I will take glucocorticoids only as ordered."

33. When an herbal laxative such as cascara or senna and herbal diuretics such as celery seed are taken with a corticosteroid, which imbalance can occur?
   a. Hypoglycemia
   b. Hypokalemia
   c. Hyponatremia
   d. Hypophosphatemia

34. Which changes may occur when ginseng is taken with a corticosteroid?
   a. Central nervous system (CNS) depression
   b. CNS stimulation and insomnia
   c. Counteraction of the effects of the corticosteroid
   d. Electrolyte imbalance

35. Which drug is known to interact with levothyroxine? **Select all that apply**.
   a. Anticoagulants
   b. Digitalis
   c. Diuretics
   d. NSAIDs
   e. Oral antidiabetics

CLINICAL JUDGMENT STANDALONE CASE STUDY

Read the scenario and answer the following questions on a separate sheet of paper.

SLO: Compare clinical manifestations of hormonal imbalances between pituitary and adrenal glands
NGN Item Type: Drop-Down Cloze
Cognitive Skills: Analyze Cues

A 35-year-old female is seen in the clinic for complaints of nervousness, muscle weakness, and lethargy. She also reports her "female cycle is not regular." The conducts an assessment and reviews the labs:

Blood pressure 84/56 mm Hg
Heart rate 125 beats per minute
Respiratory rate 24 breaths per minute
Oxygen saturation 96% on room air
Skin bronzy-brown and cool and clammy
Muscle strength 4 on a scale of 0–5 in all extremities
Total white blood cell count (WBC) 7800/mm^3
Hemoglobin 10 g/dL
Hematocrit 32%
Serum sodium 128 mEq/L
Serum potassium 5.3 mEq/L
Serum calcium 9.9 mg/dL
Serum albumin 4.9 g/dL
Blood urea nitrogen (BUN) 25 mg/dL
Serum creatinine 1.9 mg/dL
Serum glucose nonfasting 65 mg/dL
Serum osmolality 325 mOsm/kg

Choose the *most likely* options for the missing information from the statements by selecting from the list of options provided.

The nurse recognizes that the patient's clinical manifestations could be a complication from ___1___ insufficiency, also known as ___2___ disease. To determine primary deficiency, ___3___ is a drug used to determine if the problem is related to the pituitary gland or the adrenal glands. Treatment for this patient's insufficiency would include __3___, such as cortisone acetate, and mineralocorticoids, such as ___3___.

Options for 1	Options for 2	Options for 3
Parathyroid	Cushing	Somatropin
Thyroid	Addison	Glucocorticoids
Adrenal	Grave's	Cosyntropin
Pituitary	Hashimoto	Fludrocortisone
		Dexamethasone

Chapter **49 Pituitary, Thyroid, Parathyroid, and Adrenal Disorders**

50 Antidiabetics

STUDY QUESTIONS

Match the term in Column I with its definition in Column II.

Column I

_____ **1.** Diabetes mellitus

_____ **2.** Insulin

_____ **3.** Hypoglycemic reaction

_____ **4.** Ketoacidosis

_____ **5.** Lipodystrophy

_____ **6.** Polydipsia

_____ **7.** Polyphagia

_____ **8.** Polyuria

Column II

a. Increased hunger

b. Increased urine output

c. Use of ketones for energy in diabetics

d. Disease resulting from deficient glucose metabolism

e. Increased thirst

f. Protein secreted from the beta cells of the pancreas

g. Changes to tissue from frequent insulin injections

h. Occurs when more insulin is administered than is needed for glucose metabolism

Complete the following.

9. Hemoglobin A1c (HbA1c) has a life span of approximately _____ months.

10. Some patients may need higher doses of insulin because of _____, _____, or _____.

11. Subcutaneous injections to the _____ absorb insulin faster than other body sites.

12. Insulin is not administered orally because _____ _____ destroys insulin.

13. Lipoatrophy and lipohypertrophy are terms used to indicate _____ due to not _____ injection sites.

14. Antibody development can cause _____ _____ and _____.

Match the terms in Column I with their definitions in Column II.

Column I

_____ **15.** NPH insulin

_____ **16.** Sulfonylureas

_____ **17.** Regular insulin

_____ **18.** Glucagon

_____ **19.** Insulin lispro

_____ **20.** Insulin glargine

Column II

a. Oral hypoglycemic drug group

b. Hyperglycemic hormone that stimulates glycogenolysis

c. Intermediate-acting insulin

d. Long-acting insulin

e. Rapid-acting insulin

f. Short-acting insulin

Complete the following.

21. All insulins can be administered subcutaneously, but only _____ insulin can be given intravenously.

22. A hypoglycemic event that usually occurs between 2:00 am and 4:00 am followed by an increase in blood glucose level by lipolysis, gluconeogenesis, and glycogenolysis is called the _____.

23. _____ on awakening or the _____ phenomenon is usually controlled by increasing the bedtime dose of insulin.

24. A major side effect of many oral antidiabetic drugs is _____.

25. Metformin, an oral antidiabetic drug in the _____ class, decreases hepatic production of _____, decreases the _____ from the small intestine, increases insulin _____ sensitivity, and increases _____ glucose uptake at the cellular level.

26. Metformin should be held for _____ _____ before and after administration of IV contrast because _____ _____ or acute renal failure can develop.

27. Incretin mimetics improve glucose control in people with _____ diabetes; they should not be given to people with type 1 diabetes.

REVIEW QUESTIONS

28. Which symptom best characterizes diabetes? **Select all that apply**.
    a. Polydipsia
    b. Polyphagia
    c. Polyposia
    d. Polyrrhea
    e. Polyuria

29. Which drug can cause hyperglycemia? **Select all that apply**.
    a. Epinephrine
    b. Hydrochlorothiazide
    c. Doxepin
    d. Prednisone
    e. Thiazolidinediones

30. Which clinical manifestation may be seen in a patient experiencing a hypoglycemic (insulin) reaction? **Select all that apply**.
    a. Abdominal pain
    b. Headache
    c. Excessive perspiration
    d. Nervousness
    e. Tremor
    f. Vomiting

31. Which clinical manifestation may be seen in a patient experiencing diabetic ketoacidosis (hyperglycemia)? **Select all that apply**.
    a. Bradycardia
    b. Dry mucous membranes
    c. Fruity breath odor
    d. Kussmaul respirations
    e. Polyuria
    f. Thirst

32. A patient has type 1 diabetes. Which medication would the patient not use to control diabetes?
    a. Insulin glulisine
    b. Insulin lispro
    c. Insulin aspart
    d. Tolazamide

33. Which information would be included in health teaching for patients taking oral antidiabetic (hypoglycemic) drugs? **Select all that apply**.
    a. Adhere to prescribed diet.
    b. Monitor blood glucose levels.
    c. Monitor weight.
    d. Participate in regular exercise.
    e. Take the drugs based on blood glucose level.

34. In which location would the patient who takes insulin daily be taught to store the opened insulin?
    a. In a cool place
    b. In the light
    c. In the freezer
    d. Wrapped in aluminum

35. Which action would be appropriate when preparing cloudy insulin before administration?
    a. Add diluent to the bottle.
    b. Allow air to escape from the bottle.
    c. Roll the bottle in the hands.
    d. Shake the bottle well.

36. The patient needs to develop a "site rotation pattern" for insulin injections. The American Diabetes Association suggests which action? **Select all that apply**.
    a. Choose an injection site for a week.
    b. Change the injection area of the body every day.
    c. Inject insulin each day at the injection site at 11/2 inches apart.
    d. Inject insulin intramuscularly (IM) in the morning and subcut at night.
    e. With two daily injection times, use the right side in the morning and the left side in the evening.

37. Which time frame would the nurse expect the patient to experience a hypoglycemic reaction to regular insulin if administration occurs at 0700 and the patient does not eat?
    a. 0800–0900
    b. 0900–1300
    c. 1300–1500
    d. 1500–1700

38. Which statement best describes insulin glargine, a long-acting insulin? **Select all that apply**.
    a. Always combine it with regular insulin for good coverage.
    b. It is given in the evening.
    c. It is safe because hypoglycemia cannot occur.
    d. It is available in a prefilled cartridge insulin pen.
    e. Some patients complain of pain at the injection site.

39. The insulin pump has become popular in the management of insulin. Which statement is true about this method of insulin delivery?
    a. It can be used with intermediate insulin as well as regular insulin.
    b. It can be used with the needle inserted at the same site for weeks.
    c. It is more effective in decreasing the number of hypoglycemic reactions.
    d. It is more effective for use by type 2 diabetic patient.

40. Which mechanism of action is correct of an oral hypoglycemic drug?
    a. It increases the number of insulin cell receptors.
    b. It increases the number of insulin-producing cells.
    c. It replaces receptor sites.
    d. It replaces insulin.

41. Metformin is used to control serum glucose among persons with type 2 diabetes mellitus. Which statement describes their mechanism of action?
    a. Causes a hypoglycemic reaction.
    b. Decreases hepatic production of glucose from stored glycogen.
    c. Increases the absorption of glucose from the small intestine.
    d. Raises the serum glucose level following a meal.

42. Herb-drug interaction must be assessed in patients taking herbs and antidiabetic drugs. Which drug-herb interaction is correct on how ginseng and garlic affect insulin or oral antidiabetic drugs?
    a. They can be taken with insulin without any effect, but they can cause a hypoglycemic reaction with oral antidiabetic drugs.
    b. Ginseng and garlic can lower the blood glucose level.
    c. They decrease the effect of insulin and antidiabetic drugs, causing a hyperglycemic effect.
    d. They may decrease insulin requirements.

43. Which drug or category of drug will interact with a sulfonylurea? **Select all that apply**.
    a. Antacids
    b. Anticoagulants
    c. Anticonvulsants
    d. Aspirin
    e. Cimetidine

CLINICAL JUDGMENT STANDALONE CASE STUDY

Read the scenario and answer the following questions on a separate sheet of paper.

SLO: Determine the nursing actions for patients experiencing glucose imbalance.
NGN Item Type: Drop-Down Cloze
Cognitive Skills: Take Action

An 18-year-old who has type 1 diabetes mellitus presents to the emergency department (ED) with confusion. According to the friend who brought the patient into the ED, the patient has recently been under increased stress studying for major exams. The patient has slurred speech and complains of a headache. The glucose level in triage reads "low" on the glucometer. While being transferred from triage to a treatment room, the patient becomes unresponsive. Other assessment data include:

Blood pressure 106/68 mm Hg
Heart rate 132 beats per minute
Temperature 97.3° F
Oxygen saturation 96% on room air

Complete blood count (CBC) unremarkable
Chemistry panel:

    Sodium 139 mEq/L
    Potassium 3.2 mEq/L
    Glucose 23 mg/dL
    Blood urea nitrogen 9 mmol/L
    Creatinine 1.3 mg/dL
    Carbon dioxide 23 mEq/L

Choose the *most likely* options for the missing information from the statements below by selecting from the list of options provided.

The nurse realizes the patient is most likely experiencing a reaction due to __1____ and notifies the attending health care provider. The nurse would anticipate administering ___2___ intravenously to stimulate glucose production and ___3___ blood sugar.

Options for 1	Options for 2	Options for 3
Migraines	Sugar-containing drinks	Increase
Hypoglycemia	Glucagon	Normalize
Hyperglycemia	Hard sugary candy	Decrease
Electrolyte imbalance	Insulin	
	Glucose	

51 Urinary Disorders

STUDY QUESTIONS

Match the drug class in Column I to the appropriate therapeutic effect in Column II. Therapeutic effect in Column II may be used more than once.

Column I

_____ **1.** Urinary stimulants

_____ **2.** Anticholinergics

_____ **3.** Urinary antiseptics

_____ **4.** Bactericidal

_____ **5.** Antimuscarinics

_____ **6.** Antiinfectives

_____ **7.** Urinary analgesics

_____ **8.** Bacteriostatic

_____ **9.** Antispasmodics

Column II

a. Inhibits bacterial growth
b. Increases urinary muscle tone
c. Relieves pain and burning
d. Prevents bacterial growth
e. Decreases urgency and urinary incontinence
f. Kills bacteria

Divide the figure of the genitourinary tract into upper tract and lower tract. Label the infectious processes to the appropriate urinary structures.

10.

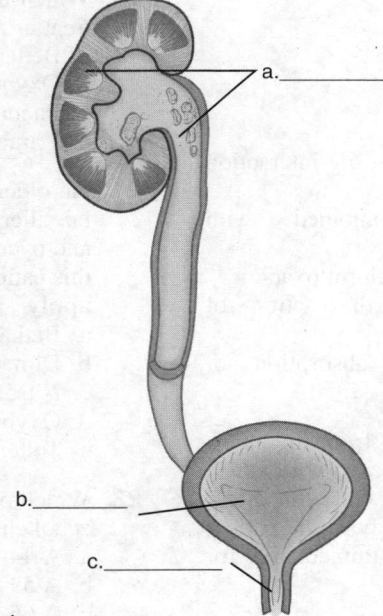

a._____

b._____

c._____

Select the best response.

11. Which complication can occur when methenamine is given with a sulfonamide?
    a. Bleeding
    b. Chest pain
    c. Crystalluria
    d. Intestinal distention

12. A patient with a urinary tract infection (UTI) has been advised to increase fluids to decrease urine pH. Which information would the nurse include in discharge teaching to help the patient meet this goal?
    a. "Drinking whole milk will help."
    b. "Cranberry juice can help acidify the urine."
    c. "Be sure to drink 12-14 8-oz glasses of water per day."
    d. "Drink prune juice four times per day to make urine alkaline."

13. An older adult patient has been prescribed flavoxate for urinary spasms. Which medical history would be of highest concern to the nurse?
    a. Dementia
    b. Glaucoma
    c. Hypoglycemia
    d. Migraines

14. A patient will be receiving ertapenem to prevent recurring UTIs. Which side effect would the nurse include in the patient teaching? **Select all that apply.**
    a. Visual disturbances
    b. Back pain
    c. Diarrhea
    d. Headache
    e. Nausea

15. Which oral urinary antiseptic drug-drug interaction is correct? **Select all that apply.**
    a. Trimethoprim can be combined with sulfamethoxazole.
    b. Antacids increase absorption of ciprofloxacin.
    c. Sodium bicarbonate inhibits the action of methenamine.
    d. Antacids can decrease the absorption of nitrofurantoin.

16. A patient who is being discharged from the emergency department after being diagnosed with a UTI is prescribed nitrofurantoin 100 mg qid with meals and at bedtime. The nurse would advise the patient to contact the health care provider immediately for which side effect?
    a. Brown urine
    b. Frequency in urination
    c. Diarrhea
    d. Dyspnea

17. For which condition would the nurse expect to see urinary analgesics prescribed? **Select all that apply.**
    a. Burning sensation
    b. Frequency
    c. Hesitation
    d. Retention
    e. Urgency

18. Which drug is commonly prescribed as a urinary analgesic?
    a. Bethanechol
    b. Flavoxate
    c. Phenazopyridine hydrochloride
    d. Trimethoprim

19. A patient who was prescribed an antiinfective and phenazopyridine for a UTI calls the clinic reporting urine color has turned reddish orange. After reviewing the patient's chart and current list of drugs, which information would the nurse tell the patient?
    a. "If you do not take the antibiotic with food in your stomach, your urine will turn orange."
    b. "Inadequate liquid intake will cause your urine to turn bright orange."
    c. "This is an indication of an allergic reaction. You need to come back to the clinic."
    d. "Bright reddish-orange urine is to be expected when taking phenazopyridine."

20. Which urinary antispasmodic is commonly used to treat urinary tract spasms?
    a. Bethanechol
    b. Oxybutynin
    c. Phenazopyridine
    d. Trimethoprim

21. An older adult patient has a history of environmental allergies, narrow-angle glaucoma, depression, and overactive bladder. Which drug, if prescribed to this patient, would concern the nurse? **Select all that apply.**
    a. Bethanechol
    b. Dimethyl sulfoxide (DMSO)
    c. Nitrofurantoin
    d. Oxybutynin
    e. Tolterodine tartrate

22. Which patient is more likely to benefit from bethanechol chloride?
    a. A 44-year-old patient with prostatitis
    b. A 53-year-old patient with paraplegia
    c. A 65-year-old patient with pyelonephritis
    d. A 70-year-old patient with overactive bladder

CASE STUDY: CRITICAL THINKING

Read the scenario and answer the following questions on a separate sheet of paper.

A young adult patient sustained an injury to the urinary tract while playing football and has been prescribed oxybutynin chloride 5 mg bid for spasms while urinating.

1. Describe the mechanism of action of oxybutynin.

2. Which persons should not take oxybutynin, and why?

3. Which side effects that can be expected?

4. What dose adjustments, if any, need to be made for this patient?

52 Pregnancy and Preterm Labor

Match the terms in Column I with the definitions in Column II.

Column I

_____ 1. Preeclampsia

_____ 2. Gestational hypertension

_____ 3. HELLP syndrome

_____ 4. L/S (lecithin/sphingomyelin) ratio

_____ 5. Eclampsia

_____ 6. Preterm birth

_____ 7. Hyperemesis gravidarum

_____ 8. Surfactant

_____ 9. Teratogens

_____ 10. Tocolytic therapy

Column II

a. New onset of seizures with preeclampsia

b. Prior to 37 gestational weeks

c. Drug therapy to decrease uterine muscle contractions

d. Severe nausea and vomiting during pregnancy

e. Decreases the incidence of respiratory distress syndrome (RDS)

f. Hypertension during pregnancy without proteinuria

g. Gestational hypertension with proteinuria

h. Substances that cause developmental abnormalities

i. Predictor of fetal lung maturity and risk for neonatal RDS

j. Hemolysis, elevated liver enzymes, and low platelet count

REVIEW QUESTIONS

Select the best response.

11. Which maternal physiologic change is seen during pregnancy that affects drug dosing? **Select all that apply**.
    a. Decreased urine output.
    b. Gastric motility is more rapid, resulting in faster absorption.
    c. Increased fluid volume.
    d. Increased glomerular filtration rate and rapid elimination of drugs.
    e. Increased liver metabolism of drugs.

12. The mechanism in which drugs cross the placenta is similar to the way drugs infiltrate which type of body tissue?
    a. Breast
    b. Liver
    c. Subcutaneous
    d. Uterine

13. Which important factor determine the teratogenicity of any drug ingested during pregnancy? **Select all that apply**.
    a. Dosage
    b. Duration of exposure
    c. Gastric motility
    d. Timing
    e. Urinary clearance

14. A patient in preterm labor (PTL) at 28 weeks is prescribed betamethasone 12 mg intramuscularly (IM) every 24 hours for 2 doses. The patient wants to know why she has to receive the drug. Which response would the nurse provide?
    a. "Betamethasone will stop your labor."
    b. "It will help the fetus' lungs mature more quickly."
    c. "It will promote closure of a patent ductus arteriosus."
    d. "This drug will promote fetal adrenal maturity."

15. The patient has been diagnosed with gestational hypertension. Which treatment goal would be appropriate? **Select all that apply**.
    a. Decrease the incidence of PTL
    b. Delivery of an uncompromised infant
    c. Ensure future ability to conceive
    d. Prevention of HELLP syndrome
    e. Prevention of seizures

16. Which patient complaint is common during pregnancy? **Select all that apply**.
    a. Heartburn
    b. Headaches
    c. Nausea
    d. Vomiting
    e. Weakness

17. A pregnant patient with iron-deficiency anemia was prescribed ferrous sulfate 325 mg bid. Which laboratory value will show the first indication that the patient is responding to the iron supplement?
    a. Increased blood urea nitrogen
    b. Increased hemoglobin
    c. Increased reticulocyte count
    d. Increased international normalized ratio

18. A pregnant patient presents to her health care provider with complaints of morning sickness. "I didn't have it with my first. I'm just not sure what to do." Which nonpharmacologic measure would the nurse suggest? **Select all that apply**.
    a. Avoid fatty or spicy foods.
    b. Avoid fluids before arising.
    c. Drink flat soda between meals.
    d. Eat crackers, dry toast, cereal, or complex carbohydrates.
    e. Eat a high-protein snack at bedtime.

19. A pregnant patient in her first trimester of pregnancy was started on a prenatal vitamin with iron. Which teaching would the nurse provide? **Select all that apply**.
    a. Antacids can be taken with the iron tablet to help with epigastric discomfort.
    b. Ensure adequate fluid and fiber intake to assist with constipation.
    c. Iron can be taken with food if necessary to prevent nausea.
    d. Jaundice is a common side effect of iron supplements.
    e. Orange juice enhances iron absorption.

20. Which food would the nurse recommend to eat to increase iron intake during pregnancy?
    a. Broccoli
    b. Cabbage
    c. Apples
    d. Potatoes

21. Which range of folic acid is the recommended daily allowance for during pregnancy?
    a. 100–400 mcg
    b. 400–800 mcg
    c. 800–1200 mcg
    d. 1200–1600 mcg

22. Which drug is the most commonly ingested nonprescription drug for pain during pregnancy?
    a. Acetaminophen
    b. Aspirin
    c. Diphenhydramine
    d. Ibuprofen

23. Which priority intervention would the nurse implement for the patient receiving a beta-sympathomimetic drug?
    a. Auscultate breath sounds every 4 hours.
    b. Encourage patient to sleep on her back.
    c. Have atropine available as a reversal agent.
    d. Monitor maternal vital signs every 5 minutes when receiving intravenous dose.

24. Which nursing intervention would be required in a patient receiving magnesium sulfate for preeclampsia? **Select all that apply**.
    a. Administer the loading dose as a bolus given by intravenous push (IVP).
    b. Continuously monitor vital signs and fetal monitor.
    c. Encourage patient to ambulate in room to prevent blood clots.
    d. Have calcium gluconate available at the bedside.
    e. Monitor deep tendon reflexes (DTRs).

25. A patient who is 38 weeks pregnant and complaining of a sinus headache takes a combination drug that contains aspirin, acetaminophen, and caffeine. Which event can occur with the use of aspirin late in pregnancy? **Select all that apply**.
    a. Decreased hemostasis in the newborn
    b. Increased maternal blood loss at delivery
    c. Increased risk of anemia
    d. Low-birth-weight infant
    e. Precipitous delivery

26. The patient is receiving magnesium sulfate for gestational hypertension. Which side effect may be expected? **Select all that apply**.
    a. Dizziness
    b. Flushing
    c. Hyperreflexia
    d. Slurred speech
    e. Urinary incontinence

CASE STUDY: CRITICAL THINKING

Read the scenario and answer the following questions on a separate sheet of paper.

A 40-year-old patient is pregnant with her fourth child. She is at 33 weeks' gestation. She has had one miscarriage and has two living children, ages 15 and 9 years. It is 2100 on Friday night, and her health care provider's office is closed, so she has left a message with the answering service. She contacts obstetric (OB) triage and states, "I think I may be having contractions, but I know I'm too early. My 15-year-old was born at 30 weeks, and I am so scared that this is happening again." She complains of lower abdominal tightening and back discomfort that comes and goes about every 8 minutes. She was instructed to come to the hospital.

1. What are some priority questions for the nurse to ask while on the phone?

2. What puts the patient at high risk for PTL?

3. What are some nonpharmacologic measures to treat PTL? What are some pharmacologic options to treat PTL?

4. What actions would the nurse anticipate would be required for the fetus at 33 weeks' gestation?

53 Labor, Delivery, and Postpartum

Label the following areas for regional anesthesia.

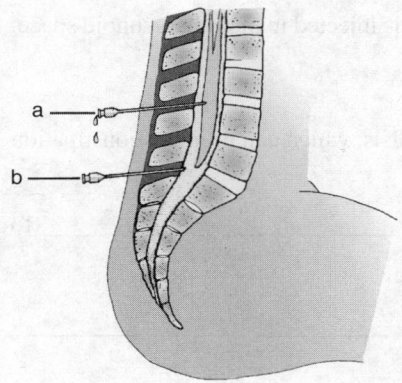

Match the term in Column I to its definition in Column II.

Column I

_____ **2.** Somatic

_____ **3.** Visceral

_____ **4.** Contraction

_____ **5.** Regional

_____ **6.** Ripening

Column II

a. Type of anesthesia for pain relief during labor and delivery without loss of consciousness

b. Type of pain caused by pressure of the presenting part and stretching of the perineum and vagina

c. Softening of the cervix

d. Type of pain due to stretching of the cervix

e. Tightening and shortening of uterine muscles

Match the labor and delivery stage in Column I with its definition in Column II.

Column I

_____ **7.** Dilating stage

_____ **8.** Pelvic stage

_____ **9.** Placental separation and expulsion

_____ **10.** Early postpartum

Column II

a. Placental separation from the uterine wall and its delivery

b. Cervical effacement and dilation occur

c. First 4 hours after delivery of the placenta

d. Complete cervical dilation and ends with delivery of the newborn

Complete the following.

11. The three *phases* of the dilating stage include _____, _____, and _____.

12. Sedative-hypnotics should be given at the onset of uterine contractions to decrease (maternal/neonatal) drug exposure. *(Circle the correct answer.)*

13. Adverse effects of opioids depend on the responses activated by the _____ and _____ receptors.

14. Barbiturates (should/should not) be given during active labor. *(Circle the correct answer.)*

15. Spinal anesthesia, also known as a/an _____ _____, is injected in the subarachnoid space.

16. A uterotropic drug, _____, stimulate(s) uterine contraction.

17. Progesterone on the smooth muscle _____ gastrointestinal peristalsis, which can promote constipation during the postpartum period.

18. A pregnant patient with Rh-negative blood should receive _____ _____ _____ to prevent fetal hemolysis in an Rh-positive fetus.

REVIEW QUESTIONS

Select the best response.

19. The patient has received spinal anesthesia for delivery. Which pathophysiological alteration would the nurse monitor?
a. Decreased hemoglobin and hematocrit
b. Palpitations
c. Pedal edema
d. Postdural headache

20. Which action is a treatment for postdural headaches after spinal anesthesia? **Select all that apply**.
a. Analgesics
b. Bed rest
c. Blood patch
d. Caffeine
e. Decreased fluids

21. A baby with respiratory depression was born within 15 minutes after the mother received opioids for pain. Which drug would the nurse anticipate administering to provide reversal of neonatal respiratory depression?
a. Calcium gluconate
b. Calcium carbonate
c. Flumazenil
d. Naloxone

22. Before administration of general anesthesia, a laboring woman is given an antacid. Which purpose of giving this drug is correct?
a. Decrease gastric acidity
b. Enhance anesthesia induction
c. Maintain a patent airway
d. Prevent nausea and vomiting

23. After a patient received an epidural the blood pressure begins to decrease. Which initial nursing action would be correct?
a. Administer oxygen.
b. Expect an order to administer 5–15 mg of ephedrine IV.
c. Expect an order to transfuse with 1 unit of packed red cells.
d. Turn her on her left side.

24. Which value on the Bishop score is associated with the most successful labor induction?
a. 5
b. 6
c. 8
d. 10

25. During which stage of labor are ergot alkaloids administered?
a. First
b. Second
c. Third
d. Fourth

26. Before administering methylergonovine, which baseline value would be measured?
a. Blood pressure
b. Fetal heart rate
c. Maternal hourly urinary output
d. Respiratory rate

27. The nurse assesses a patient receiving a regional anesthesia for side effects. Which side effect would the nurse monitor? **Select all that apply**.
    a. Dizziness
    b. Hypertension
    c. Metallic taste in mouth
    d. Nausea
    e. Palpitations

28. Which baseline data would the nurse collect on a patient who is being inducted at 41+ weeks with intravenous (IV) oxytocin? **Select all that apply**.
    a. Deep tendon reflexes
    b. Fetal heart rate
    c. Pulse rate and blood pressure
    d. Type and crossmatch for blood
    e. Uterine activity

29. The patient is complaining of labor pain due to the pressure of the presenting part and stretching of the perineum and vagina. This pain is experienced in which stage of labor? **Select all that apply**.
    a. First
    b. Latent
    c. Second
    d. Transition
    e. Third

30. Which type of anesthesia can be used for cesarean deliveries? **Select all that apply**.
    a. Caudal block
    b. Epidural anesthesia
    c. General anesthesia
    d. Pudendal anesthesia
    e. Spinal anesthesia

31. Which drug is most commonly used for the relief of perineal pain resulting from episiotomy or laceration? **Select all that apply**.
    a. Benzocaine
    b. Erythromycin
    c. Mineral oil
    d. Witch hazel compresses

32. A patient with a repaired fourth-degree laceration postdelivery has benzocaine topical spray. The patient asks if a heat lamp on the perineum can be used for additional comfort. Which response would be the nurse's best answer?
    a. "No, the heat lamp will increase the incidence of bacteria growth."
    b. "No, use of a heat lamp with benzocaine may cause tissue burns."
    c. "What a good idea; it will decrease pain while improving healing."
    d. "Yes, you can use a heat lamp to augment the action of benzocaine."

33. At which time frame is the best time to administer the standard dose of $Rh_0(D)$ immune globulin?
    a. After chorionic villus sampling and at 38 weeks' gestation
    b. At 28 weeks' gestation and again within 72 hours after delivery
    c. Before amniocentesis and at 38 weeks' gestation
    d. Only at 28 weeks' gestation

34. A client at 3 weeks postpartum is seen in the clinic for postpartum depression and is prescribed zuranolone. For which patient teaching would the nurse provide? **Select all that apply**.
    a. "Do not drive until you know how this drug affects you."
    b. "If you are breastfeeding, it is recommended to hold breastfeeding."
    c. "Take the medicine on an empty stomach for better absorption."
    d. "This medication may make you sleepy."
    e. "You will need to take this medication for 1 year."
    f. "You may start breastfeeding one week after your last dose."

CLINICAL JUDGMENT STANDALONE CASE STUDY

Read the scenario and answer the following questions on a separate sheet of paper.

SLO: Determine appropriate nursing actions for patients receiving intravenous oxytocin
NGN Item Type: Drop-Down Table
Cognitive Skills: Take Action

A 22-year-old female who is at 38 weeks' gestation is seen by her obstetrician. During her routine perinatal visit, the ultrasound revealed intrauterine growth retardation (IUGR). The patient is scheduled for induction. After appropriate cervical ripening, oxytocin intravenously was started to enhance labor.

For each Potential Complication listed in the second column, indicate which Nursing Action listed in the far-left column is *most* appropriate for the patient receiving intravenous oxytocin. Note that not all nursing action will be used.

Nursing Action	Potential Complication	Appropriate Nursing Action for the Complication
Have oxygen readily available	Uterine rupture	
Review labs for any electrolyte imbalance	Maternal hypoxia	
Increase the infusion rate of oxytocin	Uterine hyperstimulation	
Ensure terbutaline is readily available	Seizures	
Administer one liter of 0.9% sodium chloride intravenously		
Monitor fetal heart rate for any decelerations		
Prepare patient for regional anesthesia		

54 Neonatal and Newborn

STUDY QUESTIONS

Complete the following.

1. _____ _____ _____ can occur because of immature lung development and low _____ level, which is needed to decrease surface tension.

2. A patent _____ tube is required to administer surfactant.

3. _____ is excessive oxygenation and _____ is decreased carbon dioxide concentration.

4. Hepatitis B immunization should be initiated during the _____ period.

5. Erythromycin ophthalmic ointment is administered to newborns to prevent _____ _____, an eye infection among newborns.

REVIEW QUESTIONS

Select the best response.

6. A baby is born at 30 weeks' gestation and is having respiratory distress. Which class of drug would ***most likely*** be administered?
   a. Antibiotics
   b. Benzodiazepines
   c. Calcium chloride
   d. Surfactant replacement

7. A nurse is preparing to assist in administering beractant intratracheally. Which action is needed in preparing the drug?
   a. Warm for 5 seconds under hot running water.
   b. Shake the vial to mix the solution.
   c. Warm at room temperature for 20 minutes.
   d. Keep it refrigerated until immediately before administration.

8. Which drug could be administered to a premature newborn to mature lung development? **Select all that apply**.
   a. Erythromycin
   b. Beractant
   c. Vitamin K
   d. Poractant alfa
   e. Calfactant

9. A nurse is assisting with administering exogenous surfactant via endotracheal tube. Which complication could occur with surfactant? **Select all that apply**.
   a. Desaturation
   b. Bradycardia
   c. Pallor
   d. Hyperoxia

10. A preterm neonate becomes cyanotic and the oxygen level decreases during surfactant administration. Which action would be most appropriate by the nurse?
    a. Gently suction through the endotracheal tube immediately to raise the oxygen level.
    b. Reposition the neonate to disperse the drug throughout the lungs.
    c. Do nothing.
    d. Increase the amount of oxygen the neonate is receiving.

11. Which substance would be administered to a neonate born to a hepatitis B carrier to provide passive protection against hepatitis B?
    a. Recombinant hepatitis B
    b. Varicella zoster
    c. Phytonadione
    d. Hepatitis B immune globulin

12. Which ophthalmic ointment is administered to the newborn immediately after birth?
   a. Bacitracin
   b. Erythromycin
   c. Gentamicin
   d. Penicillin

CASE STUDY: CRITICAL THINKING

Read the scenario and answer the following questions on a separate sheet of paper.

A patient who is Gravida 1, Para 0 is in active labor and is anxious. Prenatal laboratory tests revealed the patient was positive for HBs-Ag. Additional blood work was positive for active hepatitis B virus (HBV). The patient is worried that the baby will also have hepatitis B.

1. How can HBV be transmitted to the neonate?

2. What is the nurse's best response to the patient's concerns?

3. Which drug would the nurse administer to the neonate for hepatitis B? Discuss the rationales for the drugs?

4. What is the immunization schedule for recombinant hepatitis B?

55 Women's Reproductive Health

STUDY QUESTIONS

Match the medical disorder in Column I with its definition in Column II.

Column I

_____ **1.** Endometriosis

_____ **2.** Dysmenorrhea

_____ **3.** Dysfunctional uterine bleeding

_____ **4.** Polycystic ovarian syndrome

_____ **5.** Premenstrual syndrome

Column II

a. Collection of cyclic physical and mood alterations

b. Abnormal location of endometrial tissue outside the uterus

c. A disorder in the metabolism of androgens and estrogens

d. A classification of irregular bleeding

e. Also called cyclic pelvic pain

Complete the following.

6. A women's reproductive life cycle begins with _____ and continues through _____.

7. Ethinyl estradiol is a synthetic _____ found in combined hormonal contraceptives.

8. Drospirenone is an analog of _____, a potassium-sparing _____.

9. If the minipill is delayed for more than 3 hours, a back-up contraceptive method should be used for _____ hours.

10. The inhibition of both FSH and LH secretion results in _____ and _____.

11. Gonadotropin-releasing hormone agonists (GnRH) inhibit the release of GnRH creating a _____ environment.

Match the term in Column I with its definition in Column II.

Column I

_____ **12.** Amenorrhea

_____ **13.** Dysmenorrhea

_____ **14.** Mittelschmerz

_____ **15.** Breakthrough bleeding

_____ **16.** Chloasma

Column II

a. Episodes of bleeding during the active pill cycle of hormonal contraceptives

b. Absence of bleeding

c. Mid-cycle pain usually associated with ovulation

d. Painful periods

e. Hyperpigmentation of the skin

REVIEW QUESTIONS

Select the best response.

17. Which individual would be contraindicated for oral contraceptives?
a. 20-year-old who is not sexually active
b. 40-year-old with diabetes
c. 38-year-old with breast cancer
d. 48-year-old with emphysema

18. In which patient would combined hormone contraceptives (CHCs) be used with caution? **Select all that apply**.
a. 37-year-old who smokes
b. 45-year-old who does not exercise
c. 38-year-old with diabetes
d. 28-year-old with epilepsy
e. 18-year-old with depression

221

19. A patient who works the night shift realized that she missed a dose of combined hormonal contraceptive (CHC). She calls the on-call nurse and asks what she should do. Which response would be most appropriate by the nurse?
   a. "It isn't a big deal. Just take one tomorrow."
   b. "Stop this pack and use alternative birth control for the next month."
   c. "Take your dose now, and then get back on schedule with the next one."
   d. "Take two now and use an alternative method of birth control."

20. A patient who has been taking conjugated estrogen for contraception reports a variety of side effects. Which clinical manifestation is due primarily to an excess of estrogen? **Select all that apply**.
   a. Acne
   b. Breast tenderness
   c. Fluid retention
   d. Leg cramps
   e. Nausea

21. Which drug would mostly have a drug-drug interaction with oral conjugated estrogen? **Select all that apply**.
   a. Aspirin
   b. Fluoxetine
   c. Folic acid
   d. Phenobarbital
   e. Topiramate

22. Which laboratory value would be monitored closely in a patient who has been taking drospirenone for contraception?
   a. Blood glucose
   b. Hemoglobin
   c. Potassium
   d. Thyroid-stimulating hormone

23. A patient who has been using ethinyl estradiol and etonogestrel transvaginal for contraception calls and reports that the device fell out. Which response by the nurse would be most correct?
   a. "Discard the current pill pack and start a new package of pills."
   b. "Do a home pregnancy test and report the results."
   c. "Rinse it off if it has been less than 3 hours and reinsert."
   d. "Throw it away and get a new one."

24. The family planning nurse would be correct to tell a patient to stop taking her combined oral contraceptive and notify her health care provider if she experiences which alteration?
   a. Increased vaginal discharge
   b. Severe headaches
   c. Lighter/shorter periods
   d. Menstrual cramping

25. Which risk factor decreases with the use of progestin in hormone therapy (HT)?
   a. Breast cancer
   b. Cervical cancer
   c. Endometrial cancer
   d. Vaginal cancer

26. A patient told the nurse that they have been taking calcium to prevent osteoporosis. The nurse recommends the patient also takes vitamin D for which reason?
   a. Decrease calcium loss from the bone
   b. Increase dietary calcium absorption
   c. Decrease calcium excretion
   d. Increase metabolism of calcium

CASE STUDY: CRITICAL THINKING

Read the scenario and answer the following questions on a separate sheet of paper.

During a gynecology intake interview with the nurse practitioner at the company's new health care clinic, A 55-year-old patient states, "I seem to be having more discomfort when I have sex. I don't lubricate when I want and need to; if my partner hurries me, it is downright painful. This is probably my problem, but my partner thinks that after a 35-year marriage, I just don't really desire to have sex anymore."

The nurse compiles a few more facts about the patient for review and consideration. In addition to dyspareunia, the patient has urinary frequency and urgency, vaginal pruritus, thinning vaginal epithelium with a glazed-looking appearance, and minimal elasticity upon speculum examination.

The patient is Caucasian, is very thin, and reports no periods for nearly 8 years. The patient has no history of vaginal infections.

1. Given this history, what would the nurse suspect is occurring, and what other history would be important to obtain regarding symptoms?

2. What treatment options can be offered to this patient?

3. What other health concerns should be discussed?

56 Men's Reproductive Health

STUDY QUESTIONS

Match the terms in Column I with the definitions in Column II.

Column I

_____ **1.** Anabolic steroids

_____ **2.** Androgen

_____ **3.** Hirsutism

_____ **4.** Spermatogenesis

_____ **5.** Virilization

_____ **6.** Antiandrogens

_____ **7.** Cryptorchidism

_____ **8.** Gynecomastia

_____ **9.** Oligospermia

_____ **10.** Priapism

Column II

a. Low sperm count
b. Undescended testis
c. Breast swelling or soreness
d. Ongoing painful erection
e. Growth of facial hair and vocal huskiness in women
f. Formation of spermatozoa
g. Steroid hormones related to the hormone testosterone
h. Testosterone
i. Blocks the synthesis or action of androgens
j. Increased hair growth

REVIEW QUESTIONS

Select the best response.

11. Which medical condition would sildenafil be contra-indicated?
a. Hepatitis
b. Seizure disorder
c. Renal insufficiency
d. Unstable angina

12. The 17-year-old patient is receiving androgen therapy for hypogonadism. He asks the nurse what androgen therapy does. Which response by the nurse would be most appropriate?
a. "It ensures the ability to respond sexually."
b. "It ensures adequate sperm production."
c. "It promotes larger stature through protein deposition."
d. "It stimulates the development of secondary sex characteristics."

13. A 16-year-old wrestler at a local high school tells the nurse during an annual sports physical that some of the athletes at the school use hormones to "bulk up" during the season. The patient wants to know if this is safe. Which response by the nurse is most correct?
a. "A safer way to bulk up is to eat an all-protein diet."
b. "As long as they don't use other street drugs, this is probably safe."
c. "This can cause serious, often irreversible, health problems even years later."
d. "This is a safe practice as long as a health care provider adjusts the dose."

14. A patient who is receiving androgen therapy takes prescribed drugs for cardiovascular disease, diabetes, and chronic obstructive pulmonary disease. Which drug-drug interaction can occur in this patient?
a. Androgens may decrease blood glucose levels, and insulin doses must be adjusted.
b. Androgens decrease the effect of anticoagulants.
c. Phenytoin potentiates the action of androgens.
d. There are no interactions with steroids.

15. Which indication would be appropriate for androgen therapy in females? **Select all that apply**.
    a. Advanced carcinoma of the breast
    b. Delayed development of sexual characteristics
    c. Endometriosis
    d. Infertility
    e. Severe premenstrual syndrome

16. A teenage male patient is receiving androgen therapy for hypogonadism. Which side effect might this patient experience? **Select all that apply**.
    a. Gynecomastia
    b. Continuous erection
    c. A rise in voice pitch
    d. Urinary urgency
    e. Visual disturbances

17. Which indication would be appropriate for antiandrogen drugs? **Select all that apply**.
    a. Advanced prostatic cancer
    b. Erectile dysfunction
    c. Male pattern baldness
    d. Menopausal symptoms
    e. Benign prostatic hypertrophy (BPH)

CASE STUDY: CRITICAL THINKING

Read the scenario and answer the following questions on a separate sheet of paper.

A male patient who has a history of diabetes and hypertension reports to their health care provider that they are frustrated in not able to "get it up" and is wanting treatment for erectile dysfunction.

1. Discuss erectile dysfunction and how it relates to the patient's history.

2. Which drug class is the patient referring to, and how does it work?

3. Discuss the common side effects associated with drugs used in treating erectile dysfunction.

4. What health teaching would the nurse provide for the patient regarding erectile dysfunction?

224

Chapter **56 Men's Reproductive Health**

57 Sexually Transmitted Infections

STUDY QUESTIONS

Match the infection in Column I to its description in Column II.

Column I

_____ **1.** Gonorrhea

_____ **2.** Primary syphilis

_____ **3.** Secondary syphilis

_____ **4.** Tertiary syphilis

_____ **5.** Bacterial vaginosis

_____ **6.** Chlamydia

Column II

a. Thin, white vaginal discharge with a strong fishy odor

b. Characterized by a skin rash that appears 2–8 weeks after the chancre

c. Second most common sexually transmitted infection (STI) that is characterized by a greenish-yellow or whitish discharge and dysuria in men

d. Most common STI in young adults and is often asymptomatic

e. A chancre at the site of the original infection caused by *Treponema pallidum*

f. Occurs as early as one year after the initial infection, causing large sores inside the body along with systemic syphilis to the cardiovascular and neurologic systems

Match the sexually transmitted infection (STI) in Column I with its appropriate drug in Column II.

Column I

_____ **7.** Herpes simplex virus

_____ **8.** Bacterial vaginosis

_____ **9.** Chlamydia

_____ **10.** Gonorrhea

_____ **11.** Syphilis

_____ **12.** Trichomoniasis

Column II

a. Benzathine penicillin G

b. Acyclovir

c. Ceftriaxone and azithromycin

d. Metronidazole

e. Doxycycline

TRUE OR FALSE. If the statement is false, rewrite the sentence to make it true.

_____ **13.** Scabies in adults is often transmitted sexually.

_____ **14.** Washing bed linens of a patient diagnosed with scabies is not necessary.

_____ **15.** Nitroimidazoles and alcohol is not contraindicated.

_____ **16.** Pediculosis pubis is treated with topical azole.

Select the best response.

17. A patient presents to the clinic complaining of dysuria and yellow-green discharge. Culture confirms *Neisseria gonorrhoeae*. Which additional test would the patient be counseled to consider?
    a. Fasting blood sugar
    b. Fertility workup
    c. Human immunodeficiency virus (HIV) testing
    d. Liver panel

18. Which advice would a nurse provide to a patient with gonorrhea to prevent further transmission of gonorrhea?
    a. Abstain or use condoms during sex.
    b. Ask partners to take antibiotics.
    c. Douche before intercourse.
    d. Only engage in anal intercourse.

19. The patient, who has a history of repeated gonorrhea, chlamydia, and human papillomavirus (HPV), asks how long to abstain from sex. Which response by the nurse would be most appropriate?
    a. "For at least two months."
    b. "Until the drugs are finished."
    c. "Until your partner finishes his treatment."
    d. "You may have sex using condoms."

20. The patient asks if gonorrhea and syphilis are the same thing. Which response by the nurse would be correct?
    a. "No, but if you have one, you should consider being tested for the other."
    b. "No, gonorrhea has no serious side effects."
    c. "No, only women get gonorrhea."
    d. "No, syphilis cannot be cured."

21. The patient would like to know how human immunodeficiency virus (HIV) is spread. Which method of transmission would be discussed with the patient? **Select all that apply**.
    a. Breast milk
    b. Contact with infected blood
    c. Vaginal secretions
    d. Sexual contact
    e. Mosquitoes

CASE STUDY: CRITICAL THINKING

Read the scenario and answer the following questions on a separate sheet of paper.

An adult patient presents to the health care provider complaining of abnormal vaginal discharge and pelvic pain that worsens during intercourse. The patient also complains of pharyngitis. On examination, the pharynx is erythematous with whitish patches. The pelvic examination revealed odiferous, whitish discharge with adnexal tenderness. The patient reports being sexually active, including oral sex, with multiple partners.

1. What is the presumptive diagnosis, and what are some of its clinical manifestations?

2. How should the patient be treated pharmacologically? What are the dosages?

3. What information regarding sexually transmitted infections would be provided to the patient?

58 Adult and Pediatric Emergency Drugs

STUDY QUESTIONS

Match the condition in Column I with the drug of choice that treats it in Column II.

Column I

_____ **1.** Anaphylactic shock

_____ **2.** Angina pectoris

_____ **3.** Opioid overdose

_____ **4.** Extravasation of dopamine

_____ **5.** Hypoxemia

_____ **6.** Torsade de pointes

_____ **7.** Frequent premature ventricular contractions (PVCs)

_____ **8.** Atrial fibrillation

_____ **9.** Increased intracranial pressure

_____ **10.** Hemodynamically significant bradycardia

_____ **11.** Paroxysmal supraventricular tachycardia (PSVT)

Column II

a. Magnesium sulfate
b. Diltiazem
c. Atropine sulfate
d. Mannitol
e. Phentolamine
f. Amiodarone
g. Nitroglycerin
h. Epinephrine
i. Oxygen
j. Adenosine
k. Naloxone

Match the drug in Column I with its classification in Column II. Classifications may be used more than once.

Column I

_____ **12.** Nitroprusside

_____ **13.** Epinephrine

_____ **14.** Lidocaine

_____ **15.** Norepinephrine

_____ **16.** Mannitol

_____ **17.** Diltiazem

_____ **18.** Albuterol

_____ **19.** Furosemide

Column II

a. Antidysrhythmic, class IB
b. Osmotic diuretic
c. Calcium channel blocker
d. Catecholamine
e. Beta-adrenergic agonist
f. Vasodilator
g. Loop diuretic

Select the best answer.

20. Sublingual nitroglycerin may be prescribed for chest pain. Which vital sign would be most important to assess before administering this drug?
    a. Blood pressure
    b. Heart rate
    c. Respiratory rate
    d. Temperature

21. Following administration of intravenous (IV) morphine to treat chest pain associated with acute myocardial infarction, which nursing action would be most important?
    a. Assessment of respiratory status
    b. Documentation of neurologic function
    c. Measurement and strict recording of intake and output
    d. Measurement of central venous pressure

22. When monitoring a patient who is receiving dobutamine infusion, the nurse must be alert to the development of adverse effects. Which side or adverse effect may require slowing or discontinuing drug administration?
    a. Bradycardia
    b. Confusion
    c. Diaphoresis
    d. Myocardial ischemia

23. Procainamide 1.4 mg/minute is infusing in a patient with supraventricular tachycardia (SVT). The nurse is closely monitoring the patient to determine if the procainamide should be discontinued. Which side or adverse effect is an end point of procainamide administration?
    a. Headache
    b. Hypotension
    c. Respiratory depression
    d. Vomiting

24. A patient post myocardial infarction complains of "heart racing" and is dyspneic. The cardiac monitor shows the patient to be in a tachyarrhythmia. Which dysrhythmia is amiodarone intravenous (IV) used to treat? **Select all that apply**.
    a. Asystole
    b. Atrial fibrillation
    c. Bradycardia
    d. Second-degree heart block
    e. Ventricular fibrillation

25. Which acid-base imbalance is the best indication for sodium bicarbonate?
    a. Metabolic acidosis
    b. Metabolic alkalosis
    c. Respiratory acidosis
    d. Respiratory alkalosis

26. The patient is admitted to the critical care unit after sustaining a severe closed head injury in a motorcycle collision. Mannitol is ordered to decrease intracranial pressure. Through which mechanism does mannitol exert its pharmacologic effects?
    a. Cerebral vasoconstriction
    b. Loop diuresis
    c. Osmotic diuresis
    d. Peripheral vasodilation

27. A patient, who is allergic to shellfish, presents to the emergency department (ED) with hives after eating soup. The patient's tongue and lips are swollen. Which drug would be appropriate to administer?
    a. Atropine
    b. Diltiazem
    c. Diphenhydramine
    d. Lidocaine

28. An unresponsive patient presents to the ED in respiratory distress. The patient's friends report the patient "using a lot of those pain pills for the back." The patient's pupils are pinpoint, and the respiratory rate is 4 breaths/minute. Which drug would the nurse prepare to administer?
    a. Diltiazem 0.25 mg/kg IV piggyback
    b. Flumazenil 2.5 mg IV push
    c. Naloxone 0.4 mg IV push
    d. Magnesium 2 g IV piggyback

29. For which type of shock would dopamine be indicated? **Select all that apply**.
    a. Cardiogenic shock
    b. Hypovolemic shock
    c. Insulin shock
    d. Neurogenic shock
    e. Septic shock

30. Through which mechanism does dobutamine elevate blood pressure?
    a. Increasing cardiac output
    b. Positive alpha effects
    c. Vasoconstriction
    d. Vasodilation

31. A patient has a diagnosis of septic shock. A norepinephrine drip is infusing through a central intravenous (IV) line. The bag of norepinephrine is almost empty. For which reason would the nurse prepare to hang another bag of norepinephrine?
    a. Hypertensive crisis can result if the infusion is interrupted.
    b. Profound hypotension can occur if the infusion is abruptly discontinued.
    c. The patient is at high risk for bradycardia and heart block.
    d. The organisms responsible for septic shock will proliferate.

32. A patient with diabetes was brought to the ED unconscious. The nurse prepares to administer dextrose 50% (D_{50}). For which conditions is D_{50} most commonly prescribed?
    a. As a maintenance infusion to keep a vein open
    b. To increase urine output
    c. To treat hyperglycemia
    d. To treat insulin-induced hypoglycemia

33. A patient was brought into the ED with SVT. The nurse is preparing to administer adenosine. Which method of administering adenosine is correct?
    a. Slow IV push over 2 minutes
    b. Diluted in 50 mL as IVPB over 30 minutes
    c. Rapid IV push as a bolus followed by saline flush
    d. Via a nebulizer

34. Which priority nursing action would be implemented after administering a total intravenous (IV) lidocaine dose of 3 mg/kg to an adult and the dysrhythmia has been suppressed?
    a. Assess the patient for confusion, drowsiness, muscle twitching, and myocardial conduction defects.
    b. A therapeutic serum level will be achieved and maintained.
    c. Additional bolus doses must be administered to achieve a therapeutic serum level.
    d. 3 mg/kg is too much, and the patient has been overdosed.

35. The nurse is preparing to administer epinephrine intramuscularly (IM) to a patient with an allergic reaction. Which concentration would the nurse select?
    a. 1:10,000 concentration of epinephrine
    b. 1:1000 concentration of epinephrine
    c. 1:100 concentration of epinephrine
    d. 1:1 concentration of epinephrine

36. The patient is in cardiac arrest. To administer epinephrine intravenously, which concentration would the nurse select?
    a. 1:10,000 concentration of epinephrine
    b. 1:1000 concentration of epinephrine
    c. 1:100 concentration of epinephrine
    d. 1:1 concentration of epinephrine

37. A patient presents to the ED with hemodynamically unstable bradycardia. The nurse prepares to administer atropine 1 mg intravenously, knowing that lower dosages can cause which adverse effect?
    a. Paradoxical bradycardia
    b. Miosis
    c. Tachycardia
    d. Increased vagal activity

38. A patient with history of panic disorder is brought to the ED from an overdose of diazepam. The nurse prepares to administer flumazenil knowing that it is effective in reversing which class of drugs?
    a. Antipsychotics
    b. Benzodiazepines
    c. Opioids
    d. Paralytic agents

39. Magnesium sulfate is indicated for the treatment of which medical condition? **Select all that apply**.
    a. Atrial dysrhythmias
    b. Hypokalemia
    c. Cardiac arrest
    d. Torsades de pointes

40. A patient with heart failure and pulmonary edema was ordered furosemide 60 mg by intravenous push (IVP). Furosemide exerts its effects on pulmonary edema through which mechanisms?
    a. Bronchodilation and diuresis
    b. Bronchodilation and antiinflammatory actions
    c. Vasoconstriction and diuresis
    d. Vasodilation and diuresis

41. Which priority nursing intervention would be implemented when caring for a patient with a nitroprusside infusion? **Select all that apply**.
    a. Always use nitroprusside with a blue or brown color to the solution.
    b. Monitor blood pressure continuously.
    c. Stop the nitroprusside immediately when blood pressure has stabilized.
    d. Protect the solution from light.
    e. Monitor thiocyanate levels.

42. Which side and/or adverse effect is associated with intravenous (IV) atropine? **Select all that apply**.
    a. Dry mouth
    b. Miosis
    c. Mydriasis
    d. Urinary retention
    e. Vomiting

CASE STUDY: CRITICAL THINKING

Read the scenario and answer the following questions on a separate sheet of paper.

An adult patient calls emergency medical services (EMS) with complaints of chest pain and shortness of breath. The patient has a history of angina, asthma, and obesity. The patient states, "It just hit me hard. I think I'm going to die." The patient has taken three nitroglycerin tablets, and was given aspirin and morphine en route to the hospital. On arrival at the hospital, an electrocardiogram is obtained. The patient is not having a myocardial infarction but is diagnosed with unstable angina and is admitted to the coronary care unit. Vital signs on admission are temperature 97.3° F, heart rate 88 beats/minute, respiratory rate 20 breaths/minute, and blood pressure 214/118 mm Hg. A nitroglycerin drip is started.

1. How does nitroglycerin work to treat a patient with angina?

2. Explain the benefit of receiving aspirin and morphine en route to the hospital? Why was the nitroglycerin drip started?
   The patient became unresponsive and developed widened QRS complex ventricular tachycardia with a ventricular rate of 190 beats/minute. Code blue was called, and a crash cart was brought into the room. The patient was shocked with 360 joules three times, without any change to the rhythm. CPR was initiated and the nurse prepares to administer emergency drugs.

3. What drug would the nurse prepare first to administer for pulseless ventricular tachycardia after unsuccessful defibrillation?

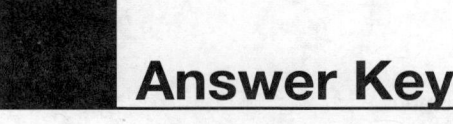

Answer Key

CHAPTER 1: CLINICAL JUDGMENT MANAGEMENT MODEL AND THE NURSING PROCESS

1. False. "Concept" focuses on the *patient-centered model of care* instead of a disease-centered model.
2. False. Concepts are related to patient's problems, the medications, or topic of care listed within the *nursing process*.
3. False. The Nursing Alliance for Quality Care (NAQC) that supports quality patient-centered health care is partnered with the American *Nurses* Association.
4. False. NAQC believes that it is *nurse's* role to cultivate successful patient and family engagement.
5. True. The purpose of developing good clinical judgment is to allow nurses to recognize changes in patient's conditions with appropriate assessment and evaluation skills.
6. False. Cues are what the nurse gathers from the patient about their health and lifestyle practices. The nurse asks direct questions and conducts physical assessment to gather data.
7. d, e, b, a, c
8. b
9. a
10. c
11. a
12. d
13. a
14. d or e
15. d
16. d
17. a
18. e
19. b. The nurse is observing that the patient is producing phlegm when coughing; this is objective data.
20. a
21. b
22. a. The patient complains of nausea. The nurse can observe vomiting, not nausea.
23. b. Even though the patient may know how to obtain heart rate, the nurse usually obtains heart rate by palpating pulse or auscultating heart sounds.
24. a
25. a
26. d. *Analyze cues and prioritize hypothesis* are based on analysis of subjective and objective data so that patient-centered care is provided.
27. a. *Recognize cues* are part of the data gathering of subjective and objective data, such as obtaining patient's baseline weight to compare with future weight, to provide patient-centered care.

28. c. Goals are set to *generate solutions* after analyzing all the data that was gathered during the assessment (*Recognize cues*) phase. Usually, an *expected outcome* statement starts with "The patient will... "
29. c. Expected outcomes are set during *generating solutions* after analyzing all the data that was gathered during the assessment (*Recognize cues*) phase. Usually, an *expected outcome* statement starts with "The patient will..."
30. b. Nurses *take action* when they provide education, drug administration, patient care, and other nursing interventions.
31. b. After taking action on the plan the nurse must *evaluate outcomes* to determine whether the outcome statements and teaching objectives were met. At this time the nurse would determine if the goal statements need revision. Patient-centered model of care is an ongoing process in which nurses recognize cues, analyze cues, prioritize hypotheses, generate solutions, take action, and evaluate outcomes.
32. d. A hypothesis statement is based on analysis of subjective and objective data so that nurses prioritize patient problems and provide patient-centered care. *Disturbed sleep* is a hypothesis based on objective data caused by diuretics.
33. b. Nurses *take action* by providing education, administering drugs, providing patient care, and other interventions. *Advising the child's parents to report adverse reactions* is educating parents.
34. c. *Analyzing cues* and *prioritizing hypotheses* are based on the analysis of subjective and objective data to provide patient-centered care. *Psychological disturbance* is a hypothesis based on objective cues that can be observed in patients on opioids.
35. c. Nurses *take action* by providing education, administering drugs, and other interventions. *Instructing patient not to discontinue drugs abruptly* is patient education.

Case Study: Critical Thinking

1. The nurse will consider the nursing process: recognize cues, analyze cues and prioritize hypothesis, generate solutions, take action, and evaluate outcomes.

    Nurses recognize cues not only by obtaining subjective and objective data, such as patient history and physical examination, but also by reviewing current medications, allergies, and results of any tests, such as laboratory work and radiographs. Reviewing current medications includes comparing the newly prescribed medication to the medications the patient is currently taking. This is called medication reconciliation, which helps in preventing drug errors. Physical examination should include physical reasons why the patient may not be able to administer the injection. Other items to assess include the home environment and, most importantly, the patient's readiness to learn and education level.

The next phase in the nursing process is to analyze cues and prioritize hypothesis. These are based on actual concerns recognized during assessment or potential problems attributable to risk factors that arise during assessment. The patient's statements suggest several potential hypotheses, including those related to anxiety, knowledge deficit, and nonadherence.

While *generating solutions*, measurable expected outcomes are established in collaboration with the patient, family, and other members of the healthcare team. The outcomes must be realistic and measurable and occur in a certain time frame. A realistic outcome for this patient could be *The patient will prepare the prescribed dose of insulin by the second day of instruction.*

During the next phase of patient-centered care, nurses would *take action* to provide the education necessary for the patient to be able to achieve the expected outcome. In this situation the teaching needs to address several areas, including the psychomotor skill of preparing and administering an insulin injection.

2. In the last phase, the nurse *evaluates outcomes* to determine the effectiveness of the teaching plan by having the patient return demonstration of injecting insulin. Adequate time for questions must be provided, as well as contact information for the healthcare provider. The nurse must ensure that the patient is ready to learn, the material is presented in an appropriate manner for learning to occur, and the materials are culturally appropriate.

Continue to assess the attainment of the hypotheses and outcomes and revise the plan to ensure success. Evaluation of the outcomes is the final step in the nursing process. The outcome must be evaluated, and changes made if necessary. Was the patient able to correctly demonstrate insulin preparation? Did the patient have problems with anxiety surrounding the preparation? Was the patient able to verbalize concerns to the healthcare provider?

CHAPTER 2: DRUG DEVELOPMENT AND ETHICAL CONSIDERATIONS

1. b
2. g
3. e
4. a
5. d
6. b
7. h
8. f
9. trade or brand
10. I
11. health information
12. FDA; health; innovative; safe; effective
13. nurse practice act
14. False. Schedule II drugs include methamphetamine, cocaine, methadone, meperidine, and oxycodone.
15. True
16. True
17. True
18. False. A nurse could be prosecuted for omitting a drug dose, giving the wrong drug, or giving the drug by the wrong route.
19. b. Beneficence is the duty to protect research participants from harm. It clearly defines the research and ensures the benefits outweigh the risks. Justice involves the selection process of research participants that is fair. Autonomy is the right to self-determination, and the nurse must allow the research participant to make decisions. Respect for persons means that all patients, including research participants, are treated as independent persons who are capable of making decisions in their own best interests.
20. a. Prior to administering *any* drugs, a nurse would verify the prescription. When administering any controlled substances, a nurse must document all wasted amount; keep all controlled drugs in a secure, locked area; and have a witness for *any* controlled drug wastages.
21. d. The *International Pharmacopeia* provides a basis for standards in strength and composition of drugs for use *throughout* the world. The *United States Pharmacopeia/National Formulary* sets the drug standards used in the United States. The *American Hospital Formulary Service Drug Information* provides complete drug information for both the healthcare provider and the consumer for drugs marketed in the United States. The *MedlinePlus* provides extensive drug information and is available on the World Wide Web.
22. c. Federal legislation's primary purpose is to ensure safety and protect the public from drugs that are impure, toxic, ineffective, or not tested.
23. d. The Kefauver-Harris Amendment requires adverse reactions and contraindications to be included in the drug's literature.
24. d. LSD and mescaline are schedule I drugs. Schedule IV drugs include alprazolam and zolpidem. Schedule III drugs include ketamine and products containing less than 90 mg of codeine. Schedule II drugs include products such as methylphenidate, cocaine, meperidine, fentanyl, and products with less than 15 mg of hydrocodone.
25. d. Schedule V drugs include cough preparation containing not more than 200 mg of codeine. Schedule

II drugs include products with less than 15 mg of hydrocodone, cocaine, meperidine, and fentanyl. Schedule III drugs include ketamine and products containing less than 90 mg of codeine. Schedule IV drugs include alprazolam and zolpidem.

26. d. All controlled substances must be stored in a locked, secured area.

27. c. All participants in a research study have the right to be informed. It is the responsibility of the health-care provider, *not the nurse*, to explain the study. In order for the participant to provide an informed consent, the person must be alert and able to comprehend the information.

28. a, c, d, e. Differences in appearance, either in the drug or in the packaging, can be an indication of a counterfeit drug. However, it is important to remember that pharmacies may change their pharmaceutical supplier, so the drug may appear as a different color or shape to the patient. This is an opportunity for the nurse and the pharmacist to work together to provide patient education.

Case Study: Critical Thinking

1. The nurse will tell the patient that the personal information will be shared with the pharmacist as it pertains to proper health care. The pharmacist will be able to discuss the drug and treatment with the patient in a separate counseling area, away from other people.

2. HIPAA sets the standard for privacy of individuals of their identifiable health information. The act allows patient more control on who has access to their health records.

CHAPTER 3: PHARMACOKINETICS AND PHARMACODYNAMICS

1. absorption, distribution, metabolism, and excretion
2. half-life
3. Pharmacodynamics
4. bloodstream; administration
5. antagonists
6. receptors
7. f
8. e
9. c
10. a
11. b
12. d
13. g
14. a
15. d
16. c
17. b
18. c. Since liquid drugs do not need to dissolute and dissolve like tablets and capsules, they are absorbed more rapidly. Absorption of drugs is the movement of the drug from the gastrointestinal (GI) tract into the bloodstream after administration. Sublingual drugs enter the bloodstream without having to be absorbed by the GI tract.

19. c. Disintegration of enteric-coated (EC) tablets occurs in an alkaline environment of the small intestine. Drugs that are EC resist disintegration in the stomach by the gastric acid.

20. b. Food usually decreases dissolution and absorption of drugs. However, there are some drugs that are irritating to the gastric mucosa. Food can decrease these irritating effects.

21. d. Absorption, distribution, metabolism, and excretion is the correct sequence of the pharmacokinetic phases. The drug must be *absorbed* from the GI tract (stomach and small intestine) into the bloodstream; drug must be *distributed* through the circulatory system to the tissues (cells), including the liver; drug must be *metabolized* into an excretable form; the drug must be *excreted*.

22. b. Drugs that are lipid soluble and nonionized can readily pass through the GI membrane. The mucous membrane lining the GI tract is composed of lipids and protein that allow lipid-soluble drugs to pass through. On the other hand, water-soluble drug needs a carrier.

23. b, c, e. For drugs to be absorbed, adequate blood flow must be present. The gastrointestinal tract is not considered vital to a patient in shock and hypotension, so blood is shunted away causing decreased drug absorption. Blood flow is also slowed because of pain and stress. Pain and stress can cause vasoconstriction, which decreases drug absorption.

24. c. Both drugs are highly protein bound. When two or more highly protein-bound drugs are taken at the same time, they compete for the protein-binding sites. The more highly bound drug could displace the lesser bound drug; therefore ampicillin/sulbactam (higher) could displace diazepam, which results in increased activity of diazepam. The drugs that are not bound result in pharmacologic effect.

25. b. The liver is the primary site for drug metabolism. Kidneys excrete the drug.

26. b. The percentage of drug (bioavailability) for therapeutic activity is greatest after intravenous administration. Factors that affect bioavailability of drugs include drug form, route of administration, gastric mucosa and motility, food or other drugs, and liver function.

27. b. The most correct description is the time required for half of the drug to be eliminated. Other factors affecting drug's half-life are amount administered, amount of drug remaining from previous dose, metabolic activity, and the ability of the body to eliminate the drug.

28. a. A drug that has a half-life of 24–30 hours will be taken once daily to maintain a steady state.

29. d. Kidneys excrete drugs that are water soluble, drugs that are not bound, and drugs that are unchanged.

30. b. A decreased eGFR indicates renal dysfunction. Decreased eGFR is expected in older adults because of their decreased muscle mass. Many drugs, including trimethoprim, are eliminated through the kidneys. To prevent toxicity the dose would need to be decreased.

31. a. Drug is more active if it is able to "fit" at the receptor site. The drug-receptor interactions are similar to the fit of the right key in a lock.

32. b. An antagonist prevents (inhibits) and/or blocks a response. An agonist activates receptors and/or produces a desired response. A cholinergic is a type of receptor or neurotransmitter. Nonspecific drug can either be an antagonist or agonist; it depends on the type of receptors the drug affects.

33. c. A nonspecific drug affects same type of receptors located throughout the body, producing both antagonist and agonist effects. On the other hand, a nonselective drug affects more than one type of receptor.

34. b. Therapeutic index, which is closely related to dose response and efficacy, describes the relationship between the therapeutic dose and the toxic dose. Therapeutic range is a range of doses that produce a therapeutic response without causing significant adverse effects. Duration of action is the length of time the drug exerts a therapeutic response. The drug half-life is the time it takes for half of the drug to be reduced in the body.

35. a. Measurements that check a drug's concentration include peak and trough levels; peak level measures the highest serum concentration, and the trough level measures the lowest serum concentration of the drug. Minimal effective concentration is the smallest amount of the drug required for a therapeutic effect. The drug half-life is the time it takes for half of the drug to be reduced in the body. Trough level is the lowest plasma concentration of a drug.

36. a, b, d, e. The nurse must be completely familiar with any drug being administered, such as contraindications, half-life, protein-binding effect, and therapeutic range. Information needs to be obtained not only on the drug but also on the specific patient's history. Drug reference books, drug pamphlets/inserts, or a pharmacist may be consulted with questions.

37. b. Side effects are secondary effects of all drugs and are often predictable. They may be desirable or undesirable. Adverse reactions, either mild or severe, are unintentional, unexpected reactions that occur at *normal* dosages. Synergistic effects occur when two or more drugs given together have a combined effect greater than the sum of their separate effects. Toxic effects are undesirable drug effects, oftentimes life threatening.

38. c. Loading dose is a larger than usual dose to obtain a quicker therapeutic effect while waiting for the steady state to be achieved.

39. a, b, c. A time-response curve shows the dose-relationship of the drug's pharmacodynamic profiles, which include onset, peak, and the duration of the drug's action.

40. a, b, d, e. The nurse would assess the patient for side effects (both desirable and undesirable) when administering drugs. This is especially important for drugs that have nonselective actions. The nurse must be familiar with the drug, including its dose range, desired effects, side effects, and adverse effects, before administration. This information can be obtained from a variety of sources including current reference books, drug inserts, and pharmacists. If the drug has a narrow therapeutic range or requires peak/trough levels, these should be evaluated before and after administration. Side effects may occur immediately or up to several days after a dose. There is no set time to wait and see if side effects disappear. The healthcare provider should be notified as soon as possible after the appearance of side effects, especially if they are undesirable.

Case Study: Critical Thinking

1. The receptor theory states that drugs bind to receptor sites to activate a receptor, produce a response, or inhibit (block) a response. Some receptor sites are specific to only one drug, whereas others may accommodate several different drugs. However, some "fit better" and are more active. The drug-binding sites are located on cell membranes and are primarily protein, glycoprotein, proteolipids, and enzymes in nature. The four receptor families are cell membrane–embedded enzymes, ligand-gated ion channels, G protein–coupled receptor systems, and transcription factors.

   Verapamil is a calcium channel blocker. Ligand-gated ion channels stretch across the cell membrane. If the channel is open, ions (usually calcium and sodium) can flow across the membrane. A calcium channel *blocker* prevents the flow of calcium. In the case of verapamil, this causes a decreased force of contraction, less spasm, and ultimately less anginal chest pain.

2. As with any new drug, the nurse would teach the patient about how to take the drug (with or without food, timing during the day), what effects to expect and how soon to expect to see results, what undesirable side effects or adverse effects to monitor for, and what to report to the healthcare provider. It is important to stress that the drug must be taken "as prescribed" even if the patient is feeling better or not feeling any changes because some drugs work immediately and some medications may take several weeks to build up to a therapeutic level.

CHAPTER 4: PHARMACOGENETICS

1. Pharmacogenetics
2. irinotecan
3. abacavir

4. CYP2C9; VKORC1
5. False. Persons with genetic variation necessary to convert clopidogrel to the active metabolite is at risk for *clot formation*.
6. False. The CYP2D6 enzyme has *90 known variants* slowing down drug metabolism, potentially leading to toxic drug concentrations.
7. False. *Not* everyone within the same ethnic group shares the same genetic variations.
8. True
9. c. Pharmacogenetics is the study of how a person's genetic makeup (genomes) affects their responses to drugs. Pharmacogenetics helps personalize medicine to optimize therapy and decrease adverse drug reactions. Pharmacodynamics studies how drugs affect the body as it relates to onset, peak, duration, and half-lives.
10. d. A patient on multiple drugs would benefit the most from the use of pharmacogenetics. Other patients who would benefit are those who are on complex treatment regimen, such as patients on multiple antivirals to treat HIV or on combination anticancer drugs.
11. a. Patients with UGT1A1 gene variations may not be able to eliminate irinotecan. Patients with a variation to the CYP2D6 are unable to metabolize codeine and tramadol, thereby not achieving pain relief. Patients with a variation to the CYP2C19 enzyme will not be able to convert clopidogrel to its active metabolite. Gene variation in TPMT can interfere with the metabolism of mercaptopurine.

Case Study: Critical Thinking

1. The first concern for the nurse would be to determine whether the patient has a variant gene for metabolizing tramadol. Persons who lack the CYP2D6 enzyme cannot metabolize opioids, including tramadol, to the active form. Since the patient is of Asian descent, the possibility of lacking the enzyme can occur.
2. The nurse needs to guard against genetic profiling. Determine if there is a family history of treatment failures by assessing family back three generations. Also determine patient's ethnicity. If genetic variations are suspected, determine patient's knowledge concerning genetics and genetic testing; explore any concerns. Consider other treatment options.

CHAPTER 5: COMPLEMENTARY AND ALTERNATIVE THERAPIES

1. e
2. b
3. a
4. d
5. c
6. plants; infusion

7. tincture
8. Extract; liniment
9. decoction
10. volatile; herb-infused oils
11. d, h
12. g, h
13. j
14. a, c
15. b, f
16. f
17. c
18. b, e
19. i
20. a. Chamomile and ginger are used for stomach or intestinal distress. They are also used for sleeplessness and anxiety. *Ginkgo biloba* can be beneficial in those with anxiety or allergies. *Echinacea* is commonly used for virus-related symptoms. St. Johns wort is used to treat mental disorders and nerve pain.
21. c. *Ginkgo biloba* is used to improve memory and prevent Alzheimer disease and other dementias. It is also used for pulmonary distress, fatigue, and tinnitus. *Echinacea* is mostly used for virus-related symptoms. Ginger is mostly used for nausea and diarrhea. Chamomile is beneficial to induce sleep.
22. a, b, c, d. Bilberry, garlic, ginseng, and licorice can interfere with anticoagulants, such as warfarin.
23. a, d, e. The nurse would intervene by discussing with the patient that ginseng can interfere with the anticoagulants and increase the chance of bleeding; therefore the patient should report any signs or symptoms of bleeding, such as bleeding of gums, black and tarry stools, and blood in the urine. Educate the patient about the potential food-drug interactions while taking an anticoagulant. The patient has a history of atrial fibrillation, and it is necessary to be on anticoagulants, such as warfarin; therefore the patient should not stop taking the warfarin.
24. b, d. Large quantities of any one herbal product can lead to an "overdosage" of that product. Because specific doses and quantities are not regulated in the United States, it is difficult to determine the correct amount. More is not necessarily better. Infants and children should not receive herbal preparations because of the lack of standardization and testing in the pediatric population.
25. c, d. Ginseng and milk thistle can have an additive effect when used with antidiabetic drugs causing hypoglycemia.
26. a, b, c, d. St. Johns wort interacts with multiple drugs including anticoagulants and antiplatelets, anticonvulsants, antidepressants, and drugs for birth control. St. Johns wort can increase bleeding time; it can cause decreased drug levels of anticonvulsants and oral contraceptives; it can increase serotonin levels, leading to serotonin syndrome.

Case Study: Critical Thinking

1. The most commonly utilized herbal preparation for depression is St. Johns wort. It may also be beneficial for those with somatic symptom disorder, obsessive-compulsive disorder, attention-deficit disorder, and hyperactivity disorder. However, St. Johns wort has many interactions with other medications.

   Lavender is commonly used for depression, anxiety, and digestive disorders. Lavender is oftentimes available as essential oil and spray. Lavender spray can be used on the bedding to reduce anxiety which can promote sleep. depression is St. Johns wort. The patient is also most likely using lavender spray to help with insomnia.

2. The mechanism of action for St. Johns wort is unknown. There are multiple herb-drug interactions with St. Johns wort. Sometimes they can be life threatening. St. Johns wort interacts with antidepressants and can cause serotonin syndrome. The nurse would assess for evidence of confusion, restlessness, or agitation. Other signs and symptoms include agitation, diaphoresis, and fever.

   Topical lavender may cause skin reactions. The nurse would educate the patient on the signs and symptoms, such as redness, itching, raised rash, or even blistering.

CHAPTER 6: PEDIATRIC CONSIDERATIONS

1. fewer; increased
2. age; health status; weight; route of administration
3. 2; 3
4. body fluid composition; tissue composition; protein-binding capability
5. 2 years; higher
6. e
7. d
8. a
9. b
10. c
11. a, b. The rate of absorption depends on the drug formulation (basic [alkalotic] or acidic). A low pH environment favors acidic drug absorption, whereas a high pH favors basic (alkalotic) drug formulations. The difference in the drug pH may hinder or enhance drug absorption. Medications in liquid formulation may be administered to infants using a bottle nipple.
12. c. The dosage for a water-soluble medication may need to be increased in this age group because their bodies are about 70% water up until age 2 years. Therefore there is more water in which the drug will be distributed.
13. d. Immature blood-brain barrier allows drugs to pass easily into the central nervous system tissue (brain), increasing the risk of toxicity. As a child matures, the blood-brain barrier becomes more impervious to drugs.

14. a. The drug will absorb faster. One of the factors in which the degree and rate of drug absorption is age. The skin of infants and young children is thinner than that of adults. Furthermore, the ratio of body surface area to body mass is proportionately higher than for adults. Topical drugs are readily absorbed and toxicity can result. Sex of a child does not influence drug absorption.
15. a, b, c, d. Pharmacokinetics includes drug absorption, distribution, metabolism, and excretion. Onset is a pharmacodynamic, not pharmacokinetic, profile.
16. a, b, c, e. In early adolescence, renal tubular function decreases, which may lead to impaired excretion and a higher risk for toxicity. Dehydration can also decrease renal function and may lead to toxicity. An alternate route, other than oral, should be considered because the patient is nauseated and vomiting. When providing care to any patient, developmental levels should be considered. Drugs administered rectally do not promote quick absorption.
17. b, c, d, f. If necessary, a child may be lightly restrained but should not be forcibly held down. The child should be praised for taking the drug. At no time should a child be threatened, forced, or made to view the medication as punishment. Depending on the developmental level of the child, explanations should be given to the child about what to expect, but the child should not be given the option of debating whether to take the drug. Herbal preparations are not usually given to children; however, cultural traditions should be respected as much as possible.

Case Study: Critical Thinking

1. Preschoolers may respond to age-appropriate explanations. They may also benefit from a familiar toy or stuffed animal as support. Allow the child to verbalize being scared or upset. Whenever possible, allow the child options and control. Do not argue with the child or tell the child that they are being punished for falling from the tree. Tell the child what will happen before it happens. Do not just surprise the child.
2. A topical anesthetic like an eutectic mixture of local anesthetics or topical lidocaine may be utilized to lessen the pain of establishing an intravenous (IV) site. The downside to using these topical anesthetics is that they must be in place 60–90 minutes before the IV can be started for anesthetic effect.
3. Answers can vary. Caregivers may be involved in child care (if they choose to be) by helping to gently restrain the child. They can also provide distraction ("What color sling would you like?" or "What should we have to eat tomorrow morning when we get up?"). Reassuring the child can also be beneficial.

CHAPTER 7: GERIATRIC CONSIDERATIONS

1. absorption, distribution, metabolism
2. lower; gradually; response
3. sensory; physical; aging
4. receptor; affinity
5. Remember the acronym BANDD CAMP: *B*eta-blockers: sotalol; *A*CEIs/ARBs: olmesartan; *N*SAIDs/opioids: all NSAIDs, meperidine; *D*iuretics: potassium-sparing diuretics, thiazide diuretics; *D*iabetic drugs: glyburide, metformin, exenatide; *C*holesterol drugs: none; *A*ntimicrobials: nitrofurantoin; *M*iscellaneous: new anticoagulants; *P*sychotropics: none, olmesartan, and new anticoagulants
6. c
7. b
8. d
9. a
10. Angiotensin-converting enzyme inhibitor (ACE-I)
11. Beta-blockers
12. Psychotropics
13. Angiotensin II-receptor blockers (ARBs)
14. False. Risk factors associated with polypharmacy *include* advanced age in addition to female sex, having multiple healthcare providers, use of herbal therapies, use of over-the-counter (OTC) drugs, multiple chronic disorders, and frequency of hospitalizations and care transitions.
15. True
16. True
17. False. Risk factors associated with polypharmacy *include* over-the-counter (OTC) drugs and herbal agents, in addition to female sex, having multiple healthcare providers, advanced age, multiple chronic disorders, and frequency of hospitalizations and care transitions.
18. False. Beers criteria is a document developed by the American Geriatric Society listing drugs *that may be inappropriate to use among adults 65 years and older.*
19. True
20. True
21. a. Normal working kidneys will have a GFR of 100–125 mL/min. It is also generally accepted that the GFR declines by 1 mL/min after 40 years of age. Aspartate aminotransferase (AST) measures the liver function. Troponin is a type of protein found in skeletal and heart muscles. Urea is a waste product.
22. b. Renal function is decreased in older adults, which can cause electrolyte imbalance. Also, decreased renal function can lead to prolonged half-life and elevated drug levels. Certain antihypertensives like ACE-I, potassium-sparing diuretics, and thiazide diuretics can worsen electrolyte imbalance.
23. a. There is no reason that the patient cannot work outside while taking digoxin, and the patient's symptoms are not related to the digoxin.

Diphenhydramine can be very sedating among older adults, and there are substitutes that are equally effective with fewer side effects. Fluoxetine, an SSRI, is prescribed for depression. Patients of all ages should be advised not to take each other's medications.

24. c. Drugs with a shorter half-life will be eliminated from the body faster than drugs with longer half-life without interfering with their therapeutic effect. Quicker elimination will decrease the risk of adverse/toxic drug effects. The more protein binding the drug has, the less active the drug is available to exert its therapeutic effect. Fat-soluble drugs have greater volume of distribution and a prolonged period of action. This can also increase the risk for toxicity.
25. a, b. BUN (blood urea nitrogen) and creatinine clearance are assessed to determine renal function. The ability of the kidneys to excrete drugs decreases with age. CBC (complete blood count) is a test that evaluates red blood cells, white blood cells, and platelets. Lipase is a pancreatic enzyme. Triglycerides are a type of fat.
26. d. Dizziness with position changes, such as going from a supine to a standing position is referred to as *orthostatic hypotension*. Although bradycardia may cause dizziness, this is not the most likely cause.
27. a. Changing positions slowly should assist in decreasing the dizziness associated with hypotension related to changes in position. Taking a deep breath and checking heart rate will not affect dizziness. Having a chair close to the bed may be beneficial if the patient feels dizzy but may also pose a safety risk; the patient may strike the chair while fainting.
28. c. When a person has been hospitalized, a drug reconciliation has been completed. Depending on the patient's responses to the drugs administered during hospitalization, drugs may be added to or subtracted from the regimen and dose adjustments (including home medications) may be made. The patient should take only those drugs that have been prescribed at discharge.
29. a. Although a family member could assist with the daily medication regimen, the patient will be able to maintain more independence using a nonchildproof cap. Using a nonchildproof cap should make the container easier for the older adult patient to grasp and open. All medicines should be kept in their original container and not in an open glass cup or envelope. An exception to this is a medication dispensing system, such as daily pill container.
30. b. Maintaining independence for as long as possible is crucial for an older adult. A patient who has visual challenges can, with assistance, fill a drug-dispensing container for the upcoming week. The patient must have assistance in the setup to ensure that the correct medicines are in each

separate compartment. Leaving the medicine bottles on the counter could lead to a mix-up if they are displaced. Writing down which medications need to be taken is not beneficial if the patient has visual challenges.

31. a, c, d, e. Of the listed factors, only height does not have a role in dosage adjustment. Older adults have more adipose tissue, so a greater amount of lipid-soluble drug would be absorbed. Protein is required for binding of some drugs, so if a patient is malnourished, there would be less protein available, leading to more free drug; this can lead to drug toxicity. Laboratory results, specifically those that assess renal and hepatic function, are important to trend, as well as those drug levels (digoxin, INR) needed to measure toxicity. As with any population, it is important to evaluate the patient for responsiveness to the drug.

32. a, b, d, e. Older adults have less protein available for binding, so it is important to know if a drug is highly protein bound. Drugs with a short half-life are less likely to cause problems for the older adults. Certain drugs (some antibiotics, digoxin, warfarin) have very narrow therapeutic ranges, so they must be monitored closely. Vital signs may vary as patient ages; therefore it is important to obtain baseline vital signs to know the patient's norm.

Case Study: Critical Thinking

1. Because both renal function and hepatic function are important in drug metabolism and excretion, and both decrease with aging, the nurse would anticipate that measurement of liver enzymes, BUN, creatinine, and creatinine clearance would be ordered. Because this patient also has diabetes, the patient's blood glucose level would be evaluated.

2. There are a variety of sleep aids besides triazolam that could be utilized. Because the patient is also taking a diuretic, it would be important to suggest taking the diuretic in the morning to prevent frequent awakenings during the night to go to the bathroom. Some nonpharmacologic measures include taking warm baths, decreasing stimulation in the evening, and eliminating caffeine intake late in the day. The patient also likes chamomile tea, which may help induce sleep. A light bedtime snack will help maintain blood sugar levels throughout the night.

3. The nurse should recognize and support the patient's desire to adhere with the drug regimen; however, the patient does need further education about "doubling up" on drugs. A variety of methods can be used to help the patient remember to take the prescribed drug. These can include using commercial pill dispensers, making a list, keeping a calendar, or setting an alarm.

CHAPTER 8: DRUGS IN SUBSTANCE USE DISORDER

1. b
2. c
3. a
4. dopamine, neurotransmitters
5. reward circuit
6. epigenetics
7. inhibits
8. methadone or buprenorphine, or naltrexone
9. GHB (gamma-hydroxybutyrate)
10. euphoria, tranquility, blocks
11. CAGE
12. personality, behavior, job performance and job attendance
13. False. Electronic cigarettes are *not* safer than tobacco products.
14. False. DHEA is found in many dietary supplements, and there is *no* evidence that DHEA slows aging, increases energy levels, or increases muscle strength.
15. True
16. b
17. a
18. d
19. c
20. a. Cocaine can cause dilated pupils (not pinpoint pupils) and restlessness. It can also cause hypertension (not hypotension), tachycardia, insomnia, erratic behaviors (not fine tremors), and tachypnea (not respiratory depression).
21. c. Methadone is a long-acting opioid that is effective in treating persons addicted to opioids by blocking the sensation of euphoria and tranquility produced by opioids, and it prevents opioid withdrawal and craving. Dronabinol is a synthetic cannabis, lorazepam is a benzodiazepine to decrease anxiety, and naloxone is a reversal agent for opioid-induced respiratory depression.
22. a, c, e. A patient must be ready and motivated to quit any addictive substance or the likelihood of success is decreased. This is a difficult process that will require the patient's commitment. Certain triggers, like places where a person smokes or times that trigger the craving for a cigarette, should be identified and alternatives determined. There are a variety of aids, both pharmacologic and nonpharmacologic, that can be utilized to help quit smoking. Ideally, a quit date of 1–2 weeks should be set so the patient stays motivated. Tobacco in any form is still addictive, so chewing tobacco or smoking tobacco in a pipe instead of a cigarette is still abusing tobacco. Although it is difficult, some patients prefer to quit smoking "cold turkey" or without the use of aids.
23. d. It is estimated that 1 in 10 nurses have a substance use disorder, including benzodiazepines, fentanyl, hydrocodone, and alcohol.

24. d. Intranasal naloxone is available as a kit that lay-people can purchase to reverse symptoms of opioid overdose, such as fentanyl, to reduce mortality related to opioid overdose. In addition to administering intranasal naloxone, the family member should provide rescue breathing, if needed, while waiting for the drug to take effect (usually 2–3 minutes after administration). 911 should be called prior to administering the intranasal naloxone. Flumazenil is an antidote for benzodiazepine overdose.

Case Study: Critical Thinking

1. Even though the patient appears to be intoxicated, other causes of unresponsiveness need to be evaluated. There is no antidote for alcohol intoxication other than supportive care. The patient's respiratory rate and saturation are insufficient, and patient's respirations must be assisted. Treatment should be aimed toward airway management and supplemental oxygenation, supportive care, and IV hydration.
2. A person with alcohol toxicity can aspirate on vomitus and asphyxiate. They can also develop severe dehydration, seizures, hypothermia, and eventually brain damage and death.
3. Disulfiram inhibits aldehyde dehydrogenase, the enzyme needed to metabolize alcohol. Disulfiram keeps patients from ingesting alcohol because of its severe unwanted side effects. It is slowly metabolized by the liver. The side effects can occur up to 2 weeks after cessation of drug therapy. Side effects can occur within 10 minutes of ingesting alcohol (including mouthwash, cough medicine, or foods containing or cooked in alcohol). Side effects include severe nausea, headache, vomiting, chest pains, dyspnea (difficulty breathing), rash, drowsiness, impotence, acne, and a metallic aftertaste.
4. Metronidazole, an antimicrobial, and paraldehyde, a sedative, when taken concomitantly with disulfiram can produce the same side effects as if the person had been ingesting alcohol.

CHAPTER 9: SAFETY AND QUALITY

1. Safety
2. Patient-family-centered care
3. Collaboration and teamwork
4. Quality improvement
5. Informatics
6. Evidence-based care
7. c
8. f
9. j
10. g
11. a
12. h
13. b
14. d
15. e
16. i
17. a
18. a
19. b
20. a
21. b
22. a
23. a. intradermal, yes; b. morphine sulfate or multiple sclerosis, no; c. every other day, no; d, drops, yes; e. kilograms, yes; f. 1 mg, no; whole numbers should not contain trailing zeros; g. milligram, yes; h. daily, no; i. keep vein open, yes; j. intravenous piggyback, yes; k. each ear, yes; while it is legal to use, it is an error-prone abbreviation. Instead, OU should be spelled out; l. discharge or discontinue, yes; while it is legal to use, it is an error-prone abbreviation. Instead, D/C should be spelled out; m. twice daily, yes
24.

Abbreviation	Meaning
CR	controlled release
ER	extended release
IR	immediate release
XR	extended release
XT	extended time

25. c. Antibiotics must be taken at regularly spaced intervals to maintain therapeutic blood levels. All antibiotics should be completed even if the patient feels better. The dosage of antibiotics should not be increased, even if the patient does not feel better.
26. b. ac is before meals and hs is at bedtime. However, it is best to not use these abbreviations.
27. c. "Tall man" letters promote safety between drugs with similar names by calling attention to differences in spelling, such as quiNIDine and quiNINE.
28. c. A nurse must never administer a dose that seems an abnormal amount without rechecking the calculations. If there continues to be a question, another nurse should double-check the dose as well.
29. a. The nurse's first action is to document the refusal immediately. It is important to remember that the refusal to take a medication is the patient's right. The nurse should investigate the patient's reasoning behind refusing to take a medication and stress the importance of the medication regimen. The healthcare provider should be notified of the refusal.
30. b, c, d, e. The "Do Not Use List" of abbreviations include q.d., U, IU, and MS. q.d. should be written as "daily"; U is to be written as "unit"; and IU as "International Unit." MS can be confused for morphine sulfate or magnesium sulfate; instead, write out the drugs. IM is an appropriate abbreviation to use.
31. d. Unused drugs should not be disposed in a manner that is connected to the sewage. Instead, it is best to

dispose of them by taking the drug to a facility that has a "take-back" program. If this is not available, then drugs should be mixed whole in an unpalatable nonfood substance, such as kitty litter or dirt prior to placing them in the regular trash. It should not be crushed prior to mixing it.

Case Study: Critical Thinking

1. The "six rights" are (1) the right patient, (2) the right drug, (3) the right dose, (4) the right route, (5) the right time, and (6) right documentation. Other "rights" include the expiration date and right education.

2. Ask the patient to state their full name and date of birth and compare these with the patient's identification (ID) band and the medication administration record (MAR).

   Many facilities have electronic health records (EHRs) that allow the nurse to directly scan the bar code from the patient's ID band. Once the band is scanned, the nurse can see the patient's medication record.

   If the patient is an adult with a cognitive disorder or a child, verify the patient's name with a family member. In the event a family member is unavailable and the patient is unable to self-identify, follow the facility's policy. Many facilities have policies that include a photo ID on the band with the patient's name and date of birth affixed to the band.

   Distinguish between two patients with the same first or last name by placing "name-alert" stickers as warnings on the medical records.

3. The nurse would check the drug with the medication administration record and physician's order to ensure they are the correct drugs. If the drugs are dispensed in a unit dose method, the drugs should be taken out of their package at the patient's bedside. Show the package to the patient. Many facilities dispense drugs using unit dose method rather than multidose to reduce drug errors.

CHAPTER 10: DRUG ADMINISTRATION

1. Enteric-coated; timed-release. Other formulations include controlled release, extended release, and immediate release.
2. fine particle
3. semi-Fowler's or high Fowler's; these are the preferred positions, but the nurse would provide patient-centered care and determine if the patient should be placed in either of these two positions.
4. 0
5. 30
6. c
7. a
8. b
9. ventrogluteal
10. vastus lateralis

11. deltoid
12. ventrogluteal
13.

a Tubercle of iliac crest

◆ Injection site
● Landmarks

Gluteus b
maximus
muscle

c Greater trochanter of femur

14. c. The oral route is contraindicated in a patient who is vomiting. Parenteral (IM or IV) or topical routes are preferred.

15. a. In children younger than 3 years old, straighten the external ear canal by pulling the auricle down and back. In older children and adults, straighten the canal by pulling the auricle upward and outward.

16. d. The ventrogluteal muscle is the preferred site for many IM injections because it is a deep muscle, situated away from major nerves and blood vessels.

17. c. Vastus lateralis is the preferred site because of easy access; however, ventrogluteal can also be used. Dorsogluteal muscle is no longer used because of the proximity of the sciatica nerve. Deltoid muscle is not developed in infants.

18. a. Over-the-counter drugs and herbal preparations may interact with prescription drugs. Patients must be encouraged to discuss the use of these preparations with their pharmacist or healthcare provider.

19. a, b, e. Nurses have the responsibility of teaching patients about their drugs. Verbal and written instructions include expected therapeutic effects, side effects, and dietary considerations. Other aspects of teaching include possible adverse drug effects, possible laboratory tests that may be required, and ensuring continuous supply of the drug, among others. c is incorrect because not all drugs are stored in the refrigerator. d is incorrect because patients do not need to know how the drug was tested and developed.

20. b. The patient should rinse out the mouth after administering a dose from a metered-dose inhaler. This will help prevent secondary infection and irritation that can be caused by medications. a is incorrect because the MDI must be used as prescribed. Overuse can increase side effects and tolerance can result. c is incorrect because the mouth is closed around the MDI with the opening toward the back of the throat so that the drug can be inhaled or it can be positioned 1–2 inches from the mouth if a spacer is not used. d is incorrect; subsequent doses should be spaced 1–2 minutes apart.

Case Study: Critical Thinking

1. 20-25 gauge needle that is 5/8–1½ inches long and 1–3 mL syringe. The size of the syringe depends on the mL (volume) drawn for the correct dose. The gauge and length of the needle are determined by the site and patient's age, weight, amount of adipose tissue, and muscle size.

2. The potential sites for IM injections include deltoid, ventrogluteal, or the vastus lateralis. The preferred site for anyone at any age is the ventrogluteal. Ventrogluteal muscle is a deep muscle that is away from major nerves and blood vessels. The deltoid is easier to access, but not all patients have developed deltoids. Deltoids are reserved for small volume of drug. Vastus lateralis would be appropriate, but it is usually hard to access.

3. Promethazine is irritating to tissue. It should be given deep IM. The best method would be to use the Z-track. The ventrogluteal is the preferred site for Z-track IM administration. Z-track seals the drug in the muscle and prevents leakage of the drug minimizing local skin irritation.

CHAPTER 11: DRUG LABELS AND DOSAGE CALCULATIONS

Metric and Household Systems

1. b
2. f
3. g
4. c
5. i
6. j
7. o
8. e
9. n
10. m
11. d
12. l
13. a
14. k
15. h
16. A. 1000 mg; B. 1000 mL; C. 1000 mcg
17. 3000 mg
18. 1500 mL
19. 100 mg
20. 2.5 L; notice the trailing zero is not included. For any digits right of a decimal point, do not include a trailing zero.
21. 0.25 L
22. 0.5 g
23. 4 pt
24. 32 fl oz
25. 48 fl oz
26. 2 pt
27. 3 mg
28. 15 mL
29. 1 fl oz
30. 3 tsp
31. 1000 mg
32. 0.5 g
33. 100 mg
34. 1 L; 1 qt
35. 8 fl oz
36. 1 fl oz; 2 T; 6 t
37. 1 t
38. 1.5 fl oz; 9 t
39. 150 mL; 10 T

Drug Calculations for Enteral and Parenteral Drugs

1. d. When calculating drug dosages, it is most helpful to convert to the system used on the drug label.

2. b, c, d, e. Parenteral routes are any routes that do not involve the gastrointestinal (GI) system; medications applied topically; and medications for ears, eyes, and nose. These routes generally bypass the first-pass effect by the hepatic system. Parenteral routes include subcutaneous, intramuscular, intradermal, and intravenous.

3. c, d. All insulins and heparinized products can be given subcutaneously. Regular insulin and fractionated heparin can be given intravenously.

4. self-sealing rubber tops; reusable if properly stored

5. a, b. Once a drug in a multidose vial has been reconstituted, the nurse would label the vial with the date and time the drug was reconstituted or when to discard the vial and their initials. The type of diluent is not needed on the label.

6. c. The body's habitus must be considered when administering IM injection. On an average adult, 19, 20, or 21 gauges with 1, 1½, or 2 inches in length are appropriate.

7. b. The needle, plunger, and inside of the barrel should remain sterile when administering medications via parenteral routes.

8. b. Subcutaneous injections can be administered at 45-, 60-, or 90-degree angles, depending on the person's body habitus.

9. c. Because the volume to be administered is less than 1 mL, a tuberculin (TB) syringe is most appropriate. A TB syringe is a 1-mL syringe. An insulin syringe is measured in units and not in mL. The 3-mL and 5-mL syringes can be used; however, the amount drawn into these syringes will be less accurate than a 1-mL syringe.

10. d. A 5-mL syringe is most appropriate to measure 3 mL of saline solution to mix the powdered drug. The solution of saline and drug will be more than 3 mL; therefore a 3-mL syringe would be too small.

11. c. Since the drugs are compatible, use one syringe to draw up the correct amount of volume from each drug and attach the syringe to a syringe pump for infusion. Total volume is 13 mL; one 20-mL syringe will suffice.

Interpreting Drug Labels

12. A. Viread;
B. a generic name is not available;
C. 300 mg/tab;
D. tab

13. A. hydrocodone bitartrate and acetaminophen;
    B. 5 mg/300 mg per tab;
    C. yes; it is a schedule II drug
    D.

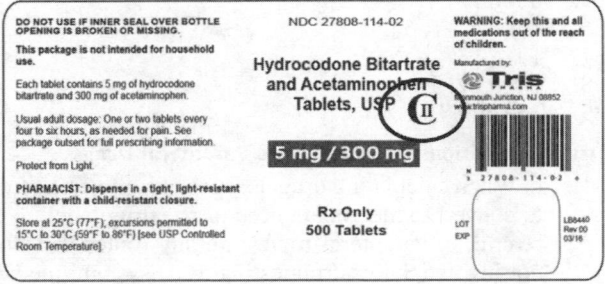

    E. Tab;
    F. controlled room temperature between 59°F and 86°F;
    G. Tris Pharma
14.
    A. phenytoin sodium;
    B. no;
    C. cap;
    D. 100 mg;
    E.

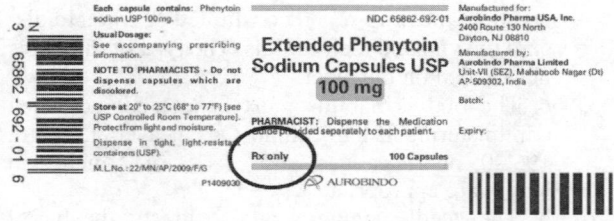

    F. in its original container at controlled room temperature and protect from light and moisture
15. A. dextromethorphan polistirex;
    B. Robitussin;
    C. no;
    D. liquid;
    E. 30 mg/5 mL;
    F. 89 mL;
    G. 10 mL q12h;
    H. approximately nine doses
16. A. influenza A (H1N1)
    B. liquid;
    C. multidose;
    D. in an environment that is 35°F–46°F;
    E. IM
17. A. interferon gamma-1b;
    B. Actimmune;
    C. refrigerated
18. A. d;
    B. d; solution in DA:

    C. $x\ tab = \dfrac{1\ tab}{100\ \cancel{mg}} \times \dfrac{1000\ \cancel{mg}}{1\ \cancel{g}} \times \dfrac{0.5\ \cancel{g}}{X}$
    $= 5\ tab$

19. A. a; B. b

20. A. d; B. b; solution:

    $x\ mL = \dfrac{5\ mL}{12.5\ mg} \times \dfrac{25\ mg}{x} = 10\ mL$

21. d
22. A. b; concentration is 350 mg/mL after reconstitution. The amount 1 g does not need to be factored into the equation since the resulting concentration is given in mg.
    B. 3-mL syringe
23. b
24. A. losartan potassium;
    B. Cozaar;
    C. 30 tab;
    D. b
25. A. a; since both tab are scored, then 10 mg can be divided into ½ tab for the ordered dose;
    B. b
26. A. furosemide;
    B. Lasix;
    C. room temperature;
    D. c
27. A. Extended-release tablet; oral liquid is not extended release, and the bioavailability will be decreased.
    B. c; The nurse cannot switch the formulation of a drug without an order from a prescriber.
    C. a; liquid solution; drugs in ER cannot be crushed; liquid solution can be given via NGT; b. 7.5 mL.
28. A. a; B. a
29. A. 1 tab; B. 2 tab
30. A. 5.7 mL; B. d
31. A. subcut;
    B. 40 mg/0.8 mL;
    C. 0.8 mL;
    D. a, c; tuberculin syringe is a 1-mL syringe. Insulin syringe is measured in units. Less accurate dosing can occur with a 3-mL syringe.
32. A. c; B. c
33. A. a and b or just a or just b;
    B. 1 tab from 2.5 mg and 5 mg; 3 tab from 2.5 mg; or 1.5 tab from the 5-mg tab.
34. A. d. This lithium level is too high, and adjustments need to be made. Withhold the dose and contact the healthcare provider.
35. A. b; B. a
36. xx
    A.

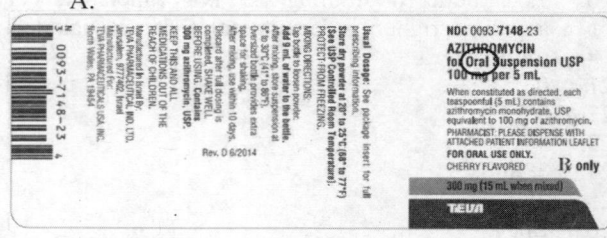

    B. d;
    C. d
37. b

38. d
39. c
40. c. The nurse would acknowledge the patient's concerns and provide an appropriate answer. The first two responses negate the patient's concerns, while the last response is incorrect.
41. a
42. d
43. A. No, Duramorph is morphine and is much weaker in strength than hydromorphone;
    B. d
44. d
45. c
46.

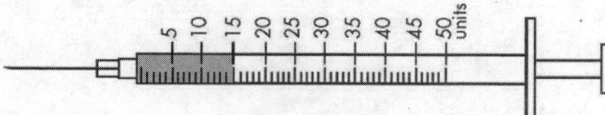

47. A. Topamax;
    B. topiramate;
    C. sprinkle capsules;
    D. 1 cap/dose

Drug Calculations Using Body Weight

48. A. b; *solution:*

$$\frac{25,000 - 90,000 \text{ units}}{\cancel{kg}} \times \frac{1 \ \cancel{kg}}{2.2 \ \cancel{lb}} \times \frac{46 \ \cancel{lb}}{4}$$

$$= 130,682 \text{ units} - 470,455 \text{ units};$$

child's dose is 200,000 units which is between this range.

B. d; *solution*:

$$mL = \frac{5 \text{ mL}}{400,000 \ \cancel{units}} \times \frac{200,000 \ \cancel{units}}{x}$$

$$= \frac{1000 \text{ mL}}{400} = 2.5 \text{ mL}$$

49. A. b, *solution*:

$$min = \frac{10 \text{ mg}}{1 \ \cancel{kg}} \times \frac{1 \ \cancel{kg}}{2.2 \ \cancel{lbs}} \times \frac{75 \ \cancel{lbs}}{24 \ \cancel{h}} \times 12 \ \cancel{h} = 170 \text{ mg};$$

$$max = \frac{15 \text{ mg}}{1 \ \cancel{kg}} \times \frac{1 \ \cancel{kg}}{2.2 \ \cancel{lbs}} \times \frac{75 \ \cancel{lbs}}{24 \ \cancel{h}} \times 12 \ \cancel{h} = 256 \text{ mg};$$

the dose of 200 mg is between the recommended dose; the question is asking if 200 mg is appropriate; therefore do not include the ordered dose of 200 mg into the equation.

B. d

50. A. a; the dose is too low; child should receive 133–150 mg/dose;
    B. a; 225 mg/d
51. c
52. A. 2.1 mL;
    B. 350 mg/mL;

C. b; *solution:*

$$mL = \frac{1 \text{ mL}}{350 \ \cancel{mg}} \times \frac{50 \ \cancel{mg}}{\cancel{kg}} \times 8 \ \cancel{kg} = 1.1 \text{ mL}$$

53. A. b; no, the dose is too low; B. d
54. A. $\dfrac{(20 \text{ mg}/1 \ \cancel{kg} \times 1 \ \cancel{kg}/2.2 \ \cancel{lb} \times 22 \ \cancel{lb})}{3 \text{ doses}}$

    $= 66.7 \text{ mg and}$

    $\dfrac{(50 \text{ mg}/1 \ \cancel{kg} \times 1 \ \cancel{kg}/2.2 \ \cancel{lb} \times 22 \ \cancel{lb})}{3 \text{ doses}}$

    $= 133.3 \text{ mg};$

    B. Yes, the dose ordered is between the minimum and maximum dosage range;
    C. b
55. A. b;
    B. b;
    C. a
56. A. 11.4 kg;
    B. 114–171 mg; range provided by using weight 11 kg (after rounding)
    Solution using dimensional analysis:

$$X \text{ mg} = \frac{10\text{-}15 \text{ mg}}{1 \ \cancel{kg}} \times \frac{1 \ \cancel{kg}}{2.2 \ \cancel{lbs}} \times \frac{25 \ \cancel{lbs}}{?}$$

$$= 113.6 - 170.5 \text{ mg} = 114 - 171 \text{ mg per rounding rule}$$

Notice with dimensional analysis, all conversion factors were included in the equation. Only the final answer had to be rounded.

C. Yes, it is within the recommended dose.

57. 523 mg; *solution:*

$$mg = \frac{50 \text{ mg}}{1 \ \cancel{kg}} \times \frac{1 \ \cancel{kg}}{2.2 \ \cancel{lb}} \times 23 \ \cancel{lb}$$

$$= 523 \text{ mg per rounding rule}$$

58. A. 2954.5 mg; *solution:*

$$mg = \frac{100 \text{ mg}}{1 \ \cancel{kg}} \times \frac{1 \ \cancel{kg}}{2.2 \ \cancel{lb}} \times 65 \ \cancel{lb} = 2955 \text{ mg}$$

B. 1477 mg; *solution:*

$$mg = \frac{2955 \text{ mg}}{2 \text{ doses}}$$

Drug Calculations Using Body Surface Area

59. All answers are approximates.
    A. 0.17–0.18 m²;
    B. 0.52 m²;
    C. 0.9–0.95 m²
60. All answers are approximates.
    A. 0.88 m²;
    B. 0.9 m²;
    C. 0.56 m²
61. A. 0.51 m²; *solution:*

$$\sqrt{\frac{25 \times 32}{3131}} = \sqrt{0.256} = 0.51 \text{ m}^2$$

B. 0.66 m²; *solution:*

$$\sqrt{\frac{58 \times 48}{3131}} = 0.94 \text{ m}^2$$

C. 0.66 m²

$$\sqrt{\frac{40 \times 34}{3131}} = 0.66 \text{ m}^2$$

62. A. 0.25 m²; *solution:*

$$\sqrt{\frac{8 \times 28.2}{3600}} = 0.25 \text{ m}^2$$

B. 1.02 m²; *solution*:

$$\sqrt{\frac{28.1 \times 133.4}{3600}} = 1.02 \text{ m}^2$$

C. 0.77 m²; *solution*:

$$\sqrt{\frac{85.5 \times 25}{3600}} = 0.77 \text{ m}^2$$

63. A. 1.06 m²;
B. 1.01 m²; *solution*:

$$\sqrt{\frac{80 \times 40}{3131}} = 1.01 \text{ m}^2$$

C. 101 mg; *solution*: 100 mg × 1.01 m² = 101 mg; note there is a 4-mg difference between the West Nomogram and square root method. The square root method is more precise.

64. A. 1.10 m²; B. 55 mg
65. A. 0.85 m²; B. 30 mg
66. A. 1.31 m²; B. 300 mg; *solution*:

$$\frac{500 \text{ mg}}{1.73 \text{ m}^2} \times \sqrt{\frac{100 \times 54}{3131}} = 379.5589 = 380 \text{ mg}$$

Note: the answer differs if using child's approximate BSA of 1.31 m²; the answer would be 378.612 = 379 mg.

67. A. 1.17 m²; B. 237 mg; *solution*: per dimensional analysis:

$$\frac{350 \text{ mg}}{1.73 \text{ m}^2} \times \sqrt{\frac{71 \times 60}{3131}} = 235.985 = 236 \text{ mg}$$

Note: the answer differs if using child's approximate BSA of 1.17m²; the answer would be 236.705 = 237 mg.

68. A. 1.46 m²; B. 5 mg
69. A. 0.78 m²; B. 273 mg
70. A. 1.45 m²; B. 247 mg

Drug Calculations for Drugs Requiring Reconstitution

71. A. 5.4 mL; 250 mg/1.5 mL; B. c
72. A. 3.4 mL; 250 mg/mL; B. b
73. b
74. c
75. d

Drug Calculations for Intravenous Drugs and Fluids

76. c; the question was asking for dosage for infusion. mL/h would be *flow rate* for infusion. gtt/min is the *flow rate* when calculating the rate for infusion using gravity and the *drop factor* is known. Dosage and flow rate are not synonymous.

77. d. Any method of dosage calculation can be used; however, dimensional analysis is the best method when conversion factors are needed. Rounding is conducted at the end.

78. d
79. a; gtt/min is the flow rate, whereas gtt/mL is the drop factor that is needed to determine the flow rate. The drop factor can be found on the IV tubing packaging.

80. c
81. a
82. b
83. d
84. 10–20 gtt/mL; 60 gtt/mL
85. keep vein open; 250-mL IV bag
86. calibrated cylinder with tubing
87. volumetric
88. uniform concentration of the drug, patient control and ownership of the pain
89. 28 gtt/min; solution:

$$\frac{\text{gtt}}{\text{min}} = \frac{10 \text{ gtt}}{1 \text{ mL}} \times \frac{1000 \text{ mL}}{6 \text{ h}} \times \frac{1 \text{ h}}{60 \text{ min}} = 28 \text{ gtt / min}$$

90. 31 gtt/min
91. 50 gtt/min; *solution:*

$$\frac{\text{gtt}}{\text{min}} = \frac{15 \text{ gtt}}{1 \text{ mL}} \times \frac{100 \text{ mL}}{30 \text{ min}} = \frac{50 \text{ gtt}}{\text{min}}$$

92. A. 1000 mL;
B. 2500 mL;
C. 104.2 mL/h; *solution:*

$$\frac{\text{mL}}{\text{h}} = \frac{2500 \text{ mL}}{24\text{h}} = 104.2 \text{ mL/h}$$

93. A. e;
B. 28 gtt/min; *solution:*

$$\frac{\text{gtt}}{\text{min}} = \frac{10 \text{ gtt}}{1 \text{ mL}} \times \frac{500 \text{ mL}}{3 \text{ h}} \times \frac{1 \text{ h}}{60 \text{ min}} = \frac{28 \text{ gtt}}{\text{min}}$$

94. A. c;
B. d
95. d; partial drops cannot be administered; therefore round 12.5 gtt/min up to 13 gtt/min.
96. A. 3.4 mL;
B. 250 mg/mL;
C. b
97. 25 gtt/min; see problem 18B for example solution.
98. 67 gtt/min
99. A. 614 mcg;
B. 307 mcg;
C. 127.5 mL/h; flow rate is based on 255 mL = 250 mL fluid + 5 mL of drug.

D. 42 gtt/min; *solution:*

$$\frac{127.5 \text{ mL}}{1 \text{ h}} \times \frac{1 \text{ h}}{60 \text{ min}} \times 20 \text{ min} = 42.5 \text{ mL infused};$$

therefore,

$$\frac{20 \text{ gtt}}{\text{mL}} \times \frac{255\text{-}42.5 \text{ mL}}{100 \text{ min}} = \frac{43 \text{ gtt}}{\text{min}} \text{ per rounding rule}$$

100. 200 mL/h
101. A. 1.6 mL;
    B. 203.2 mL/h; add 1.6 mL of diluent to the total fluid amount to equal 101.6 mL.
102. 84.2 mL/h
103. 100 gtt/min
104. 50 gtt/min
105. A. 1250 units/h; *solution*

$$\frac{\text{units}}{\text{h}} = \frac{30000 \text{ units}}{1 \text{ day}} \times \frac{1 \text{ day}}{24 \text{ h}} = 1250 \text{ units / h}$$

    B. 25 mL/h; *solution:*

$$\frac{\text{mL}}{\text{h}} = \frac{250 \text{ mL}}{12500 \text{ units}} \times \frac{1250 \text{ units}}{\text{h}}$$

106. A. 81.8 kg;
    B. 6544 units;
    C. 14.7 mL/h; *solution:*

$$\frac{\text{mL}}{\text{h}} = \frac{250 \text{ mL}}{25000 \text{ units}} \times \frac{18 \text{ units}}{1 \text{ kg}} \times \frac{81.8 \text{ kg}}{\text{h}}$$

$$= 14.7 \text{ mL / h}$$

107. A. 10.1 mL/h; *solution:*

$$\frac{\text{mL}}{\text{h}} = \frac{1 \text{ mL}}{100 \text{ unit}} \times \frac{18 \text{ unit}}{1 \text{ kg}} \times \frac{1 \text{ kg}}{2.2 \text{ lb}} \times \frac{123 \text{ lb}}{\text{h}}$$

$$= 10.1 \text{ mL / h}$$

    B. 2236.4 units; 11.2 mL/h
108. A. 11.3 mL/h;
    B. 2520 units; 12.6 mL/h
109. A. 25.2 mL/h;
    B. 21 mL/h
110. A. 39 mg; *solution:* $(0.25 \text{ mg} \times 65 \text{ kg}) + (0.35 \text{ mg} \times 65 \text{ kg}) = 39 \text{ mg}$
    B. 10 mL/h
111. 7.6 mL/h (NOTE: Both mcg and mg measurements are provided. Use the mcg measurement when calculating dosage.); *solution:*

$$\frac{\text{mL}}{\text{h}} = \frac{1 \text{ mL}}{1000 \text{ meg}} \times \frac{2 \text{ meg}}{1 \text{ kg}} \times \frac{63 \text{ kg}}{1 \text{ min}}$$

$$\times \frac{60 \text{ min}}{1 \text{ h}} = 7.6 \text{ mL / h}$$

112. A. 23.4 mL/h (NOTE: Both mcg and mg measurements are provided. Use the mcg measurement when calculating dosage.)
    B. 32.8 mL/h
113. 16.7 mL/h (NOTE: No conversion factors are needed.)
114. 75 mL/h
115. 33 mL/h

116. 10.4 mL/h; *solution:*

$$\frac{\text{mL}}{\text{h}} = \frac{250 \text{ mL}}{500 \text{ mg}} \times \frac{1 \text{ mg}}{1000 \text{ meg}} \times \frac{5 \text{ meg}}{1 \text{ kg}} \times \frac{1 \text{ kg}}{2.2 \text{ lb}}$$

$$\times \frac{152 \text{ lb}}{1 \text{ min}} \times \frac{60 \text{ min}}{\text{h}} = 10.4 \text{ mL / h}$$

117. 14.3 mL/h
118. 11.1 mL/h
119. 11.3 mL/h
120. 8 mL/h
121. A. 4 mg/min; *solution:*

$$\frac{\text{mg}}{\text{min}} = \frac{1000 \text{ mg}}{1 \text{ g}} \times \frac{2 \text{ g}}{250 \text{ mL}} \times \frac{30 \text{ mL}}{1 \text{ h}} \times \frac{1 \text{ h}}{60 \text{ min}}$$

$$= \frac{4 \text{ mg}}{\text{min}}$$

    B. 30 mL/h. (NOTE: The flow rate is already provided in the question.)
122. A. 3 mcg/kg/min per rounding rule; *solution:*

$$\frac{\text{mcg}}{\text{kg / min}} = \frac{1000 \text{ mcg}}{1 \text{ mg}} \times \frac{100 \text{ mg}}{250 \text{ mL}} \times \frac{29 \text{ mL}}{1 \text{ h}}$$

$$\times \frac{1 \text{ h}}{60 \text{ min}} \times \frac{2.2 \text{ lb}}{1 \text{ kg}} \times \frac{1}{143 \text{ lb}}$$

    B. 29 mL/h

CHAPTER 12: FLUID VOLUME AND ELECTROLYTES

1. d
2. f
3. b
4. e
5. a
6. c
7. b
8. a
9. c
10. d
11. a. Oral potassium supplements can be irritating to the stomach and should be taken with at least 8 oz of fluid and/or with a meal. The patient is correct in that the tablet should not be chewed.
12. d. IV potassium must be given using a rate-controlling device and cannot be allowed to run freely. In many hospitals the nurse does not prepare this medication, and it is either mixed in the pharmacy or comes prepackaged from the manufacturer. IV potassium is never given as a bolus (IVP).
13. d. Potassium is very irritating to the vein. If the site has become reddened and swollen, the IV should be discontinued immediately and another IV site should be started. The rest of the potassium is then infused. If another peripheral IV access is not possible, the healthcare provider should be contacted for possible central venous access.
14. b, c. Hyperkalemia can cause cardiac dysrhythmia, such as tachycardia. Other clinical manifestations

of hyperkalemia include paresthesia to the face, tongue, and extremities; gastrointestinal hyperactivity (nausea, vomiting, and abdominal cramps), and acidosis may be present. Patient with hyperkalemia will most likely have hyperglycemia, not hypoglycemia.

15. d. Administering sodium bicarbonate intravenously (IV) (50 mEq/L) as a one-time dose may help temporarily by driving potassium back into the cell. A patient with hyperkalemia will most likely have hypermagnesemia. Saline will not help move the potassium back into the cell. $D_{10}W$ is high in glucose, and glucose pulls the potassium out of the cell which will worsen hyperkalemia.

16. a, b, d, e. A patient who is taking a potassium supplement orally should be taught the signs and symptoms of both hypo- and hyperkalemia and when to notify the healthcare provider. Since there is a narrow range for potassium level, the patient should anticipate routine blood work to evaluate if the potassium level is in the expected range. Because potassium is irritating, the supplement should be taken with a meal or a full glass of liquid and the patient should remain upright for a minimum of 30 minutes to prevent esophagitis.

17. b. Normal serum osmolality (isoosmolar) is 275–295 mOsm/kg. Levels below 275 mOsm/kg are considered hypoosmolar. Levels greater than 295 mOsm/kg are considered hyperosmolar.

18. c. 285 mOsm/kg is normal (isoosmolar). Levels below 275 mOsm/kg are considered hypoosmolar. Levels greater than 295 mOsm/kg are considered hyperosmolar. Patient has normal serum osmolality, not in a dehydrated state.

19. b. 3% saline is considered to be a hypertonic solution. Any solution that is greater than 0.9% sodium chloride is considered hypertonic. Hypotonic fluid has less than 0.9% saline, such as 0.45% sodium chloride.

20. b. Around 80%–90% of potassium is excreted in the urine. 8% is excreted in feces.

21. a, c. A patient with pancreatitis will most likely have hypocalcemia due to calcium shifting into cells and hypomagnesemia.

22. b. Vitamin D helps the absorption of calcium from the small intestine, primarily in the ileum. Products in the large intestine are waste. Kidneys do help with resorbing calcium, but not with the help of vitamin D. Liver does not absorb calcium.

23. b. Most of the calcium is located in bones and teeth. Of the remaining calcium, 50% is bound to protein. The other 50% is circulating free (ionized calcium) to assist with cellular functions.

24. b. D_5W and $D_51/2NS$ are considered crystalloids. Crystalloids help maintain and/or temporarily correct hydration; they cause early plasma expansion. They do not contain proteins. Colloids contain protein, lipids, and/or carbohydrates and are given to increase serum osmolality; they are also called plasma expanders. Examples of colloids are albumin and dextran. Lipids are fats and are considered colloids. Parenteral nutrition (PN) is intravenous nutrition containing protein, fats, and many minerals and electrolytes. PN is considered colloids.

25. b. $D_51/2NS$ a is hypertonic solution. But, once it is in the body, it becomes hypotonic since the body metabolizes the glucose rather quickly, leaving free water and 0.45% saline.

26. a. Dextran is a colloid (volume expander) made from glucose. It is given to persons with major burns to temporarily restore circulating volume. No other drugs, including blood, should be infused in the same line as dextran.

27. a. Plasma has similar electrolyte content as lactated ringers.

28. c, d, e. This patient is hypokalemic. Early signs of hypokalemia usually do not occur until serum K^+ level falls below 3 mEq/L and may include muscle weakness, anorexia, nausea, and vomiting. Untreated hypokalemia can lead to cardiac arrest and death.

29. a. Decreased magnesium (hypomagnesemia) is associated with hypocalcemia. Other electrolyte imbalance associated with low magnesium is hypokalemia.

30. a. A potassium level of 3.2 mEq/L is considered hypokalemia and may require a supplement. Potassium supplements are taken over an extended period and not just a few days. Hypokalemia is rarely caused by inadequate intake. This response is also accusatory and is not therapeutic. Gastrointestinal (GI) losses attributable to vomiting and diarrhea may lead to hypokalemia; constipation will not.

31. c. A sodium level of 150 mEq/L is considered hypernatremia. The normal range for serum sodium is 125–135 mEq/L. All other electrolytes are in normal range.

32. a, d, e. Gastrointestinal (GI) disturbances, such as abdominal cramps; paresthesia of the face, hands, and feet; and arrhythmias are commonly seen with hyperkalemia.

33. c, d, e. Insulin moves the potassium back into the cells while exogenous glucose maintains serum glucose level. Sodium polystyrene sulfonate binds with potassium, then it is excreted in feces while sorbitol maintains serum glucose level. Sodium bicarbonate shifts potassium intracellularly, while calcium gluconate decreases myocardial irritability.

34. a, b, e. Serum calcium level of 7.2 mg/dL is low; therefore the patient has hypocalcemia. Clinical manifestations of hypocalcemia include anxiety, irritability, tetany, seizures, hyperactive deep tendon reflexes, and carpopedal spasms.

Case Study: Critical Thinking

1. The patient is in hemorrhagic shock from massive blood loss as indicated by the vital signs. Stab wounds to the chest and abdomen can penetrate

vital organs, causing large blood loss and risk of death. The priority assessment for this patient is homeostasis, which includes circulation and airway. Circulation and airway are always a priority. During a systematic assessment of the patient, two large-bore IVs (14 or 16 gauge) should be established in large veins to replace fluids rapidly. Another option is to assist the healthcare provider in placing a central line for rapid fluid resuscitation with colloids and crystalloids.

2. The patient needs to be resuscitated with blood and blood products (colloids) and crystalloids.

3. Whole blood may be more beneficial for this patient because it contains all the components (plasma, platelets, and RBCs); however, uncrossmatched packed red blood cells (PRBCs) may be easier to obtain in the emergent setting of trauma. Volume can be expanded using volume expanders.

CHAPTER 13: VITAMIN AND MINERAL REPLACEMENT

1. a
2. b
3. b
4. a
5. a
6. a
7. a
8. a
9. b
10. b
11. a
12. d
13. c
14. e
15. a
16. b
17.

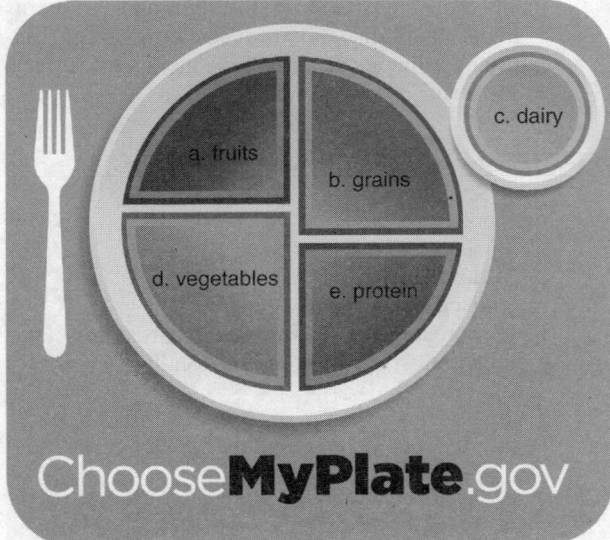

18. d. Vitamin D is needed to regulate calcium and phosphorous. It is also necessary for calcium absorption from the small intestines. Vitamin A is essential for bone growth and maintenance of epithelial cells. Vitamin B_{12} is essential for DNA synthesis, conversion of folic acid to its active form, and maintenance of the integrity of the nervous system, among others. Vitamin C is absorbed in the small intestine and aids in the absorption of iron and conversion of folic acid.

19. c. Vitamin K is needed to help the blood to clot. Newborns are vitamin K deficient at birth, and it is a common practice in the United States to administer a one-time dose of vitamin K to prevent hemorrhagic disease of the newborn, which can present up to 6 months after birth.

20. c. Vitamin E has antioxidant properties to protect red blood cells from hemolysis and cellular components from being oxidized. Vitamin A aids in the formation of the visual pigment needed for night vision, bone growth/development, and promoting integrity of the epithelial cells. Vitamin D is needed to regulate calcium and phosphorous. It is also necessary for calcium absorption from the small intestines. Vitamin K is needed for synthesis of prothrombin and various clotting factors.

21. a. Folic acid is very important during the first trimester of pregnancy to prevent neural tube defects such as anencephaly or spina bifida. All females who may become pregnant should be encouraged to take folate 600 mcg/day, since frequently a female does not know she is pregnant until well into the first trimester. Multivitamin with iron should be taken *during* pregnancy according to the RDA recommendations.

22. c. Iron is essential for hemoglobin (Hgb) regeneration. Bleeding decreases the number of Hgb, and vitamin A can assist in increasing Hgb. Chromium is needed for proper metabolism of carbohydrates, lipids, and other essential nutrients. Copper is needed for formation of red blood cells (RBCs), not hemoglobin regeneration. Selenium is needed for protection from oxidative damage and infection, among other functions.

23. b. Vitamin B_1 is also known as *thiamine*. Thiamine deficiency is evident in Wernicke encephalopathy, which, if left untreated, leads to Wernicke-Korsakoff syndrome and irreversible brain damage. Thiamine should be administered before dextrose. Vitamin B_6 deficiency can also be seen in alcohol abusers but does not necessarily create the above symptoms.

24. a. Vitamin C is a water-soluble vitamin that is needed for collagen synthesis, aiding in absorption of iron, and assisting in converting folic acid to its active form. Vitamin D, a fat-soluble vitamin, helps in absorption of calcium. Iron, a mineral, is needed for hemoglobin regeneration. Zinc, a mineral, is important for growth, appetite, and skin integrity, among others.

25. c. Antacids will decrease the absorption of iron from the intestines. They do not help each other to do their job. Iron must be taken daily, not every other day. Iron does not decrease the effectiveness of the antacids; instead, antacids decrease the absorption of iron.

26. d. Liquid iron can discolor teeth; therefore taking liquid iron through a straw can decrease the discoloration. Liquid iron does not cause bleeding gums, esophageal varices, or corroded tooth enamel.

27. b. Vitamin A deficiency can be seen in patients with biliary and pancreatic disorders. Celiac disease damages the lining of the intestine and impairs absorption of vitamin A.

28. b. Vitamin A, a fat-soluble vitamin, is excreted in urine and feces.

29. a, b, c, d. Vitamin A is a fat-soluble vitamin and is stored in the liver. Toxicity can occur. Any dose changes should be discussed with the healthcare provider before changes are made. Symptoms of hypervitaminosis A include nausea, vomiting, anorexia, lethargy, peeling skin, hair loss, and abdominal pain. Alcohol ingestion will decrease the absorption of vitamin A.

30. b. Pyridoxine or vitamin B_6 might be considered beneficial for a patient with neuritis from INH therapy. Signs and symptoms of neuritis include numbness, tingling, "pins and needles" feeling, and difficulty gripping an object. Niacin can be used to alleviate pellagra and elevated cholesterol. Riboflavin can be used for dermatologic disorders. Thiamine is appropriate for persons with Wernicke-Korsakoff syndrome with central nervous system disorder. Wernicke-Korsakoff syndrome is usually associated with alcoholism, not due to drug therapy.

31. d. Patients who are receiving parenteral nutrition (PN) are at risk for zinc deficiency. Zinc will also be crucial for this patient for wound repair and tissue healing. With continued PN, deficiencies of copper and iron can also occur.

32. c. Chromium is needed for metabolizing carbohydrate, fats, and nucleic acid. It might help normalize glucose in those with type 2 diabetes. Vitamin E has been used for Alzheimer disease. Vitamin C has been used to treat the "common cold." Vitamin B3, niacin, might be useful for Raynaud phenomenon.

33. d. Shellfish is rich in copper. Other foods with rich copper include liver, nuts, seeds, legumes, and cocoa. Broccoli is rich in vitamin K. Grapefruit would be high in vitamin C. Lamb is rich in zinc.

34. d. Vitamin K is needed for synthesis of prothrombin and the clotting factors VII, IX, and X. Vitamin K_1 (phytonadione) is the only form that is available to treat an overdose of an oral anticoagulant.

Case Study: Critical Thinking

1. Vitamin A is a fat-soluble vitamin necessary for bone growth and for maintenance of epithelial tissues, eyes, and hair and has antioxidant properties. Excessive dosages can be toxic, causing alopecia, anorexia, abdominal pain, lethargy, nausea, and vomiting. Vitamin C is a water-soluble vitamin absorbed from the small intestine. Vitamin C helps absorb iron, assists in carbohydrate metabolism, and is involved in collagen, protein, and lipid syntheses. Toxicity from vitamin C is rare since excess dosages are excreted unchanged by the kidneys. Too much vitamin C can cause GI upset. Vitamin E is a fat-soluble vitamin with antioxidant properties, protecting the red blood cells from hemolysis. Excessive amounts of vitamin E may include fatigue, weakness, nausea, GI upset, headache, bleeding, and breast tenderness. Vitamin E may prolong the prothrombin time (PT). Patients on warfarin and vitamin E should have their PT monitored closely.

2. Vitamins C and D and certain foods can affect warfarin. Vitamin C has an antagonistic effect to oral anticoagulants; on the other hand, vitamin D has a synergistic effect. Vitamin K increases the synthesis of prothrombin, which is necessary for clotting. Vitamin K promotes clotting and is used as an antidote for warfarin. Foods high in vitamin K include dark green leafy vegetables, liver, cheese, egg yolk, and tomatoes. If consumed, the therapeutic effects of warfarin will decrease.

3. Advise the patient to consult with the healthcare provider if the patient wants to continue taking vitamins and eating fresh fruits and vegetables. The dose of anticoagulant may need adjustment. Explain the potential effects of the vitamins on the anticoagulant; complications of the atrial fibrillation can occur. Explain to the patient that a well-balanced diet usually negates the need for vitamin supplements. Educate patients on the signs and symptoms of hypervitaminosis. Also educate how certain vitamins and minerals can affect the therapeutic effects of warfarin.

CHAPTER 14: NUTRITIONAL SUPPORT

1. metabolic processes
2. 50%
3. hydration; electrolyte
4. multidisciplinary team approach
5. PEG (percutaneous endoscopic gastrostomy); surgically; endoscopically; radiologically
6. True
7. True
8. False. Parenteral nutrition is delivered IV, and enteral nutrition is delivered into the GI system.
9. True

10.

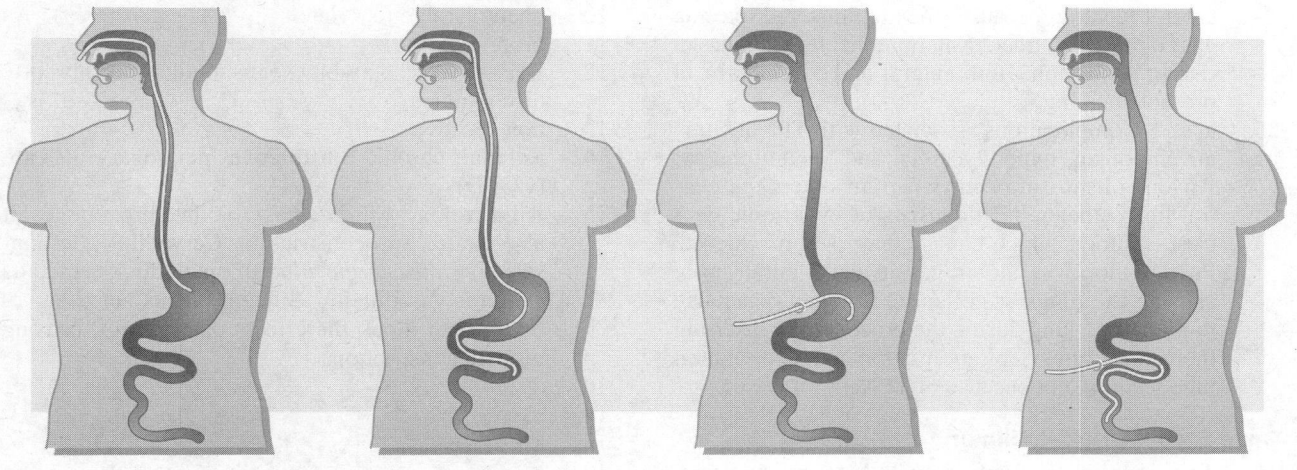

Nasogastric   Nasoduodenal/nasojejunal   Gastrostomy   Jejunostomy

11. d. It is best used for ambulatory patients so that they are not connected to tubings.
12. a
13. b
14. c
15. a. The enteral nutrition of choice for a diabetic patient is specialty formula for diabetes. It has modified macronutrient to promote glycemic control. Polymeric formula mimics macronutrients with fiber and used as supplements for persons without malabsorptive disorders. Immune modulating formula is a specialty formula that contains pharmacologically active substances aimed at modulating the immune response for improved outcome. Modular formula contains single macronutrient (carbohydrates, protein, or lipids).
16. d. Enteral tube feeding is best if the patient has a functioning GI system. However, a patient who is at risk for aspiration needs enteral feeding that will deliver the food below the pyloric sphincter or below the stomach; enteral via jejunostomy is the best answer. Nasogastric tube is placed in the stomach which is above the pyloric sphincter. Parenteral nutrition is reserved for those whose GI system is not functioning.
17. d. Intermittent enteral feeding occurs over short time every 3–6 hours. It mimics when person usually eats. Bolus feeding is given usually in less than 15 minutes with a syringe. Enteral feedings can occur by gravity or by infusion pump.
18. b. Patients with burns have a higher calorie requirement than most other types of patients. In the acute phase, this is due to a hypermetabolic state. The patient requires nutritional support to assist in wound healing. Total parenteral nutrition (TPN) would be an option; however, there is an increased risk of infection. The best response is cyclic tube feeding in which the nutrition is administered over

8–16 hours, allowing the patient to be ambulatory and active during that time.
19. d. Because of the irritation to the veins from the high glucose content, TPN must be administered through a central venous line. Central lines are usually accessed through the subclavian vein or internal jugular vein. The brachiocephalic vein is used for peripherally inserted central catheter (PICC) for parenteral nutrition for short-term therapy (less than 4 weeks).
20. d. TPN provides 60%–70% of carbohydrates. It provides 3.5%–20% of protein and about 30% of fat.
21. b. Continuous enteral feedings occur over 24 hours. Enteral feedings over 30–60 minutes are considered intermittent feedings. Enteral feedings to be administered over 15 minutes are considered bolus feedings. Enteral feedings over 8–16 hours are considered cyclic feedings.
22. a, b. Diarrhea and constipation are a common side effect associated with enteral tube feedings due to multiple reasons. Other complications include dehydration and aspiration.
23. c. If a patient is receiving continuous enteral nutrition, residuals should be checked every 2–4 hours. A residual greater than 150 mL indicates potential delay in gastric emptying. If the residual is more than 150 mL, stop the infusion for 30 minutes to 1 hour and then recheck. If the residual continues to be high, stop the feeding and contact the healthcare provider. Some studies suggest withholding if greater than 500 mL. However, it is always prudent for the nurse to assess the patient regarding the tolerance of enteral tube feeding.
24. a, c, d. Enteral nutrition is the preferred method if there is a functioning GI tract. It tends to be much less expensive than TPN and has a lower risk of infection, since TPN must be administered through

central access. There is no risk of central line–associated bloodstream infection (CLABSI) from enteral feeding, because it is administered into the gastrointestinal tract. Enteral tube feeding has a risk of aspiration. Both enteral and parenteral can promote healing.

25. a, c, d. Complications associated with TPN include air embolism, hyperglycemia, and pneumothorax. Air embolism can occur when air enters the central line catheter. TPN consists of hypertonic dextrose solution which can increase serum glucose. Pneumothorax is air or gas in the pleural space causing the lungs to collapse. This can occur due to punctured lung during the procedure in inserting the central line. Aspiration can occur with enteral tube feeding, not because of TPN.

Case Study: Critical Thinking

1. Transitioning a patient from TPN to enteral nutrition is common when the patient has a long-term need for nutritional support. Certain steps must be followed for a successful and safe transition. The first step is to see if the patient is ready for enteral feeding and how much the patient can tolerate. This is accomplished by giving small amounts of feeding at a slow rate while the TPN rate is gradually reduced. TPN can be discontinued when the patient is able to tolerate taking approximately 75%–80% of caloric needs by the enteral method. It is important to remember that a critically ill patient may require between 3000 and 5000 calories/day.

2. A patient who requires long-term enteral nutrition will likely require a gastrostomy tube. Before that time the patient may have received nutrition via a nasogastric or orogastric tube. Aspiration is a serious risk for those receiving tube feedings and may lead to aspiration pneumonia. Elevating the head of the bed between 30 and 45 degrees when possible may be beneficial. This is not an option if there is a question of spinal cord injury. The nurse would aspirate to check for residual before administering the next feeding and every 4 hours between feedings.

CHAPTER 15: ADRENERGIC AGONISTS AND ANTAGONISTS

1. c. Alpha$_1$ blocker causes vasodilation. Alpha$_2$ blocker causes vasoconstriction.
2. d. Beta-blockers can decrease heart rate. Beta$_1$ affects the heart, whereas beta$_2$ affects bronchioles, uterus, and glycogenolysis.
3. b. Has greater affinity for certain receptors
4. e. The *sympathomimetic mimics* the sympathetic nervous system.
5. a. Blocks action of sympathetic nervous system
6. effector
7. adrenergic
8. do
9. sympatholytics
10. phentolamine mesylate
11. propranolol
12. Beta-blocker; beta-blockers should not be abruptly discontinued.
13. nonselective
14. asthma; chronic obstructive pulmonary disease (COPD)
15. Albuterol is a *beta$_2$ agonist* to dilate bronchioles. It also causes vasoconstriction. Carvedilol is a nonselective *adrenergic blocker*, including beta2. Its action is vasodilation. Since it blocks beta$_2$, carvedilol could block the effects of albuterol, causing bronchoconstriction.
16. d
17. a, c
18. a
19. a
20. b
21. d
22. c
23. d
24. b
25. b. Albuterol increases the patient's heart rate, which may cause a feeling of nervousness and not an ease of breathing. It has no effect on urinary output. Albuterol causes smooth muscle dilation, not constriction or contraction. Bronchodilation and relaxation of smooth muscles will improve airflow into the lungs.
26. a. Ensuring a patent airway is the first step in providing care to any patient. There is no indication currently for an electrocardiogram. Although epinephrine is beneficial in allergic reactions, 1 mg of 1:1000 exceeds the subcutaneous dosage. Establishing an IV would not be the first action to take.
27. d. Although all pieces of information are important, the nurse would ask the patient how many puffs of the inhaler were taken to determine that the patient did not overdose on the drug. Other side effects of albuterol, besides shaking and trembling, include sweating, nausea, headaches, blurred vision, and flushing.
28. b, c, e. Albuterol is a beta agonist, and amphetamine is a sympathomimetic.
29. c. Dopamine is a vasopressor (adrenergic agonist) that acts on dopaminergic receptors and alpha$_1$- and beta$_1$-receptor sites. Dopamine can cause tissue necrosis. Phentolamine mesylate is an adrenergic antagonist and is an antidote to stop further tissue necrosis. Dobutamine and epinephrine are also adrenergic agonists that can cause tissue necrosis. Although reserpine is an adrenergic neuron antagonist, it is used to treat hypertension.
30. a, b, c. Carvedilol is an adrenergic blocker. The other three drugs are adrenergic agonists. Adrenergic agonists are contraindicated in narrow-angle glaucoma.

31. b. Many OTC drugs, such as nasal decongestion, contain pseudoephedrine, which is a sympathomimetic; they can worsen hypertension.

32. b. Dopamine acts primarily on dopaminergic receptors that are located in renal, mesenteric, coronary, and cerebral arteries. These dopaminergic receptors are primarily activated by dopamine. When these receptors are stimulated, vasodilation and increased blood flow occur, which can increase renal flow.

33. c, e. Beta$_1$ receptors are primarily located in the heart and in the kidneys.

34. a. St. Johns wort can decrease the hypotensive effects of reserpine.

35. b. The proper dosage for timolol is initially 10 mg bid., with a maximum dose of 60 mg/day. The above-ordered dose is 10 times the initial starting dose.

36. a. Catecholamines are substances that can produce a sympathomimetic response. Endogenous catecholamines include epinephrine, norepinephrine, and dopamine. Exogenous catecholamines are isoproterenol and dobutamine.

Clinical Judgment Unfolding Case Study
Phase 1
Question 1

- Blood pressure 88/48 mm Hg
- Heart rate 62 beats/min
- IV site to left forearm with redness and pain
- Lungs with faint crackles to the bases on auscultation
- Patient's complaint of "difficulty breathing"
- Peripheral pulses palpable but weak
- Urine output in urine drainage bag with 20 mL of amber-colored urine

Rationale:

Epinephrine and dopamine are adrenergic agonists used to stimulate the sympathetic nervous system. The expected responses with these agonists are for the blood pressure and heart rate to increase. Dopamine was ordered to maintain a systolic blood pressure of 100 mm Hg. The patient's blood pressure is 88/48 mm Hg and an increase in dopamine is warranted. However, the intravenous site for the dopamine is red and painful. Dopamine is irritating to the skin and extravasation of dopamine can cause tissue damage and necrosis within 12 hours of starting the infusion. The nurse would need to discontinue the current IV site and resume the dopamine infusion at another site. Adrenergic agonists, such as epinephrine and dopamine, can cause dyspnea and patient may complain of difficulty breathing. Also, crackles on auscultation could be an early indication of pulmonary edema due to fluid overload from receiving IV fluids at 125 mL/h. Pulmonary edema is a life-threatening reaction that requires emergent attention. Urine output of 20 mL in 3 hours can indicate decreased renal perfusion, further causing fluid overload. A normal urine output is 30 mL/h. Also, epinephrine and dopamine

produce a sympathomimetic response by influencing several adrenergic receptors. The response of these receptors can cause the bladder to relax preventing it from emptying. All other findings are considered within normal parameters. Once adequate blood pressure is achieved, the peripheral pulses will become stronger.

Reference

McCuistion, L.E., DiMaggio, K.V., Winton, M.B., & Yeager, J.J. (2025). Pharmacology: A patient-centered nursing process approach, 12th ed. St. Louis, MO: Elsevier. pp. 175–186.

Question 2

Options for 1	Options for 2	Options for 3	Options for 4
Increase	27 mcg/kg per minute	Phentolamine mesylate	Fluid overload

Rationale:

Based on the blood pressure of 88/48 mm Hg, which is hypotensive, the nurse would most likely increase the rate of dopamine to 27 mcg/kg per minute as ordered to attain a systolic blood pressure of at least 90 mm Hg. Redness and pain at the IV site are indicative of infiltration. Dopamine can damage tissue and cause necrosis within 12 hours and phentolamine mesylate is the antidote for infiltration of dopamine infusion. The drug would be further diluted in 10–15 mL of normal saline and instilled into the site of infiltration. The signs (crackles) and symptoms ("difficulty breathing") can indicate fluid overload from receiving 0.9% sodium chloride at 125 mL/h.

Reference

McCuistion, L.E., DiMaggio, K.V., Winton, M.B., & Yeager, J.J. (2025). Pharmacology: A patient-centered nursing process approach, 12th ed. St. Louis, MO: Elsevier. pp. 175–186.

Phase 2
Question 3

__X__ a. Complaints of "difficulty breathing" and "chest discomfort"

__X__ b. Decreased renal function

_____ c. Blood pressure 102/64 mm Hg

_____ d. Heart rate 98 beats/min

__X__ e. Oliguria

_____ f. Respiratory rate of 22 breaths/min

__X__ g. Crackles to the bases of the lungs on auscultation

Rationale:

Patients can develop complications from dopamine. Dopamine is a nonselective adrenergic agonist which stimulates alpha, beta, and dopaminergic receptors. The commonly associated side effects of dopamine include urinary retention, dyspnea, and hypertension. Other side effects include tachycardia, palpitations, restlessness, tremors, dizziness, nausea, and vomiting, in addition to angina and headache. The nurse would further investigate the patient's complaints of "difficulty breathing" and "chest discomfort" for evidence of angina and/or dysrhythmias because of dopamine's vasoconstrictive properties. When patient receives too much adrenergic agonist, blood flow can decrease to vital organs, such as the kidneys, thereby lowering renal function as evidenced by oliguria. Adequate urine output is 30 mL/h. This patient's urine output is 15 mL/h. Since blood flow decreases, fluid buildup can cause peripheral edema. In rare cases, dopamine can cause pulmonary edema, causing crackles to be heard on auscultation to the lung fields.

Reference

McCuistion, L.E., DiMaggio, K.V., Winton, M.B., & Yeager, J.J. (2025). Pharmacology: A patient-centered nursing process approach, 12th ed. St. Louis, MO: Elsevier. pp. 175–186.

Question 4

Potential Order	Anticipated	Contraindicated
12-lead electrocardiogram (ECG)	X	
Chest x-ray	X	
Decrease sodium chloride infusion to 30 mL/h	X	
Furosemide 10 mg IV once	X	
Increase intravenous fluids		X
Monitor blood pressure and heart rate every 5 min	X	
Oxygen 2 L per nasal cannula	X	
Titrate dopamine down	X	

Rationale:

Dopamine is a nonselective adrenergic agonist which stimulates alpha, beta, and dopaminergic receptors. The commonly associated side effects of dopamine include urinary retention, dyspnea, and pulmonary edema. Other side effects include tachycardia, hypertension, palpitations, restlessness, tremors, dysrhythmias, dizziness, nausea, and vomiting, in addition to dyspnea, angina, and headache. The nurse would further investigate patient's complaints of "difficulty breathing" and "chest discomfort" for evidence of pulmonary edema and/or dysrhythmias because of dopamine's vasoconstrictive properties. When patient receives too much adrenergic agonist, blood flow can decrease to vital organs, such as the kidneys, thereby lowering renal function as evidenced by oliguria. Normal urine output is 30 mL/h. This patient's urine output is 15 mL/h. Since blood flow decreases, fluid buildup can occur resulting in pulmonary and peripheral edema. The nurse would anticipate the following orders: 12-lead ECG (chest discomfort and occasional PVCs), chest x-ray (difficulty breathing and crackles to lung's bases), decreasing sodium chloride infusion (crackles to lung's bases and peripheral edema), furosemide 10 mg (crackles to lung's bases and peripheral edema, oliguria), monitoring blood pressure and heart rate every 5 minutes (titrating dopamine down), oxygen 2 L per nasal cannula (oxygen saturation 92%), and titrating dopamine down. Increasing intravenous fluids would be contraindicated in this patient because of pulmonary and peripheral edema.

Reference

McCuistion, L.E., DiMaggio, K.V., Winton, M.B., & Yeager, J.J. (2025). Pharmacology: A patient-centered nursing process approach, 12th ed. St. Louis, MO: Elsevier. pp. 175–186.

Phase 3
Question 5

Nurse's Response	Patient's Questions	Appropriate Nurse's Response
	"Can I stop taking this medicine if my blood pressure is good?"	"Stopping the medicine abruptly can cause severe high blood pressure or severe chest pain."
	"Will the medicine prevent me from enjoying sex?"	"Metoprolol can cause erectile dysfunction."
	"Can I take my nasal decongestant when I get home?"	"Nasal decongestants can decrease the effectiveness of metoprolol."
	"What do I need to do if I become dizzy when getting out of bed?"	"When getting out of bed, change your position slowly to prevent a sudden drop in blood pressure."
	"My job requires me to work odd hours. Can I take both doses when I first wake up?"	"Take the medicine twice daily, one in the morning and one just before you go to bed."

Rationale:

Metoprolol is a selective β_1 antagonist and has greater affinity to β_1 receptors in the heart and vasculature to decrease heart rate and blood pressure. Beta-blockers should not be abruptly stopped, even if the blood pressure is normal for several days. If metoprolol needs to be discontinued, it should be tapered to prevent tachycardia, hypertension, severe angina, dysrhythmia, and myocardial infarction. Metoprolol can cause erectile dysfunction. The patient should be taught to not stop the drug but notify their healthcare provider if the dysfunction is bothersome. Placing an ice pack to their genitalia will not help with the dysfunction. Decongestants are adrenergic agonists and can decrease the effectiveness of metoprolol (adrenergic antagonist) if taken concurrently. Beta$_1$ antagonists lower blood pressure and can cause dizziness when changing positions, such as getting out of bed. Patient should be taught to change their position slowly to prevent a sudden drop in blood pressure. The usual dosing of metoprolol is twice daily. The nurse would teach the patient to take their medicine one in the morning and one just before they go to bed.

Reference

McCuistion, L.E., DiMaggio, K.V., Winton, M.B., & Yeager, J.J. (2025). Pharmacology: A patient-centered nursing process approach, 12th ed. St. Louis, MO: Elsevier. pp. 175–186.

Question 6

b. "I need to stand from a sitting a position slowly."
d. "The medicine increases oxygen to the heart."
e. "I will call my doctor if I have trouble breathing."
g. "My blood pressure can decrease if I take a nitroglycerin."

Rationale:

Metoprolol is a beta$_1$-selective antagonist. It is used to manage hypertension, angina, heart failure, and acute myocardial infarction and reduces cardiovascular mortality by blocking the beta receptors of the heart and vasculature. It can cause hypotension, especially with position changes; therefore patients should stand from a sitting position slowly to decrease the risk of dizziness and falls. Metoprolol decreases the oxygen demand to the heart by decreasing blood pressure and heart rate, thereby increasing oxygen to the heart. Even though metoprolol is a selective beta$_1$ blocker, pulmonary edema and heart failure can occur. Patients who have trouble breathing should contact their healthcare provider. Nitroglycerin, a vasoactive drug, can further lower the blood pressure effects of metoprolol. Decongestants found in nasal sprays contain an adrenergic agonist, which can decrease the effectiveness of metoprolol; therefore patients should not use nasal sprays without consulting their healthcare provider. Nonsteroidal antiinflammatory drugs, such as ibuprofen, can lower the hypotensive effects of metoprolol. Metoprolol is effective in preventing anginal pain; however, patients should not take extra dose for chest pain since they do not have an immediate effect. Instead, patients would need nitroglycerin sublingual to relieve chest pain.

Reference

McCuistion, L.E., DiMaggio, K.V., Winton, M.B., & Yeager, J.J. (2025). Pharmacology: A patient-centered nursing process approach, 12th ed. St. Louis, MO: Elsevier. pp. 175–186.

CHAPTER 16: CHOLINERGIC AGONISTS AND ANTAGONISTS

1. c
2. e
3. g. Also known as acetylcholinesterase inhibitors
4. d
5. h
6. a
7. b
8. f. Direct acting acts like cholinergic agonists. Indirect acting acts like cholinesterase inhibitors.

9.

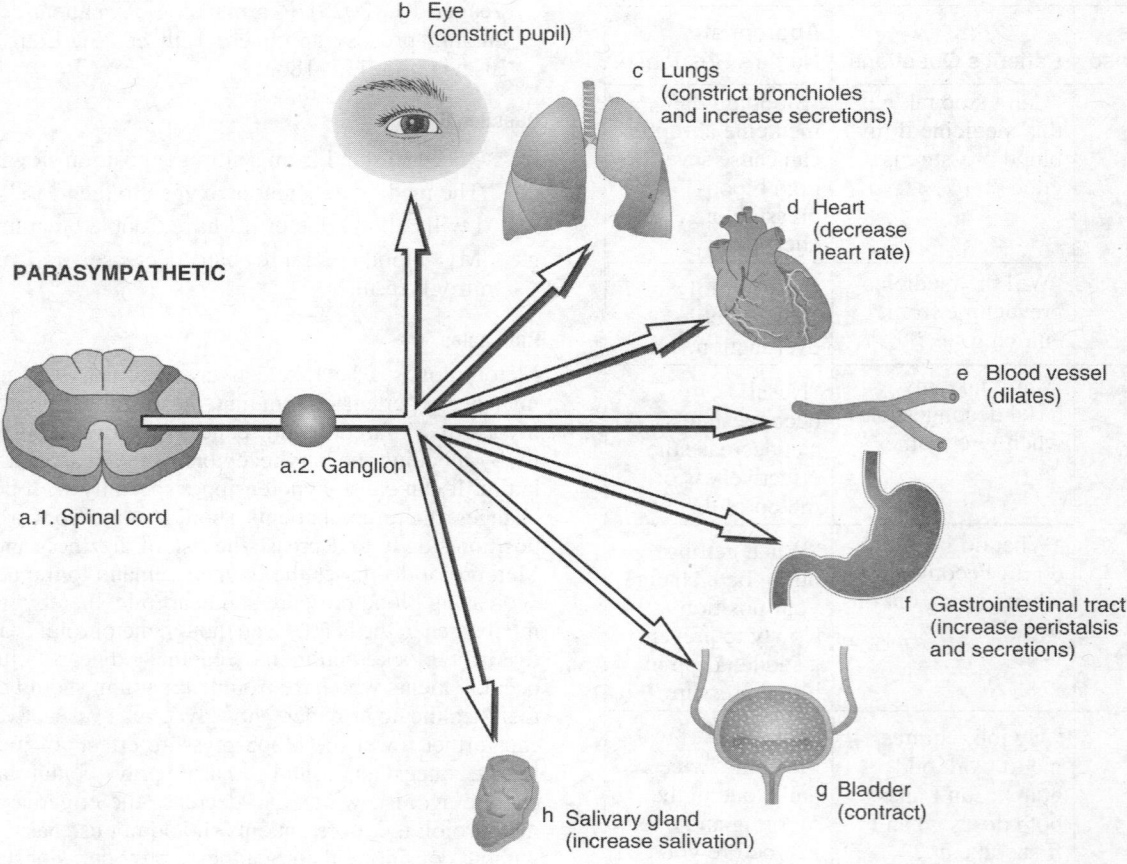

PARASYMPATHETIC

a.1. Spinal cord

a.2. Ganglion

b Eye
(constrict pupil)

c Lungs
(constrict bronchioles
and increase secretions)

d Heart
(decrease
heart rate)

e Blood vessel
(dilates)

f Gastrointestinal tract
(increase peristalsis
and secretions)

g Bladder
(contract)

h Salivary gland
(increase salivation)

10. d. Pralidoxime chloride is an anticholinergic that inhibits the actions of acetylcholine. It is given for cholinesterase inhibitor toxicity and organophosphate pesticide toxicity. Bethanechol is a direct-acting cholinergic agonist and is used to treat urinary retention. Metoclopramide, a direct-acting cholinergic agonist, is used to treat gastrointestinal (GI) symptoms.

11. a. Bethanechol, a direct-acting cholinergic agonist, is used to treat urinary retention. Metoclopramide, a direct-acting cholinergic agonist, is used to treat gastrointestinal (GI) symptoms. Neostigmine bromide is used to treat myasthenia gravis.

12. b. Anticholinergics inhibit the acetylcholine receptors and include muscarinic and nicotinic receptors. Anticholinergic eyedrops cause pupils to dilate (mydriasis). Cholinergic agonists will constrict pupils. Direct-acting cholinergic agonists will decrease intraocular pressure.

13. c. Anticholinergic drugs are contraindicated in a patient with glaucoma because they increase the intraocular pressure. Therefore the nurse would hold the drug and contact the prescriber.

14. b. Bethanechol is a direct-acting cholinergic agonist. Agonists promote tissue response.

15. c. Bethanechol, a direct-acting cholinergic agonist, works on the muscarinic receptor. Nicotinic receptors work on skeletal muscles. Anticholinergics inhibit muscarinic and nicotinic receptors.

16. c. Bethanechol, a direct-acting cholinergic agonist, stimulates the muscarinic receptors to contract bladder which increases urination.

17. a, c. Cholinergic drugs are parasympathomimetics in that they mimic the parasympathetic responses. One response is the dilation of blood vessels, which decreases blood pressure. Other responses include pupillary constriction (miosis), bronchoconstriction and increased bronchial secretions, decreased heart rate, increased gastrointestinal peristalsis and secretions, bladder contraction, and increased salivation.

18. d. Bethanechol is used to treat urinary retention but will not be effective and should not be used in the case of a mechanical obstruction. If this patient was prescribed bethanechol for urinary retention and the urine output is decreasing, the healthcare provider should be notified to investigate another cause.

19. d. Bethanechol is a cholinergic agonist. The patient is experiencing an adverse response, and the treatment of choice is atropine. The nurse would obtain an order to administer atropine, the antidote for cholinergic overdose. The nurse would also document the patient's experiences, but it is not the best action by the nurse. Abdominal cramps are due to the action on the muscarinic receptors, not due to constipation. Increasing fluid intake will not relieve the side effects of bethanechol.

20. c. Neostigmine bromide is used to *treat* myasthenia gravis (MG). Bethanechol is used to treat urinary retention. Pilocarpine is used to treat glaucoma. Edrophonium chloride is a medication to assist in the diagnosis of myasthenia gravis.

21. a, b. Atropine would be beneficial as a preoperative drug to help control oral secretions. It is also used for patients who are symptomatic with a heart rate less than 50 beats/min and is symptomatic of decreased cardiac output. Bethanechol is for urinary retention. Benztropine is for paralytic ileus. Propantheline bromide is used to treat gastric ulcers.

22. d. Atropine and atropine-like drugs should not be administered to patients with narrow-angle glaucoma because they will increase the intraocular pressure.

23. c. Because of the decrease in gastrointestinal motility that can be associated with propantheline, the patient would be encouraged to eat foods that are high in fiber and drink adequate amounts of liquid to prevent constipation.

24. a, b, c, e. Hyoscyamine is an anticholinergic drug that will have similar side effects to the prototype drug atropine. Adequate fluid intake will help prevent constipation. Vision may be blurry, and the patient would be advised not to drive until the effects of the drug on the vision are known. Sucking on hard candy or sugar-free ice pops, as well as increased fluid intake, may help with dry mouth. The patient should be educated as to baseline heart rate and advised to report tachycardia (rates above 100 beats/min) to the healthcare provider. Increased sweating is not a common side effect.

25. a, c, d. Anticholinergic drugs block the normal parasympathetic responses of the pupils, lungs, heart, blood vessels, gastrointestinal tract, bladder, and salivary glands. Therefore anticholinergic drugs are contraindicated in those with any heart disease and diabetes mellitus.

26. d. Anticholinergics, such as biperiden and benztropine, are used to treat early Parkinson. Anticholinesterases, not anticholinergics, are used to treat myasthenia gravis.

27. b, c, d, e. Common side effects of anticholinergic drugs, like benztropine, may include dry mouth, constipation, and urinary retention. Dizziness and hallucinations should be reported to the healthcare provider because these may become dangerous to the patient. Because there is a decreased ability to perspire, life-threatening hyperthermia may develop. Palpitations may be due to tachycardia.

Case Study: Critical Thinking

1. Tolterodine tartrate blocks cholinergic receptors selectively in the bladder to decrease the incidence of incontinence.

2. The common side effects are those associated with other cholinergic drugs and may include dizziness, vertigo, dry mouth, nausea, vomiting, weight gain, and urinary retention. Adverse drug effects include angioedema, chest pain, and dementia.

3. Tolterodine is contraindicated in patients with glaucoma, gastric paresis, and urinary retention.

4. Besides discussing side effects and adverse reactions the patient should be encouraged to take the drug on an empty stomach since absorption is delayed with food. Grapefruit juice should also be avoided because it decreases drug levels. Before taking any other drugs the healthcare provider should be consulted because this drug interacts with several other classes of drugs such as phenothiazines, macrolides, and antifungals.

CHAPTER 17: STIMULANTS

1. brain; spinal cord
2. dysregulation
3. norepinephrine; dopamine
4. stimulant; suppress appetite
5. analeptics
6. a, c, d. CNS stimulants, such as amphetamines, analeptics, and anorexiants, are approved to treat ADHD, narcolepsy, and PTSD.
7. a, b, c, d. Methylphenidate is a stimulant to treat ADHD and narcolepsy. Patients taking methylphenidate should not operate hazardous equipment they should avoid other stimulants, such as caffeine; and the nurse should instruct patients that nervousness or tremors can occur. The drug should be taken before meals. Weight loss, not weight gain, can occur.
8. b. Analeptics stimulate the brainstem and medulla to stimulate respiration. Anorexiants stimulate the satiety center in the hypothalamic and limbic areas of the brain. Amphetamines stimulate the cerebral cortex.
9. a, b, c, d, f. Methylphenidate can cause euphoria, headache, hypertension, irritability, and vomiting. Hypotension is an adverse effect, not a common side effect.
10. b. An immediate-release drug can be taken in two or three divided doses. An extended-release drug should be taken once daily.
11. a. Phentermine hydrochloride should not be taken within 14 days of monoamine oxidase inhibitors (MAOIs) such as selegiline. Combinations of the

two drugs intensify the stimulation and vasopressor effects of phentermine that can cause severe cardiovascular and cerebrovascular responses. Therefore the nurse would contact the healthcare provider to verify the prescription.

12. d. Phentermine-topiramate is used for short-term weight management.

13. b. The nurse would include that counseling should be obtained while on methylphenidate. Diarrhea, not constipation, is a common side effect. Methylphenidate is usually prescribed long term and should not be stopped abruptly. Weight loss, not gain, can occur.

14. a, b, e. Methylphenidate and MAOIs taken together can increase hypertensive crisis. Methylphenidate can increase the effects of anticoagulants. The effects of methylphenidate can be increased by caffeine.

15. c. Hemorrhagic stroke is the most likely diagnosis of those listed. There is a high risk for hemorrhagic stroke attributable to hypertensive crisis in patients taking stimulants, such as appetite suppressants (anorexiants). Pregnancy-induced hypertension is a possibility, but the patient has been trying to lose weight, not become pregnant. However, a pregnancy test should be obtained; anorexiants are contraindicated in pregnancy. Hypotension, not hypertension, most likely occurs with cardiac arrest and food poisoning.

16. a, d, e. CNS stimulants are absolutely contraindicated in patients with angina, uncontrolled hypertension, and glaucoma. There is no contraindication for stimulants in those with diabetes or hypothyroidism. Hyperthyroidism, not hypothyroidism, is a contraindication.

17. a. Caffeine can stimulate the respiratory system to help the neonate breathe better. It will not cause the baby to gain weight and increase body's temperature.

Case Study: Critical Thinking

1. Methylphenidate is absorbed from the GI tract and is taken before breakfast and lunch. It should be given at least 6 hours before sleep since it can cause insomnia. Methylphenidates decrease hyperactivity and improve attention span.

2. The drug is a CNS stimulant that is used in conjunction with appropriate counseling for treatment of ADHD. The best time to give the drug is 30–45 minutes before meals, so the nurse would need to review the lunch schedules of the students and plan accordingly on how best to administer the drugs.

Baseline height, weight, and vital signs should be obtained and monitored throughout the course of treatment. A record of the students' complete blood count, including a white blood cell count with differential and platelet count, should be on file. Routine vital signs should be assessed since these drugs can cause an elevation in heart rate and blood pressure, especially if taken in conjunction with caffeine. Students should also be monitored for an increase in hyperactivity.

Health teaching is important not only for the student but also for the family and the teachers on staff. The goals of these drugs are to increase focus and attention and decrease impulsiveness and hyperactivity. The student and family should be encouraged to eat three nutritious meals per day along with healthy snacks because anorexia may be a side effect. Dry mouth may also occur, and if possible, within school policy, the student should be allowed to chew gum or suck on hard candy. The importance of avoiding caffeinated beverages and foods, including chocolate, sodas, and energy drinks, must be stressed because high plasma levels of caffeine can be fatal.

Drug administration at school must be handled with tact and ease. If possible, the school nurse's office should not be open to any common areas or exposed to the main hall. Privacy is crucial.

CHAPTER 18: DEPRESSANTS

1. rapid
2. rapid
3. slow
4. rapid
5. rapid
6. sedative-hypnotics; general anesthetics; analgesics; opioid and nonopioid analgesics; anticonvulsants; antipsychotics; antidepressants
7. rapid eye movement; nonrapid eye movement
8. sedation
9. may
10. short
11. central nervous; pain; consciousness
12. surgical; analgesia; excitement or delirium; medullary paralysis
13. spinal
14. respiratory distress or failure
15. saddle block
16. are
17. short
18. zolpidem tartrate and daridorexant (also eszopiclone, zaleplon, and ramelteon)
19. flumazenil
20. esters; amides
21. d
22. f
23. e
24. a
25. b
26. c
27. c. Sedative-hypnotics are commonly prescribed to treat sleep disorders. Analeptics are CNS stimulants. Anesthetics are CNS depressants and are not prescribed for sleep. Triptans help with migraines.

28. b. Long-acting barbiturates, such as phenobarbital, are used to control seizures. Short-acting barbiturates, such as secobarbital and pentobarbital, may be used for sedation. Ultra-short-acting barbiturates, such as methohexital sodium, are used for anesthesia induction. *Note: Do not confuse PHENObarbital with PENTObarbital.*

29. c, d. Postdural-puncture headache can occur because of a decrease in pressure due to fluid leakage from the cerebrospinal space. Maintaining the patient flat in bed for 24–48 hours and encouraging adequate oral fluid intake as tolerated may help prevent a spinal headache. The patient may also require IV fluids to supplement oral intake.

30. c. By explaining the reason for positioning (either seated with an arched back or fetal position), the patient will feel more control. The nurse can reassure the patient that assistance in maintaining the proper position will be provided.

31. d. Zolpidem may be ordered. It is a nonbenzodiazepine for short-term treatment of insomnia. Flumazenil is an antidote for benzodiazepine overdose. Phenobarbital, a long-acting barbiturate, is used to treat seizures. Triazolam is a benzodiazepine. While this class of drug can help with insomnia, a nonbenzodiazepine is a better choice.

32. d, e. Lidocaine is used for local and spinal anesthesia that has a rapid onset with its effects long lasting.

33. a. Antihistamines, such as diphenhydramine, a nonscheduled drug, are the primary ingredient in over-the-counter sleep aids. All other classes of drugs are scheduled drugs.

34. a, b, c, e. Older adults may have more problems with stage 3 and stage 4 nonrapid eye movement (NREM) sleep and awaken frequently. Establishing a bedtime routine, maintaining a schedule of going to bed and arising in the morning, and avoiding caffeine and alcohol at bedtime may help. Although it sounds intuitive to take naps, they may hinder a patient from obtaining a good night's sleep if the naps last longer than 20–30 minutes. Diuretics should be taken in the morning and fluids should be limited at bedtime to prevent frequent trips to the bathroom, which may interrupt sleep.

Case Study: Critical Thinking

1. Benzodiazepines are frequently prescribed before surgery. They increase the action of the inhibitory neurotransmitter gamma-aminobutyric acid (GABA) to the GABA receptors and reduce the excitability of the neurons. Drugs such as alprazolam or lorazepam might be prescribed for anxiety.

2. Balanced anesthesia includes many parts leading up to surgery. By using a variety of agents, less general anesthetic is needed, fewer cardiovascular side effects occur, less nausea and vomiting occur, pain is decreased, and a quicker recovery is promoted.

This is also true if utilizing a laparoscopic approach instead of an "open" approach to this surgery.

The night before the surgery, a medication such as zolpidem might be prescribed to ensure a good night's sleep. After the patient has arrived in the preoperative area and approximately 1 hour before surgery, a combination of an opioid or anxiolytic and an anticholinergic such as atropine might be given. The purpose of the anticholinergic is to decrease secretions and therefore the risk of aspiration. Once the patient is transferred to the operating room, a short-acting sedative such as pentothal, propofol, or etomidate may be given, and the patient will be given inhaled anesthetics. This procedure will require some general anesthesia, so the patient will also receive a muscle relaxant to facilitate endotracheal intubation and maintain neuromuscular blockade.

CHAPTER 19: ANTISEIZURE DRUGS

1. d
2. a
3. e
4. b
5. c
6. electroencephalogram (EEG)
7. idiopathic
8. generalized; partial
9. preventing; do not
10. are not
11. phenytoin
12. over-the-counter
13. intramuscular
14. a, c. Carbamazepine and diazepam are given for tonic-clonic seizures. Pregabalin is a GABA analog and is beneficial for partial seizures, neuropathic pain, and fibromyalgia. Ethosuximide and acetazolamide are indicated for absence seizures.
15. b. Although it is important to know the patient's medical history regarding seizures, the best response is asking about the drugs that have been prescribed. Most antiseizure drugs have teratogenic properties. Females with seizure history are at increased risk for seizures during pregnancy. The risks versus the benefits of antiseizure drugs need to be discussed. Abruptly stopping antiseizure drugs can also increase the risk of seizures.
16. a, c, d. Hydantoins (e.g., fosphenytoin), barbiturates (e.g., phenobarbital), and benzodiazepines (e.g., diazepam and lorazepam) are used for status epilepticus. Diazepam is the drug of choice. Carbamazepine and topiramate are indicated for tonic-clonic and partial seizures.
17. b. Phenytoin prevents sodium from entering the cells. This reduces the activities of cells. Antiseizure drugs inhibit neurotransmitters; they do not destroy them. Antiseizure drugs suppress entry of calcium; they do not increase the influx.

18. a, b, d. Valproic acid is taken in divided doses. Doses start at 10–15 mg/kg per day and increase to a maximum of 60 mg/kg per day until seizures are controlled. Frequent labs are needed to monitor serum levels and liver functions. Antiseizure drugs control the frequency and severity of seizures; they do not cure. One of the most common side effects is nausea. Valproic acid can be taken with food to minimize the risk of nausea.

19. b, c, d. Glucose, cardiac rhythm, blood pressure, and IV site should be assessed before administering IV phenytoin. An absolute contraindication is heart block and bradycardia. Caution is advised for patients with hypoglycemia and hypotension. IV phenytoin should be administered through a large-bore IV or a central line. Phenytoin is very irritating to the tissue and sloughing could occur if the drug infiltrates. Phenytoin is excreted in small amounts in the urine. Urine output should be monitored, but not hourly.

20. d. Intravenous phenytoin is irritating to the tissue, and the nurse would discontinue the IV and restart the infusion at a different site. It is recommended that a central line or peripherally inserted central catheter (PICC) line and an in-line filter be used. The healthcare provider does not need to be notified immediately to change the medication to oral form. Continuing the infusion, even with a saline flush, may cause sloughing of the tissue.

21. a. Although a variety of antiseizures may be utilized over a patient's lifetime, at this time, there is no cure for seizure disorders. The patient will most likely need to take an antiseizure for their lifetime.

22. b. 18 mcg/mL is within the therapeutic range of 10–20 mcg/mL for bound phenytoin and 1–2 mcg/mL for unbound/free drugs. 8 mcg/mL is below the therapeutic range and the patient may be at risk for seizure. 28 and 38 mcg/mL are too high, and toxicity can occur.

23. a, b, d, e. Documenting the types of movements (tonic/clonic), the duration of seizure activity, and the locations where the movements started and progressed are important pieces of gathering the history of the seizure event. It is important to know, if possible, what the patient had been doing before the event and if the patient reported any warning before the seizure. The patient is unable to stop true seizure activity voluntarily.

24. c. Nosebleeds and sore throats may be a sign of blood dyscrasias and should be reported to the healthcare provider. A reddish-pink discoloration of the urine may be expected. To prevent injury to the gums a soft toothbrush should be utilized. Orthostatic hypotension is not associated with phenytoin use.

25. a. Gingival hyperplasia is a common side effect of phenytoin. Excessive thirst and weight gain are not common with phenytoin.

26. a. The first-line drug of choice for acute status epilepticus is diazepam. Midazolam, propofol, and high-dose phenobarbital are administered for continued seizures.

27. a, b, c. Up to 33% of females with history of seizures can have increased seizure activity during pregnancy. Many antiseizure drugs have teratogenic properties. Antiseizure drugs increase the excretion of folic acid; therefore pregnant individuals should take daily folate supplement. Antiseizure drugs inhibit vitamin K, contributing to bleeding.

28. c. Valproic acid and topiramate are indicated for migraine. Diazepam can be used additionally for those with spasms, anxiety, and alcohol withdrawal. Clorazepate can be used for anxiety and alcohol withdrawal.

Clinical Judgment Unfolding Case Study
PHASE 1
Question 1

- 12-lead electrocardiogram (ECG) showed atrial fibrillation with ventricular rate of 135 beats/min.
- Serum sodium 130 mEq/L.
- Chest x-ray with ground-glass opacities bilaterally.
- Abdomen distended.
- Arterial blood gas revealed pH 7.28, pCO_2 52 mm Hg, and HCO_3 18 mEq/L.

Rationale:

Patients who drown require careful assessment of possible complications, such as hypoxemia and acidosis (McCall & Sternard, 2020); elevated pCO2 (35–45 mm Hg), decreased HCO3 (22–28 mEq/L), and decreased oxygen saturation (96%–100%) indicate acidemia and hypoxemia. Cardiac dysrhythmias may ensue (McCall & Sternard, 2020); therefore a 12-lead ECG is warranted. Any dysrhythmia, such as atrial fibrillation, needs further investigation. Electrolyte abnormalities can also occur (McCall & Sternard, 2020). Serum sodium of 130 mEq/L is below the normal range of 135–145 mEq/L and may indicate water ingestion. Distended abdomen can also be indicative of water ingestion. Any abnormal chest x-ray would need a follow-up. Ground-glass opacities within the lung field could indicate inhaled water (McCall & Sternard, 2020). Acidosis, hypoxemia, and electrolyte imbalance could all be risk factors for seizure activity. All other test results are normal.

References

McCall, J.D., & Sternard, B.T. (2020). Drowning. *StatPearls [Internet]*. Retrieved from https://www.ncbi.nlm.nih.gov/books/NBK430833/

McCuistion, L.E., DiMaggio, K.V., Winton, M.B., & Yeager, J.J. (2025). Pharmacology: A patient-centered nursing process approach, 12th ed. St. Louis, MO: Elsevier. pp. 220–228.

Question 2

Options for 1	Options for 2	Options for 3	Options for 4
drowning	tonic-clonic	Diazepam	2373
		phenytoin	

Rationale:

Even though emphysema and diabetes can cause acidosis, the most likely cause of this patient's current acid-base imbalance is related to her drowning with continued acid-base imbalance causing the patient to experience seizure activities. Seizure activities are classified by their characteristics. Muscle contractions that are dysrhythmic bilaterally and sustained indicate the patient is experiencing tonic-clonic (grand mal seizure) seizure activities. Tonic seizure is when there is sustained muscle contraction without being dysrhythmic. Clonic seizure is when the dysrhythmic muscle contractions are not sustained. Myoclonic seizure is an isolated clonic contractions or jerks that last 3–10 seconds and can be focal or massive myoclonia. Partial seizure involves one hemisphere of the brain with unilateral muscle involvement. Diazepam is an example of a benzodiazepine, and phenytoin is a hydantoin. The total amount of phenytoin the patient would receive is 2373 mg [(174/2.2) × 30] = 2373 mg.

Reference

McCuistion, L.E., DiMaggio, K.V., Winton, M.B., & Yeager, J.J. (2025). Pharmacology: A patient-centered nursing process approach, 12th ed. St. Louis, MO: Elsevier. pp. 220–228.

PHASE 2:
Question 3

c. Aspiration

e. Falls

f. Hyperglycemia

g. Myocardial infarction

h. Respiratory depression

i. Sepsis

j. Tissue hypoxia

Rationale:

Priority complications the nurse would monitor the patient for include aspiration, tissue hypoxia, myocardial infarction, hyperglycemia, respiratory depression, sepsis, and falls. Persons who sustained drowning are at risk for tissue hypoxia and aspiration pneumonia (McCall & Sternard, 2020). Patients with aspiration can develop pulmonary infection and, if not treated, can progress into sepsis. Sepsis can exacerbate tissue hypoxia. Tissue hypoxia to the brain can cause cerebral damage, and hypoxia to the cardiac muscles can result in myocardial infarction. Persons with continued seizure activity are at

risk for further injury, such as falls. Phenytoin and diazepam can suppress respiratory center in the brain further exacerbating tissue hypoxia. Hyperglycemia can be an adverse drug reaction from phenytoin, which is exacerbated by the patient being a diabetic.

References

McCall, J.D., & Sternard, B.T. (2020). Drowning. *StatPearls* [*Internet*]. Retrieved from https://www.ncbi.nlm.nih.gov/books/NBK430833/

McCuistion, L.E., DiMaggio, K.V., Winton, M.B., & Yeager, J.J. (2025). Pharmacology: A patient-centered nursing process approach, 12th ed. St. Louis, MO: Elsevier. pp. 220–228.

Question 4

Nurse's Response	Patient's Question	Appropriate Nurse's Response
	"I really do not want to take more medicine for the seizures."	"The antiseizure medications help prevent abnormal electrical impulses in your brain."
	"How long will I need to be taking the medicine?"	"Usually, persons with seizures are on antiseizure medicines for the rest of their life. But, if the person has been seizure free for 3–5 years, the doctor may stop the medicine."
	"Will I be able to get pregnant while on the medicine?"	"Be sure to discuss this with your doctor. Phenytoin can harm the fetus so a different antiseizure medication may be needed"
	"Will I need to decrease my insulin while on this medicine?"	"Phenytoin can cause blood sugars to increase, not decrease. You may need to increase your insulin dose."
	"My urine is reddish in color. Does this medicine cause me to bleed?"	"Phenytoin can cause your urine to turn pinkish-red or reddish-brown in color. This is normal and does not indicate you are bleeding."

Rationale:

Seizure disorder is due to abnormal electrical discharges from the brain causing involuntary, uncontrolled movements. The antiseizure medications help prevent abnormal electrical impulses in the brain. Antiseizure drugs are usually taken for the duration of one's life, but there are occasions when the person has been seizure free for 3–5 years, the doctor may taper off the medicine. Some of the side effects of phenytoin include hyperglycemia, cephalgia, dizziness, drowsiness, and insomnia, among others. The patient may need to increase their insulin dose. Also, urine may turn pinkish-red or reddish-brown in color. Patients who are contemplating pregnancy or become pregnant should discuss with their healthcare provider on alternative antiseizure drug. Phenytoin is teratogenic.

Reference

McCuistion, L.E., DiMaggio, K.V., Winton, M.B., & Yeager, J.J. (2025). Pharmacology: A patient-centered nursing process approach, 12th ed. St. Louis, MO: Elsevier. pp. 220–228.

PHASE 3:

Question 5

Discharge Teaching	Indicated	Contraindicated
"Decrease your insulin dosage by 4 units since phenytoin can cause hypoglycemia."		X
"Have dental checkups on a regular basis. Phenytoin can cause overgrowth of your gums."	X	
"You will need routine labs to monitor the drug level."	X	
"It is normal if you develop nosebleeds."		X
"You will need to eat a high-fat diet while you are on phenytoin for better drug action."		X
"Check your blood sugars more frequently."	X	

Rationale:

Teaching patients to lower their insulin dosage is contraindicated. Phenytoin can cause hyperglycemia, not hypoglycemia. Therefore patients may need to increase, not decrease, their insulin dosage. Teaching patients to have regular dental checkup while on phenytoin is indicated. Phenytoin can cause gingival hyperplasia or reddened gums and can bleed easily. Also, teaching them about the need for frequent lab work is indicated. For effective seizure control, therapeutic range for phenytoin is 10–20 mcg/mL. If it is outside this range, the dosage may need to be adjusted. Decreased therapeutic range can increase the risk of seizures, whereas higher than normal therapeutic range can cause adverse drug reactions, such as pancytopenia and liver failure. Patients should notify their healthcare provider if they develop nosebleeds. Nosebleeds or unusual bruises could indicate hematologic toxicity or blood dyscrasia. There is not enough information regarding patient's work environment. Teaching them to eat high-fat foods is contraindicated. Phenytoin is highly protein bound and must have adequate protein to prevent toxic level. Patients on phenytoin should be taught to check their blood sugars more frequently since phenytoin can prevent release of insulin from the pancreas.

Reference

McCuistion, L.E., DiMaggio, K.V., Winton, M.B., & Yeager, J.J. (2025). Pharmacology: A patient-centered nursing process approach, 12th ed. St. Louis, MO: Elsevier. pp. 220–228.

Question 6

Assessment Finding	Effective	Ineffective
Fingerstick blood sugar 98 mg/dL	X	
Patient states "I do not need to worry about getting pregnant since I am on the pill."		X
Blood pressure 94/50 mm Hg		X
Phenytoin drug level 17 mcg/mL	X	
Abdomen nondistended, active bowel sounds and nontender	X	
Gait even, smooth, and controlled	X	

Rationale:

Glucose of 98 mg/dL indicates effective control of blood glucose. Phenytoin can cause hyperglycemia. Persons prescribed phenytoin, especially those who have diabetes, should monitor their blood sugar more often. Patients may need to increase their insulin dose while on phenytoin. Ineffective teaching occurs when a female patient states they do not need to worry about pregnancy since they are on oral contraceptives. Phenytoin is teratogenic to the fetus. Female patients who are of childbearing age should use additional contraceptive method. Phenytoin drug level of 17 mcg/mL is within the therapeutic range of 10–20 mcg/mL indicating patient is receiving proper dose. Levels greater than 20 mcg/mL indicate toxicity. A blood pressure of 94/50 is hypotensive. Hypotension could be a later sign of phenytoin toxicity. Side effects of phenytoin include constipation, nausea, and vomiting. Abdomen that is nondistended and has active bowel sounds and nontender are normal expected findings for patients not experiencing gastrointestinal side effects. Noticing patient's gait as even, smooth, and controlled is effective finding. Ataxia and nystagmus are initial symptoms of phenytoin toxicity.

Reference

McCuistion, L.E., DiMaggio, K.V., Winton, M.B., & Yeager, J.J. (2025). Pharmacology: A patient-centered nursing process approach, 12th ed. St. Louis, MO: Elsevier. pp. 220–228.

CHAPTER 20: DRUGS FOR PARKINSONISM AND ALZHEIMER DISEASE

1. c
2. a
3. d
4. e
5. b
6. dopamine; acetylcholine
7. dopamine
8. levodopa
9. carbidopa
10. donepezil or rivastigmine
11. enhance
12. selegiline
13. carbidopa, levodopa, entacapone
14. trihexyphenidyl (also benztropine)
15. irreversible
16. Acetylcholine
17. Acetylcholinesterase inhibitors
18. IgG1 monoclonal antibody
19. a. Dizziness is a common side effect of carbidopa-levodopa. Constipation is a side effect, not diarrhea. Anxiety and nasal stuffiness are not a side effect of carbidopa-levodopa.
20. b, c, d, e. Carbidopa-levodopa may make the patient's movements smoother, although at high doses, dyskinesia may be noted. Jaundice will not result from missing doses. Extended-release drugs should not be crushed or cut; if the patient is unable to swallow tablets, then other preparations, such as liquid or oral disintegrating tablets, are available. Nausea and vomiting are side effects, so taking the drug with meals may be beneficial. There is no indication that carbidopa-levodopa affects glucose levels.

21. a, b, e. Tyramine-rich foods should be avoided, such as aged cheeses, chocolate, and yogurt. These foods should be avoided when taking selegiline to prevent a hypertensive crisis from occurring. Peanut butter and wheat bread are not high in tyramine.

22. d. An order for tricyclic antidepressant should be questioned. Tricyclic antidepressants decrease the effect of rivastigmine.

23. c. The nurse understand that levodopa will be decreased. When taken with levodopa, COMT inhibitors like entacapone will increase the levodopa combination in the brain.

24. a. Anticholinergic drugs are contraindicated in persons with glaucoma. Extreme caution is warranted for persons with heart problems and those with urinary retention, not urinary frequency. Shingles and diabetes are not contraindications.

25. a, c. Most medications used to treat persons with Parkinson disease can cause hallucinations. The dopamine agonists stimulate the dopamine agonist receptors and provide relief from Parkinson disease symptoms. Bromocriptine and pramipexole are two drugs that are classified as dopamine agonists. Selegiline is a monoamine oxidase B inhibitor and tolcapone is a catechol-*O*-methyltransferase inhibitor.

26. c. Memantine is prescribed for the treatment of mild to severe Alzheimer disease. Increased wandering and hostility can indicate that the disease is progressing and an increase in the dose may be beneficial. The maximum dose for memantine is 20 mg/day.

27. a. Sucking on hard candy or chewing sugarless gum may help with dry mouth associated with anticholinergic drugs such as benztropine mesylate. This drug is initially taken at bedtime and twice per day in divided doses as a maintenance dose. The nurse would remind the patient that all drug adjustments need to be made by the healthcare provider. Urinary retention is a side effect of anticholinergic drugs; however, the nurse would encourage the patient to urinate when the urge is felt and not on a set schedule.

Clinical Judgment Unfolding Case Study
Question 1

- History of three falls in the last 6 months with ecchymoses with various stages of healing to legs and arms
- Masked facial expressions
- Mild resting tremors to hands bilaterally
- Patient reports his feet "drags the floor"
- Positive for cogwheel rigidity

Rationale:

Falls, especially among older adults, need further investigation to determine the cause of the falls. Variegated skin colors indicate different stages of healing. Older ecchymoses would have yellowish tinge, while new ecchymoses are red. Masked facies, resting tremors, cogwheel rigidity, and feet dragging the floor can indicate Parkinson disease. Major features of Parkinson disease include rigidity (abnormal increased muscle tone), bradykinesia (slow movement), gait disturbances, and tremors. Rigidity increases with movement. Postural changes caused by rigidity and bradykinesia include the chest and head thrust forward with the knees and hips flexed, a shuffling gait, and the absence of arm swing. Other characteristic symptoms are masked facies (no facial expression), involuntary tremors of the head and neck, and pill-rolling motions of the hands. The tremors may be more prevalent at rest.

Reference

McCuistion, L.E., DiMaggio, K.V., Winton, M.B., & Yeager, J.J. (2025). Pharmacology: A patient-centered nursing process approach, 12th ed. St. Louis, MO: Elsevier. pp. 229–243.

Question 2

Options for 1	Options for 2	Options for 3	Options for 4	Options for 5
Dopamine	Acetylcholine	Decreased	Increased	Gamma-aminobutyric acid

Rationale:

Two main neurotransmitters within the brain that control movement are dopamine and acetylcholine (ACh). Some of the motor neurons, which are dopaminergic neurons, of the brain have degenerated resulting in an imbalance between dopamine and acetylcholine. Dopamine is an inhibitory neurotransmitter, while ACh is an excitatory neurotransmitter. The degeneration of the motor neuron results in a decreased level of dopamine. Dopamine "controls" and maintains ACh. Without dopamine, ACh level and its activities are not hindered. With less DA production, the excitatory response of ACh exceeds the inhibitory response of dopamine. An excessive amount of ACh stimulates neurons that release gamma-aminobutyric acid (GABA). With increased stimulation of GABA the symptomatic movement disorders of Parkinson disease occur.

Reference

McCuistion, L.E., DiMaggio, K.V., Winton, M.B., & Yeager, J.J. (2025). Pharmacology: A patient-centered nursing process approach, 12th ed. St. Louis, MO: Elsevier. pp. 229–243.

PHASE 2
Question 3

- Falls
- Functional ability
- Gastrointestinal distress
- Hypotension

Rationale:

Parkinson disease is a disorder that primarily affects the motor neurons. Carbidopa-levodopa is a dopaminergic drug that enhances the dopamine levels in the brain. Some of the side effects of this drug include dizziness and orthostatic hypotension, which can cause falls. Since the patient also takes lisinopril and hydrochlorothiazide for hypertension, carbidopa-levodopa can enhance the action of the antihypertensives, further exacerbating the risk for falls. As Parkinson disease progresses, the functional capability declines. Also, the dopaminergic can cause worsening involuntary movements and dyskinesia. Carbidopa-levodopa can cause gastrointestinal distress, such as nausea and vomiting. It has the tendency to cause constipation, not diarrhea. Fluctuations of blood glucose are not a common side effect of carbidopa-levodopa.

Reference

McCuistion, L.E., DiMaggio, K.V., Winton, M.B., & Yeager, J.J. (2025). Pharmacology: A patient-centered nursing process approach, 12th ed. St. Louis, MO: Elsevier. pp. 229–243.

Question 4

- Administer the medication with small amount of food.
- Assess for orthostatic hypotension.
- Observe patient's ability to perform activities of daily living, such as brushing teeth.
- Place patient as "high fall risk."

Rationale:

Since the patient is complaining of "nausea 30 minutes after taking the medicine," it would be logical for the nurse to provide a low-protein snack to take with the drug. Food high in protein can decrease the absorption of levodopa, thereby decreasing nausea. Carbidopa-levodopa can cause orthostatic hypotension. The nurse would not administer antinausea medication since it is not known if the patient has antinausea medication prescribed. The nurse would need to assess the patient's blood pressure for hypotension, especially with position changes. It is common for sweat and urine to become dark when exposed to air while taking carbidopa-levodopa. It is not necessary for the patient to notify the nurse. However, the patient should be informed clothing can be stained because of darker sweat and/or urine. It is not necessary to obtain fingerstick blood sugar prior to administering carbidopa-levodopa. Patients with Parkinson disease have difficulty in motor coordination, which includes having shuffling gait, involuntary tremors of the limbs, rigidity of muscles, and slowness of movement that can increase their risk to falls. These patients should be designated as "high fall risk." Additionally, nurses would need to assess the ability of patients to perform their activities of daily living, such as brushing teeth. The involuntary tremors and rigidity of muscles should decrease within 30 to 60 minutes of dosing, thereby improving their function.

Reference

McCuistion, L.E., DiMaggio, K.V., Winton, M.B., & Yeager, J.J. (2025). Pharmacology: A patient-centered nursing process approach, 12th ed. St. Louis, MO: Elsevier. pp. 229–243.

PHASE 3:
Question 5

Nursing Action	Potential Complication	Appropriate Nursing Action for Complication
	Patient reports increased dizziness	Check blood pressure with position changes (orthostasis)
	Falls	Consult case worker to assess home environment
	Darkened area to clothing around the axillary region	Inform the patient this is harmless
	Patient reports of increased head bobbing	Notify healthcare provider
	Increased nausea with medicine	Provide small low-protein snack

Rationale:

Carbidopa can enhance the effects of antihypertensives, such as lisinopril and hydrochlorothiazide. Patient and his daughter should be informed what signs and symptoms, such as dizziness, to report to their healthcare provider. Dizziness can indicate orthostatic hypotension and the dose of the antihypertensives may need to be decreased. Changing positions slowly is important to prevent orthostasis hypotension, thereby reducing incidences of falls. Consulting a case worker to assess home environment may be necessary. Persons with Parkinson disease are at an increased risk of falls due to mobility issues. Home environment should be assessed and potential obstacles should be decreased, such as area rugs, to minimize falls. Carbidopa-levodopa may cause patients to sweat more and/or the color of their sweat may become dark and can stain clothing. Patients and family members must

be informed that this is harmless and is nothing to be concerned about. To maximize absorption of carbidopa-levodopa, it is best for patients to take the medicine on an empty stomach. However, a common side effect of carbidopa-levodopa is gastrointestinal distress. If this occurs, the medication can be taken with a small amount of food. Sugar-free candy can be encouraged to relieve dry mouth due to a common side effect from carbidopa-levodopa.

Reference

McCuistion, L.E., DiMaggio, K.V., Winton, M.B., & Yeager, J.J. (2025). Pharmacology: A patient-centered nursing process approach, 12th ed. St. Louis, MO: Elsevier. pp. 229–243.

Question 6
Progress Notes:

- Preparing protein shakes
- Sitting blood pressure 132/88 mm Hg and pulse 64 beats/min; standing blood pressure 110/62 mm Hg and pulse 80 beats/min. Patient needing moderate assistance to stand. Flat facial expression, "pill-rolling" bilaterally, and head bobbing noted while in sitting position
- Apical pulses irregular with 60-84 beats/min

Rationale:

Carbidopa-levodopa should be taken on an empty stomach. If gastric distress, such as nausea, occurs, then the medication can be taken with small amount of low-protein food. High-protein diet, such as protein shakes, decreases the rate of absorption which would decrease the amount of available drug for therapeutic effects. Changes in the blood pressure from sitting to standing indicate orthostatic hypotension. This finding in addition to continued signs of Parkinson disease would need to be provided to the healthcare provider. Symptoms of parkinsonism usually decrease within 30–60 minutes of dosing with carbidopa-levodopa. Continue masked facies, "pill-rolling," and head bobbing are indications that carbidopa-levodopa is not effective. Cardiac dysrhythmia as indicated by an apical pulse being irregular with 60–80 beats/min can be a sign of cardiac toxicity. The patient most likely will need an alternative antiparkinson drug.

Reference

McCuistion, L.E., DiMaggio, K.V., Winton, M.B., & Yeager, J.J. (2025). Pharmacology: A patient-centered nursing process approach, 12th ed. St. Louis, MO: Elsevier. pp. 229–243.

CHAPTER 21: DRUGS FOR NEUROMUSCULAR DISORDERS AND MUSCLE SPASMS

1. b
2. d
3. a

4. c
5. traumatic; debilitating disorders
6. hyperactive; antiinflammatory
7. decrease; increase
8. Myasthenia gravis is an autoimmune disorder that involves an antibody attacking the acetylcholine receptor (AChR) sites, eventually decreasing the number of the receptor sites for acetylcholine (ACh). ACh is a neurotransmitter that transmits nerve impulses to the muscles. Without proper transmission, muscle contractions become ineffective leading to muscle weakness. Drugs used to treat myasthenia gravis (MG) are the acetylcholinesterase (AChE) inhibitors (cholinesterase inhibitors and anticholinesterase), such as neostigmine or pyridostigmine. They inhibit the action of AChE, which allows more activation of the cholinergic receptors. One of the newest monoclonal antibodies is a neonatal Fc receptor blocker, such as rozanolixizumab. When the antibodies bind to the neonatal Fc receptor, circulating antibodies decrease.
9. Multiple sclerosis (MS) is an autoimmune disorder that attacks the myelin sheath of the nerve fibers of the central nervous system, resulting in plaques. Drugs used to treat MS include corticosteroids and immunomodulators, such as teriflunomide, alemtuzumab, and glatiramer acetate. A new monoclonal antibody, ublituximab, binds to CD20 receptor on B lymphocytes causing cell lysis.
10. b. Pyridostigmine increases muscle strength in patients with myasthenia gravis. Increased salivation and miosis are signs and symptoms of overdose. Bradycardia, not tachycardia, can be an adverse drug effect.
11. b. Drooling, excessive tearing, sweating, and miosis are signs of a cholinergic crisis, an overdose of AChE inhibitors.
12. a. Atropine, an anticholinergic, is the antidote for AChE inhibitor, such as pyridostigmine. Diazepam is a benzodiazepine used to treat muscle spasms. Neostigmine and pyridostigmine are AChE inhibitors; they will worsen cholinergic crisis.
13. c. Multiple sclerosis is difficult to diagnose. MRI, assessing brain's electrical activity, or analysis of cerebrospinal fluid can aid in confirming the diagnosis.
14. d. There is an increased toxicity when taken with tetracycline. AChE inhibitor can cause gastrointestinal distress. Histamine₂ blocker can decrease these side effects. Another side effect of AChE inhibitor is bradycardia. Risk of bradycardia increases when taking propranolol; the nurse would need to monitor more closely the patient's heart rate. There is no concern with cephalosporin and AChE inhibitors.
15. c. Azathioprine is an immunosuppressant, and interferon-β is an immunomodulator. Both decrease the inflammatory process of the nerve fibers. Interferon-β delays neurological deterioration.

Decreased inflammation and delaying of deterioration will decrease spasticity and hopefully muscular movement will improve. They do not form new neurons and axons nor will they stop the progression of the disease, but they can delay the deterioration.
16. b. Centrally acting muscle relaxant, such as baclofen, has actions to the neuronal activities in the brain and spinal cord. They suppress hyperreflexia and muscle spasms that do not respond to other forms of therapy. By suppressing the spasms, pain is decreased, which allows increased movement.
17. a, c. Centrally acting muscle relaxants, such as methocarbamol, can cause drowsiness and change the color of the urine. Other side effects include dizziness, lightheadedness, headaches, altered taste, and anorexia, not increased appetite.
18. b. Diazepam can increase intraocular pressure and is contraindicated in narrow-angle glaucoma.

Clinical Judgment Standalone Case Study
Answer:

Health History	Nurses' Notes	Vital Signs	Laboratory Results
1520: Postop day 1. Splint to right leg dry and intact. 3 × 6 cm pinkish slightly wet area noted to right splint anteriorly mid foreleg. Toes pink with brisk cap refill. C/o "just feeling weak" and "no energy." Lungs clear throughout area. No chest pain. Speech slightly slurred. "My vision seems to be blurry." PERRL.			

Health History	Nurses' Notes	Vital Signs	Laboratory Results
1020: Temp: 100.9°F BP: 92/58 left brachial HR: 54 bpm, regular, left radial RR: 14 bpm SpO2: 91% RA			

Rationale:

The patient is exhibiting myasthenic crisis due to being NPO and missing doses of pyridostigmine, in addition to increased stress (trauma and surgery) on the body. Persons with myasthenia gravis have the inability to manage autonomic changes to the body due to lack of ACh. Therefore people with MG have difficulty in muscle contractions. MG affects the voluntary muscles, such as those that control eye and eyelid movement, facial expression, chewing, and swallowing, causing blurry vision and slurred speech.

MG can also affect the respiratory muscles causing shortness of breath, which causes low oxygen levels. BP and HR variability can also occur with myasthenic crisis. The nurse would need to notify the healthcare provider immediately and replace the missing glucocorticoids.

The drainage is an expected finding 1 day after surgery.

CHAPTER 22: ANTIPSYCHOTICS AND ANXIOLYTICS

1. e
2. d
3. f
4. g
5. a
6. h
7. b
8. c
9. thought processes; behaviors; dopamine
10. dihydroindolones; thioxanthenes; butyrophenones; dibenzoxazepines
11. drowsiness
12. pruritus; photosensitivity
13. decrease
14. are not
15. tolerance
16. sedative-hypnotics
17. c
18. a
19. a
20. b
21. b
22. c
23. c. Neuroleptics are considered antipsychotics that modify psychotic behaviors and exert antipsychotic effects. Anxiolytics treat anxiety and insomnia. Antidepressants treat depressive disorders; antipsychotics worsen depression.
24. b. The nurse would inform the patient that antipsychotic drugs can take 3–6 weeks before full therapeutic effects occur. While psychotherapy may help, it is not required for antipsychotics to have therapeutic effects. Even though the onset may be minutes to hours, its full therapeutic effect does not occur until weeks later.
25. b. Orthostatic hypotension may occur with phenothiazines and nonphenothiazine drugs within this class. The patient should be encouraged to change positions slowly to prevent orthostatic hypotension. Patients should abstain from alcohol while on antipsychotics; they can worsen drowsiness, dizziness, and hypotension. Any antipsychotic should not be abruptly stopped.
26. d. Pseudoparkinsonism, major side effect of typical antipsychotics, is a symptom similar to Parkinson disease. Shuffling gait is one example of EPS. Other EPS include mask-like facies, rigidity, tremors at rest (not intentional tremors), pill-rolling, motions of the hands, and bradykinesia.

27. a. Benztropine is an anticholinergic antiparkinson drug. Bethanechol is an antispasmodic for urinary retention. Buspirone is an anxiolytic. Doxepin is an antidepressant.
28. b. Fluphenazine belongs to the piperazine subclass of phenothiazines. Chlorpromazine is an aliphatic phenothiazine. Thioridazine is a piperidine. Thioxanthene is a nonphenothiazine.
29. c, d, e. There are numerous side effects associated with fluphenazine, including dizziness, headache, and nausea; the patient should be encouraged to notify the prescriber if any of these symptoms occur. The drug is to be taken daily. Alcohol should not be consumed while on any antipsychotics. Either hypo- or hypertension may be an indication of an adverse reaction. Although it may be safe to take some herbal medications while taking fluphenazine, taking kava can increase dystonic reactions.
30. c. Because of less effective hepatic and renal function, doses of antipsychotics should be decreased by 25%–50% in older patients.
31. d. Overdose of phenothiazines can cause respiratory compromise. Maintaining a patent airway is a priority. Once airway is patent, then establishing an IV and administering activated charcoal and anticholinergics may be necessary.
32. a. Haloperidol has a sedative effect on patients. Haloperidol is contraindicated in patients with liver dysfunction. In older adults the dosage may need to be decreased. Like other neuroleptics, it can cause extrapyramidal syndrome.
33. c. Atypical antipsychotics, such as risperidone and clozapine, block serotonin and dopaminergic receptors. Butyrophenones, phenothiazines, and thioxanthenes are typical antipsychotic drugs.
34. c. D_2 antagonists can cause EPS. Atypical antipsychotics have a weak affinity to these receptors, thus decreasing the amount and severity of EPS.
35. d. Atypical antipsychotics have a strong affinity for D_4 and they block serotonin receptors.
36. b. Hyperglycemia is a side effect of taking risperidone. Blood glucose levels should be obtained at baseline and monitored carefully.
37. b. Alprazolam is a benzodiazepine. Benzodiazepines are used for severe or prolonged anxiety.
38. a, b, c, d. Patients with glaucoma, liver damage, subcortical brain damage, and any continued blood dyscrasia should not take fluphenazine.
39. a, b, d, e. Lorazepam is a frequently prescribed anxiolytic and is also indicated for patients with alcohol withdrawal, anxiety with depression, preoperative induction (lessen anxiety), and status epilepticus.

Case Study: Critical Thinking

1. Clonazepam is a benzodiazepine that is in the same family as diazepam, lorazepam, and alprazolam. It

is used for anxiety associated with depression and seizures.

2. Benzodiazepines enhance the action of gamma-aminobutyric acid (GABA), an inhibitory neurotransmitter. It has a rapid mechanism of action and is readily absorbed from the gastrointestinal tract.

3. Side effects include drowsiness, dizziness, and coma if taken in large doses. The action of benzodiazepines is potentiated when taken with alcohol.

4. The patient may have taken an overdose. A respiratory rate of 8 breaths/min and an O_2 saturation of 78% require immediate action by the nurse. Maintaining an airway is the priority intervention. Oxygen should be administered, and an airway adjunct should be inserted. Ventilation should be assisted with a bag mask and high-flow oxygen until the airway is secured. An IV will need to be established and flumazenil, a benzodiazepine antagonist, administered. Flumazenil has a quick onset but is only effective for benzodiazepine overdoses. An emetic is not an option for this patient because the patient is unresponsive. Gastric lavage is the intervention of choice. Blood pressure may need to be supported with IV vasopressors.

CHAPTER 23: ANTIDEPRESSANTS AND MOOD STABILIZERS

1. False. Herbal supplements, such as St. Johns wort, decrease reuptake of the neurotransmitters, such as serotonin, norepinephrine, and dopamine.
2. True
3. False. Serotonin modulators, such as selective serotonin reuptake inhibitors (SSRIs) and serotonin-norepinephrine reuptake inhibitors (SNRIs), are considered first-line therapy for depression. MAOIs are used for patients who do not respond to tricyclic antidepressants.
4. False. Amitriptyline is a tricyclic antidepressant (TCA).
5. True
6. 2–4 weeks
7. increase; increase; decrease
8. St. Johns wort
9. second-generation antidepressants; dopamine, norepinephrine, serotonin
10. stimulate; central nervous system
11. Lithium; bipolar affective
12. narrow; 0.8–1 mEq/L
13. increase; caffeine; loop; decrease
14. generalized anxiety disorder and social anxiety disorder
15. grapefruit juice; toxicity
16. b, c
17. c
18. b, c
19. b, c
20. c
21. b, c
22. a, b, c
23. a
24. a
25. b
26. d
27. c
28. b
29. c. Imipramine, a tricyclic antidepressant (TCA), is also indicated for enuresis, involuntary urination while sleeping.
30. d. The maximum daily dose of phenelzine is 90 mg. The initial dose is 15 mg/day in three divided doses.
31. b. Orthostatic hypotension is a frequent side effect of tricyclic antidepressants (TCAs). The patient should be encouraged to change positions slowly to avoid this side effect. Amitriptyline can cause tachycardia, not bradycardia. The onset of amitriptyline is 1–3 weeks, not 12 hours. Since amitriptyline has an anticholinergic action, it should be taken at night, not during the day.
32. a, b, e. Foods high in tyramine, such as bananas, chocolate, and wine, are contraindicated in a patient who is taking a monoamine oxidase inhibitor (MAOI), such as isocarboxazid. Other foods that are high in tyramine include aged cheeses, processed meats, and soybeans or soy products. These foods have sympathomimetic-like effects and can cause hypertensive crisis.
33. d. St. Johns wort is a common herbal remedy for depression. St. Johns wort, when taken in combination with selective serotonin reuptake inhibitor (SSRI) drugs, such as fluoxetine, can precipitate serotonin syndrome, which presents as headache, sweating, and agitation. Ephedra and ginseng can cause palpitations, heart attack, and hypertensive crisis when taken with MAOIs, not SSRIs.
34. c. SSRIs have less sedative effect. They also do not cause hypotension, anticholinergic effects, or cardiotoxicity. However, SSRIs can cause sexual dysfunction.
35. c. Monitoring the patient is one of the most important roles of the nurse. Trending vital signs, weight, and lab work will be important to the patient's ongoing care. Polyuria (excess urination) is a common side effect and can be an early sign of lithium toxicity. Polyuria causes excess thirst and weight loss. The patient needs to maintain a fluid intake of 2–3 L of fluid/day initially and must be especially vigilant to maintain an adequate intake in hot weather. Patients during manic phase frequently stop taking their drug when they feel better. They must be advised to continue taking the drug even if they feel better.
36. a. Monitoring renal function in a patient taking lithium should be completed with weekly blood work, which includes BUN and creatinine level measurements.
37. b. The patient's lithium level is still subtherapeutic, and the patient remains in a manic phase.

Therapeutic range for lithium is 0.8–1.2 mEq/L. Any lithium value over 1.5 mEq/L should be immediately reported to the healthcare provider.

38. a. The patient needs further education regarding the purpose of the drug. Lithium may be used in bipolar disorder as a mood stabilizer, but its effect is on the manic phase. The drug should be taken with food. Tyramine-rich foods, such as caffeine, should be avoided.

39. d. Desvenlafaxine is a serotonin-norepinephrine reuptake inhibitor (SNRI). Side effects of desvenlafaxine may include drowsiness, insomnia, photosensitivity, and ejaculatory dysfunction, among others. Taking St. Johns wort while taking desvenlafaxine increases the risk of serotonin syndrome or neuroleptic malignant syndrome.

Case Study: Critical Thinking

1. SSRIs block the reuptake of the neurotransmitter serotonin at the nerve terminal. One of the possible causes of depression is a lack of circulating serotonin. By preventing the reuptake, more serotonin is available and depression is lessened. SSRIs may be effective in the treatment of depression in cases where the patient was nonresponsive to a TCA. Additional benefits of SSRIs are prevention of migraine headaches.

2. In the initial interview the nurse would inquire about medical history, prescription and OTC drugs, allergies, and past coping behavior. The nurse would ask direct questions about suicidal thoughts. The use of herbal products should also be investigated. A thorough psychiatric history should be obtained with a specific focus on past episodes of depression and treatments. Vital signs should be obtained as well as weight. Baseline laboratory work needs to be reviewed, since fluoxetine is used with caution in patients with a history of renal or liver problems.

3. Discharge teaching includes recommendations for counseling, since studies have shown that drug and counseling together are more successful than either modality alone. Support groups have also shown benefit. The nurse would teach the patient to take fluoxetine as prescribed and inform the patient that it may take 2–4 weeks for the onset of action. Alcohol should be avoided while taking SSRIs. Fluoxetine should be taken with food. Dry mouth may be a side effect that can be relieved somewhat with sucking on hard candy or chewing gum. If the patient feels suicidal at any time, she should contact the healthcare provider or suicide hotline or go to the emergency department immediately. Even though SSRIs can have additional benefits in the prevention of migraine headache, they can precipitate headache. Since the patient is postmenopausal, she needs to be taught that sexual dysfunction can increase.

CHAPTER 24: ANTIINFLAMMATORIES

1. d
2. c
3. e
4. h
5. b
6. a
7. f
8. g
9. i
10. injury; infection
11. redness (erythema); swelling (edema); heat; pain; loss of function
12. delayed
13. does
14. higher (or increased)
15. arthritic
16. d. The vascular phase of the inflammation is associated with vasodilation and increased vascular permeability. This allows leukocytes and other substances to filter into the inflamed tissue.
17. a, c, d, e. Heartburn can be a side effect of NSAIDs. Taking NSAIDs with food may help decrease heartburn. Dark, tarry, or bloody bowel movements are an indication of GI bleeding, which is an adverse effect of NSAID use. The dosage range for NSAIDs varies from drug to drug, but large doses may cause erosive esophagitis, which would cause indigestion-type pain. There are many types of heartburn, including those associated with acute myocardial infarction. Not all heartburn is of GI origin attributable to a drug effect.
18. b. NSAIDs inhibit the production of prostaglandin, thereby decreasing inflammation and pain. Ibuprofen is not a COX-2 inhibitor. Ibuprofen does not bind to opiate receptor sites, and it does not promote vasodilation.
19. a. Warfarin is an anticoagulant that may be taken by patients with atrial fibrillation. Aspirin displaces warfarin from its protein-binding site. This increases the anticoagulant effect and may lead to excessive bleeding, which may initially be indicated by bruising. Although the other drugs may have drug-drug interactions, they do not cause increased anticoagulant effects, as evidenced by the bruising.
20. d. Aspirin should not be given to young children due to the risk of Reye syndrome, which can be fatal. Hypersensitivity reactions, such as ringing in the ears, can occur in any person, but they are not the most concerning. Side effects, such as GI distress, can occur in anyone taking NSAIDs, but they are not the most concerning.
21. c. Sulfasalazine, a salicylate derivative, can cause bronchospasms in a patient with asthma; therefore its use is contraindicated to those with known sensitivity.

22. a. Ibuprofen is a propionic acid derivative, which has a decreased risk of GI disturbances. Ibuprofen should be taken with food. It has a short half-life and is highly protein bound. There are many drug-drug interactions. Ibuprofen can increase bleed time when taken with warfarin. When taken with aspirin, the effects of the ibuprofen are decreased.

23. b. Since ibuprofen is excreted in the urine, adequate fluid intake and urine output should be maintained. Ibuprofen can have negative consequences during early pregnancy and is contraindicated during third trimester. It can cause GI upset and diarrhea.

24. c. Piroxicam has a long half-life (50 hours). Because of its long half-life, it is taken once daily. Like other NSAIDs, it can cause GI irritation. It has many drug-drug interactions, and its onset is delayed.

25. a. Colchicine inhibits the migration of leukocytes to the inflamed area, thereby decreasing inflammation. Colchicine does not inhibit the synthesis of uric acid nor does it block the reabsorption or remove uric acid. Colchicine does not block the release of prostaglandins.

26. b. Probenecid is used for the inhibition of the reabsorption of uric acid in the kidneys, thereby increasing the excretion. Its primary action is not the retention of urate crystals. Ureters are tubes for the pathway of urine; it is not the primary action of probenecid.

27. a. Etanercept neutralizes tumor necrosis factor (TNF). This neutralizing alters the inflammatory process. Anakinra, not etanercept, inhibits IL-1 from binding to interleukin receptors found in bones and cartilages. Celecoxib inhibits COX-2 receptors to alter the inflammatory process. Uricosurics, such as probenecid, block the reabsorption of uric acid.

28. c. Steroids should be tapered over 5–10 days.

29. a, c, d. Corticosteroids may be used for a variety of disease processes including flare-ups of arthritic conditions. They have a long half-life and are usually taken once a day in a large prescribed dose and then the dose is tapered for 5–10 days. Lengthy corticosteroid therapy is never stopped abruptly. They may be given in combination with other drugs including prostaglandin inhibitors.

30. b, c, d, e. Fluid intake should be increased to promote uric acid excretion. Avoiding alcohol is important because alcohol causes an overproduction, as well as an underexcretion, of uric acid. Purine is required to synthesize uric acid. Taking the drug with food will help avoid GI upset. Some studies have shown that vitamin C may help increase uric acid elimination; however, large doses of supplemental vitamin C are not recommended, and since vitamin C is an acid, there is a higher risk of kidney stone formation.

31. d. Although side effects of infliximab may include headache, dizziness, cough, nausea, and vomiting, an adverse reaction to the drug is severe infection attributable to immunosuppression. A fever of 101.9°F in an adult who is taking infliximab needs to be evaluated.

Case Study: Critical Thinking

1. The normal therapeutic dosage is 325–650 mg q4h as needed, up to a maximum of 4 g/day. If the patient takes 975 mg every 4 hours as stated, this patient will be taking 5850 mg/day, which exceeds the maximum daily dose.

2. Side effects may include anorexia, nausea, vomiting, dizziness, abdominal pain, and heartburn.

3. Signs of overdose or adverse reactions include tinnitus, GI bleeding, blood dyscrasias including thrombocytopenia and leukopenia, and liver failure.

4. The patient appears to be hypotensive, tachycardic, and tachypneic. These vital signs could be indicative of a hypovolemic state, potentially attributable to a GI bleed. Interpretation of the vital signs is compounded because of the use of caffeine with the aspirin. Metabolic acidosis due to aspirin overdose can also cause tachypnea.

CHAPTER 25: ANALGESICS

1. gate, nociceptors
2. endorphins
3. peripheral, prostaglandins
4. increased
5. c
6. f
7. e
8. a
9. b
10. d
11. central nervous system; peripheral nervous system
12. respiration; coughing
13. antitussive; antidiarrheal
14. head injury; respiratory depression (shock and hypotension are also acceptable answers)
15. side effect; healthcare provider
16. IV
17. c
18. b
19. e
20. a
21. f
22. g
23. d
24. a. A major side effect of meperidine is decreased blood pressure (hypotension). All opioids have the potential to decrease (not increase) pulse rate, respiratory rate, and urine output.
25. c. Opioid toxicity will cause pinpoint pupils, not dilation. Respiratory depression, nausea, vomiting, constipation, and urinary retention can also occur with opioid overdose.

26. b. Monitoring fluid intake is the least important. Assessing bowel sounds helps identify constipation, a common side effect of opioids. The patient's pain should be frequently assessed using a pain scale. Other assessments include vital signs, noting rate and depth of respirations for future comparisons. Opioids commonly decrease respirations and systolic blood pressure.

27. b, c, d, e. There are no dietary restrictions associated with the use of opioids. The patient should not exceed the recommended dosage. Adequate fluid intake and inclusion of fiber in the diet will assist with constipation. Patients should always be taught the side effects to report.

28. d. Drugs with long duration of action (long half-life) are more beneficial to patients dealing with chronic pain. If chronic pain needs treatment, nonopioid drugs are preferred over opioids. If opioids are used, in addition to long duration of action, they should be oral or transdermal formulation, not injectable.

29. b. An opioid antagonist is naloxone. Flumazenil is an antagonist to benzodiazepines. Butorphanol and pentazocine are opioid agonist-antagonists.

30. b. Opioid agonist-antagonists may be used to decrease substance use disorder. Opioid agonist-antagonist can cause renal failure and respiratory depression. There is still a potential to cause dependence. They are indicated for acute moderate to severe pain.

31. b. Withdrawal symptoms attributable to physical dependence can result 24–48 hours after the last opioid dose and include irritability, diaphoresis, restlessness, muscle twitching, tachycardia, and hypertension.

32. c. Controlled-released morphine has 8–12 hours of pain relief. Other types of morphine have a duration of action of 3–6 hours.

33. b, d, e. The best people to assess how a child is acting are those who are with the child the most. Ask the parents or other caregivers how the child usually acts due to pain. Utilizing developmentally appropriate communication skills and pain scales should yield the best result for the nurse treating a child's pain. Opioids are appropriate to utilize if nonopioid methods are ineffective.

34. b. Cholestyramine will decrease the effectiveness of acetaminophen. An alternative nonopioid would be an option for the patient instead of stopping the cholestyramine.

35. d. A priority assessment for a patient taking opioid agonist-antagonist is respiratory depression. While opioids can cause constipation and dysuria, they are not a priority over respiratory system. A patient effectively managed on opioids can have hypotension, not hypertension.

36. b. The best action by the nurse would be to administer the dose and contact the healthcare provider. Dose should be withheld for respiratory rate of 10 and below, not 12. Since the patient is not in respiratory distress, the dose should not be withheld due to inadequate pain relief. The dose should be given, then the healthcare provider should be contacted.

37. c. The dose may be too high for the patient. Older adults should use a lower dose fentanyl transdermal patch to avoid severe side effects. Side effects from the use of opioids are more pronounced in older adults. The rates of metabolism and excretion of drugs are decreased; thereby, drug accumulation may occur.

38. c. Alcohol must be avoided while taking opioid pain medications. Alcohol can intensify the CNS effect of the opioid. The patient should take the drug as prescribed and should avoid other drugs, including over the counters, that contain NSAIDs. Opioids can cause constipation and laxatives may be warranted.

39. c. Ketorolac is used for short-term pain management and should not be taken for more than 5 days.

40. a, b, d. Nonopioid pain drugs, such as acetaminophen, ibuprofen, and aspirin, are appropriate for minor injuries such as abrasions and minor aches and pains. Some nonopioids, such as aspirin and ibuprofen, have antiinflammatory effects that can further lessen pain and swelling. But, aspirin also has an antiplatelet effect and should not be taken concomitantly with other antiplatelets or anticoagulants. Hydrocodone and morphine are opioids and should not be taken for mild pain.

Clinical Judgment Standalone Case Study
Answers:

Options for 1	Options for 2	Options for 3
Hyperexcited	Elevated	Altered taste

Rationale:

The etiology of migraine headache is unknown, but a common theory is that a series of cerebral neurovascular events initiate the headache. The neurons in the cerebral cortex become hyperexcited. Unrelieved pain can elevate blood pressure, heart rate, and respiratory rate. Treatment for migraine headache includes analgesics, opioid analgesics, ergot alkaloids, and triptans. Sumatriptan, a triptan, is a 5-HT receptor agonist and is prescribed to relieve migraine headache. Common side effects include altered taste (dysgeusia), dizziness, and nausea.

Reference

McCuistion, L.E., DiMaggio, K.V., Winton, M.B., & Yeager, J.J. (2025). Pharmacology: A patient-centered nursing process approach, 12th ed. St. Louis, MO: Elsevier. pp. 303–320.

CHAPTER 26: PENICILLINS, OTHER BETA-LACTAMS, AND CEPHALOSPORINS

1. f
2. b
3. g
4. e
5. a
6. h
7. c
8. d
9. i·
10. d. Superinfection is a secondary infection caused by the disturbance of the normal microbial flora during antibiotic therapy. Common signs and symptoms of superinfection include vaginal itching and discharge due to fungal overgrowth. While poor hygiene can cause infection, the patient has been taking antibiotics. It is less likely the infection is due to poor hygiene. Hypersensitivity reactions usually include rash and difficulty breathing, not infection. Kidney infection is usually exhibited with dysuria and hematuria, not vaginal itching.
11. a. The nurse will teach the patient that ceftriaxone is given via IM or IV. It is not given orally. About 10% of population who has hypersensitivity to penicillin has cross-reaction to cephalosporin, such as ceftriaxone. Ceftriaxone, when taken concomitantly with anticoagulants, increases risk of bleeding. Ceftriaxone can increase liver enzymes and international normalized ratio (INR).
12. b. Cefprozil monohydrate is given for skin infections. The usual dosage range for adults is 250–500 mg/d, with a maximum dose of 1 g/d. Patients with CrCl <30 mL/min adjust dose by half; therefore the maximum dose would be 500 mg/d.
13. c. The appropriate dose for aztreonam would be 1500 mg q8h. The range for an adult dose is 1–2 g q8h–q12h, with a maximum dose of 8 g/d. The amount and frequency of drugs should be considered to obtain therapeutic response and a steady state. 500 mg q8h is too low of a dose to achieve therapeutic response. 500 mg q6h is too low of a dose. 2000 mg daily will result in low serum level.
14. c. Loop diuretics, such as furosemide, can cause nephrotoxicity when taken concomitantly with ceftriaxone. Other class of drugs that can cause nephrotoxicity include intravenous calcium salts. ACEI, antidysrhythmics, and NSAIDs are not implicated in causing nephrotoxicity when taken with ceftriaxone.
15. a. Loss of appetite, diarrhea, nausea, and vomiting are common side effects of cephalosporins, such as ceftriaxone. These side effects could cause weight loss. The nurse would encourage the patient that when the antibiotic is completed, appetite will resume and weight loss will stop. It is possible that GI bleeding can occur, but the patient is concerned about weight loss, not bleeding. Ceftriaxone is administered IM or IV, not orally; therefore absorption problem is not a concern. It is possible the patient will begin to eat more and regain weight as the illness resolves; however, the antibiotic is what is causing the side effects, not the illness.
16. b. Acidic fruits or juices, such as orange juice, may make dicloxacillin less effective. Abdominal pain is a possible side effect. The entire course of antibiotics must be completed to prevent the development of resistance. Rashes can be associated with dicloxacillin but may also be an indication of an allergic reaction. The patient would need to be evaluated for other indications of an allergic reaction, such as difficulty breathing or hives.
17. d. Uricosurics, such as probenecid, compete for renal tubular clearance which can decrease the excretion of cefotetan. Intravenous calcium salts are contraindicated when taking some cephalosporin; they can deposit crystals in the lungs and kidneys. They do not increase serum levels of cefotetan. Laxatives do not increase levels of cephalosporins. Opioid solutions that contain alcohol can have disulfiram-like reactions if coadministered with cefotetan; they do not increase the serum levels of cefotetan.
18. b. Penicillin's beta-lactam ring structure inhibits bacterial cell-wall synthesis. Penicillins, including penicillin V, can be both bacteriostatic and bactericidal. Amphotericin B and polymyxin alter membrane permeability. Aminoglycosides and tetracyclines are some drugs that inhibit protein synthesis. Sulfonamides and trimethoprim are some antibiotics that interfere with cellular metabolism.
19. c. Antibiotics, especially penicillins, may make oral contraceptives less effective, so an alternate method of birth control should be utilized. The patient does not need to increase dietary calcium or stop fexofenadine. While some antibiotics can increase photosensitivity, wearing sunscreen at all times is not necessary. Sunscreens should be worn when being exposed to sun is likely.
20. a, c, d. Ideally, culture and sensitivity should be obtained before starting antibiotics. Allergic reactions are a possibility with any antibiotic. Because cephalosporins are eliminated in the urine, monitoring for adequate urine output is important. Ceftazidime is administered q8h, not daily. Fluid intake is encouraged, not restricted, since the drug is excreted in urine.
21. c. Caution is advised in administering amoxicillin to patients with asthma. Use in pediatric population and patients with diabetes is not contraindicated. Amoxicillin is generally safe during pregnancy.
22. c. A dose of IR 750 mg every 8 hours would be too much. The standard dose for adults is 250–500 mg q8h for immediate release or 500 mg q12h for extended release.

Case Study: Critical Thinking

1. Amoxicillin has a broad spectrum of activity and is effective against many gram-positive and gram-negative organisms.

2. Broad-spectrum antibiotic can be effective against many gram-positive and gram-negative organisms and is generally prescribed when the offending organism is unknown.

3. Cefadroxil is a cephalosporin; more specifically, it is a first-generation cephalosporin. First-generation cephalosporins are effective against most gram-positive bacteria and are destroyed by beta-lactamases. Second-generation cephalosporins are effective against gram-positive and some gram-negative bacteria. Third-generation cephalosporins are resistant to beta-lactamases. They have broad-spectrum antibacterial activity and are effective against *Pseudomonas aeruginosa*. The fourth-generation cephalosporin has broad-spectrum activity, is highly resistant to beta-lactamases, and has good penetration to cerebrospinal fluid. The fifth-generation cephalosporins are broad-spectrum drugs that are effective against resistant strains such as methicillin-resistant *Staphylococcus aureus* (MRSA).

4. (Answers may vary) The nurse would explain the importance of completing the course of antibiotics, even if symptoms resolve. Not completing the treatment plan leads to the development of resistant strains of bacteria. Also, encourage the patient to consume food that contains active cultures such as buttermilk or yogurt to prevent superinfection. Advise patients to take the medication with food if they experience gastrointestinal distress, such as nausea. However, the patient should contact their healthcare provider for continued nausea and or vomiting. Other concerns to report to the healthcare provider include dizziness.

CHAPTER 27: MACROLIDES, OXAZOLIDINONES, LINCOSAMIDES, GLYCOPEPTIDES, AND LIPOPEPTIDES

1. b
2. d
3. a
4. a
5. c
6. a
7. b. A trough of 5.9 mcg/mL is usually achieved by the third dose. The units are in mcg/mL, not mg/mL.
8. a. Acid-resistant salts, such as stearate, decrease gastric acid from destroying the antibacterial into smaller particles (dissolution). By decreasing the dissolution the amount of the drug that is absorbed in the small intestine is increased, not decreased. The salts do not minimize the risk of superinfection. The salts decrease, not assist, in dissolving the drug in the stomach.

9. a, b, c, e. Many antibiotics, including clindamycin, can cause gastrointestinal distress such as diarrhea. Superinfections, which occur when normal bacteria are destroyed, are common with the use of antibiotics. Clindamycin should be taken with a full glass of water to prevent esophageal irritation. All antibacterials, including clindamycin, should be completed to decrease the risk of resistant strains of organisms. Clindamycin does not cause urinary urgency.

10. d. Erythromycin is the drug of choice in treating Legionnaires disease. Even though azithromycin and clarithromycin are macrolides, they are not the drug of choice in treating Legionnaires disease. Vancomycin is a glycopeptide, not macrolide.

11. b. Azithromycin can cause hepatotoxicity (damaged liver). Drugs that are also hepatotoxic, such as acetaminophen, can exacerbate hepatotoxicity. Azithromycin can also cause leukopenia, not leukocytosis; thrombocytopenia, not elevated platelets (thrombocytosis); and increased, not decreased, bilirubin (hyperbilirubinemia).

12. c. Pseudomembranous colitis with *Clostridium difficile* is a superinfection due to antibacterial use. Oral vancomycin is the drug of choice. Oral vancomycin is a glycopeptide and can be given by two routes: oral and intravenously. Vancomycin administered orally does not absorb systemically and is excreted in feces; it is the drug of choice for *C. difficile* colitis. Vancomycin is administered intravenously for systemic infections (sepsis). Telavancin is a glycopeptide used to treat respiratory infections, especially against resistant strains, such as MRSA. Daptomycin is a lipopeptide used to treat skin infection with resistant strain organisms, such as MRSA. Clarithromycin is a macrolide whose side effect includes *C. difficile*.

13. c. The best action by the nurse is to contact the healthcare provider. Vancomycin is nephrotoxic, and a decrease in urine output can be an early indication of renal damage. Decreasing renal function is also a part of normal aging, putting an older adult patient at higher risk for renal failure. While increasing fluids (orally and intravenously) can improve renal output, it is not the best action. Every assessment, such as decreased urine output, should be documented, but it is not the best answer.

14. c. Conjunctivitis is a possible side effect of azithromycin. If this occurs, the patient should not wear contact lenses. Photosensitivity is not a side effect of this drug. Taking azithromycin with food may help prevent nausea. If a headache occurs as a side effect, drugs such as ibuprofen or acetaminophen are not contraindicated.

Case Study: Critical Thinking

1. Azithromycin is a macrolide that binds to the 50S ribosomal subunits and inhibits protein synthesis. At low to moderate drug doses, macrolides have a bacteriostatic effect, and with high drug doses, their effect is bactericidal.

2. Side effects and adverse reactions to macrolides include GI disturbances such as nausea, vomiting, diarrhea, and abdominal cramping. Severe diarrhea occurs when antibacterials kill normal flora, allowing an overgrowth of *C. difficile*. This superinfection is called *C. difficile*–associated diarrhea (CDAD), also known as pseudomembranous colitis.

3. Loose watery stools could indicate the patient has pseudomembranous colitis with *C. difficile*, a superinfection in the colon in which the bacteria releases toxins in the colon causing inflammation and possibly bleeding in the colon lining. This condition causes severe abdominal cramping, five or more watery diarrheal stools per day, and bloody stools. The nurse would be concerned about fluid, electrolytes, and anemia.

4. Vancomycin is given orally for treatment of staphylococcal enterocolitis and antibiotic-associated pseudomembranous colitis due to *C. difficile*. When vancomycin is given orally, it is not absorbed systemically and is excreted in the feces. Vancomycin is also given intravenously for septicemia; for severe infections due to MRSA; and for bone, skin, and lower respiratory tract infections that do not respond or are resistant to other antibiotics. When patients are on intravenous vancomycin, drug levels should be monitored. The trough is 5–20 mcg/mL, and the peak is 30–40 mcg/mL.

CHAPTER 28: TETRACYCLINES, GLYCYLCYCLINES, AMINOGLYCOSIDES, AND FLUOROQUINOLONES

1. aminoglycoside
2. children
3. loop diuretics or methoxyflurane
4. DNA gyrase; DNA
5. increase
6. d
7. b
8. a
9. b
10. c
11. a
12. a. Levofloxacin dosing is daily, not twice daily. All other fluoroquinolone dosing are appropriate.
13. b, e. Ototoxicity is a serious adverse effect of gentamicin. Elevated renal function tests may indicate a decrease in renal function, which increases the risk of nephrotoxicity. Nausea, headache, and photosensitivity may be side effects; however, they are usually not considered serious.

14. d. Peak blood levels are drawn 45–60 minutes after a drug has been administered. Gentamicin is administered intravenously over 30–60 minutes. Therefore peak drug level should be checked at 10:30 p.m. Gentamicin will still be infusing at 9:15 a.m. and 9:15 p.m. 10:00 a.m. is 30 minutes or less after the drug has completed infusing.

15. b. The correct trough level for gentamicin is less than 1–2 mcg/mL. The healthcare provider should be contacted before administering the dose because it is elevated, which can cause an adverse reaction such as nephrotoxicity. The drug should not be administered because of high trough level. Diphenhydramine can decrease risk of reaction, but the patient is not having a reaction; instead, the trough level indicates toxicity.

16. c. Superinfection or secondary infection, such as vaginitis, can occur resulting from antibacterial therapy. The patient could have been exposed to other infectious agents, but since the patient has been on antibiotics, a superinfection is most likely. An allergic reaction is a hypersensitivity and would most likely manifest itself as rash, swelling, or respiratory difficulty. A drug-drug interaction is not able to be determined since the patient is on one drug.

17. a, b, c. Because gentamicin can cause hepatotoxicity, liver enzymes (AST and ALT) would need to be monitored for signs of liver failure. Gentamicin can also be nephrotoxic; therefore urine characteristics, such as color and clarity, are necessary. Ototoxicity can occur with gentamicin, causing hearing loss. Gentamicin usually does not affect vision.

18. c, d, e. Doxycycline should be taken with food or milk for improved absorption. There are no restrictions regarding eggs.

19. a, b, c, e. Outdated drugs of any kind should be discarded; however, tetracycline will break down into toxic by-products so it must be assured it is discarded. Superinfections, which occur when normal bacteria are destroyed, are common with the use of antibiotics. Tetracycline should not be taken during the first and third trimesters of pregnancy because of possible teratogenic effects. Tetracycline increases photosensitivity and sunscreen should be used when exposed to sun or limit sun exposure. Tetracycline does not cause urinary urgency.

20. a, b, c, e. Iron, which is found in prenatal vitamins and antacids, prevents absorption of doxycycline. Studies have shown that the effects of warfarin may be increased by taking doxycycline, placing the client at higher risk for bleeding. Cautious use should be exercised in a client taking doxycycline and a proton pump inhibitor like omeprazole. There are no known interactions with doxycycline and morphine.

21. b, c, d, e. Drugs in the tetracycline family should be stored away from light to prevent breakdown. Cautious use is recommended in clients with renal and/ or liver disease. Baseline levels should be assessed and reevaluated as needed. Because of mutations within the strains of various sexually transmitted infections, a culture and sensitivity should be obtained before starting treatment. It is also possible that various sexually transmitted infections could be present at the same time, and it would be beneficial to the client if the most effective antibiotic is prescribed for each. Tetracyclines may make oral contraceptives less effective, so additional contraceptive should be used.

22. c. Aminoglycosides, such as gentamicin, can cause tinnitus, ringing of the ears. Tinnitus is a high-pitch sound due to damage to cranial nerve VIII. Other side effects are pruritus and muscle cramps. Tinnitus is not related to allergy or sex.

23. a. Common side effect of doxycycline is gastro-intestinal distress, which includes nausea, vomiting, and diarrhea. These side effects could cause a decrease in serum potassium due to potassium loss. Serum calcium, platelets, hemoglobin, and hematocrit are not commonly affected by doxycycline.

Clinical Judgment Standalone Case Study
Answers:

Nursing Action	Indicated	Contraindicated
Advise the patient to stop taking the medications once the pain is relieved		X
Tell the patient to not take over-the-counter antacids	X	
Inform the patient that tetracycline can be kept in the car		X
Teach patient proper oral care to avoid mouth ulcers	X	
Instruct the patient to take the medication with food or glass of milk		X
Teach the patient to use sun block and wear protective clothing during sun exposure	X	

Rationale:

Antibiotics, such as tetracycline, should be continued for the entire course of therapy, even if the patient feels better. Discontinuing antibiotics early promotes antibiotic resistance. Antacids can decrease the absorption of tetracycline. Also, tetracycline should be taken 1 hour before or 2 hours after meals with a full glass of water. If gastric distress occurs, then small amount of non-dairy food can be taken with the medicine. Tetracycline should be kept in a cool, dry place. Tetracycline can decompose in light and heat. Patients should be instructed on proper oral care to avoid the development of mouth ulcers. If mouth ulcers do develop, their healthcare provider should be notified; this could indicate a superinfection. Patients on tetracycline should be encouraged to wear sunblock or protective clothing during sun exposure because tetracycline is associated with photosensitivity.

Reference

McCuistion, L.E., DiMaggio, K.V., Winton, M.B., & Yeager, J.J. (2025). Pharmacology: A patient-centered nursing process approach, 12th ed. St. Louis, MO: Elsevier. pp. 339–347.

CHAPTER 29: SULFONAMIDES AND NITROIMIDAZOLES ANTIBIOTICS

1. folic acid
2. penicillin
3. trimethoprim
4. are not
5. is not
6. liver; kidneys
7. bacteriostatic
8. increases
9. b
10. b
11. a
12. d. Silver sulfadiazine and mafenide are sulfonamides that are available in cream form to treat burns. Sulfadiazine is used for prophylactic treatment in patients with rheumatic fever. Sulfasalazine is used to treat irritable bowel disease, such as ulcerative colitis. Sulfacetamide sodium is for ophthalmic disorders.
13. b, c, d, e. TMP-SMZ is contraindicated while breastfeeding. It is possible that there is cross-sensitivity between sulfonamides, so it is important to determine if the patient is allergic to any other antibiotics. There are a variety of etiologies for kidney stones; however, crystallization of the urine may occur with sulfonamides, which can lead to kidney stone formation. Some patients are more prone to kidney stones than others. TMP-SMZ has a

variety of interactions with several drugs, including warfarin, oral hypoglycemic agents, ACE inhibitors, digoxin, phenytoin, and potassium-sparing diuretics.

14. a, b, c, d. To prevent crystallization in the urine, fluids should be encouraged. Urine output should be carefully monitored since this medication is excreted in the urine. Undesired side effects are possible and include abdominal pain, nausea, vomiting, diarrhea, and anorexia. A desired effect of TMP-SMZ will be resolution of the bronchitis as evidenced by decreased coughing and clear lung sounds.

15. b. The usual adult dose of TMP-SMZ is 160 mg TMP/800 mg SMZ every 12 hours. Its half-life is 6–12 hours; thus it must be administered twice a day.

16. c. Sulfonamides are not obtained from biological sources. They are bacteriostatic and, depending on the dose, can be bactericidal. They are effective against bacteria, not viruses and fungi.

17. d. Insomnia is a common side effect from TMP-SMZ. Other side effects include anorexia, nausea, vomiting, diarrhea, depression, and headache, among others. Confusion, constipation, and fever are not common.

18. a. The maintenance dose for sulfasalazine is 500 mg every 6 hours, with a maximum dose of 4 g/day. While 1000 mg every 6 hours is within the maximum dose, it is not the best answer. 1250 mg/d and 1500 mg/d are too small of a dose.

19. a. It is appropriate to use quinupristin-dalfopristin, a combination drug containing two streptogramin antibacterials, for life-threatening infection caused by vancomycin-resistant *Enterococcus faecium* (VREF). Other bacteria the drug is appropriate for include *S. aureus* and *Streptococcus pyogenes*.

Case Study: Critical Thinking

1. TMP-SMZ is a sulfonamide that is bacteriostatic. Trimethoprim and sulfamethoxazole inhibit the bacterial synthesis of folic acid, which is required for bacterial growth. The standard oral dosage is 160 mg of TMP/800 mg of SMZ q12h.

2. Patient and/or caregiver teaching will include the need for adequate fluid intake to maintain a urine output of more than 600 mL/d to prevent crystalluria. The drug should be taken on an empty stomach. The nurse will educate on the potential side effects of anorexia, nausea, vomiting, diarrhea, and abdominal pain. Other side effects include headache, fatigue, vertigo, and insomnia. The patient should be advised to ask for help when getting out of bed or ambulating because of the potential

for vertigo and risk of falling. Other plan of care instructions include teaching to monitor for any rash or bruises and, if observed, to notify the provider. TMP-SMZ can increase the effects of warfarin. The blood glucose level should be monitored more closely because of increased risk for hypoglycemia.

3. The nurse would need to be aware of the potential for increased effects of anticoagulation, such as bruising and bleeding, because of the interaction between warfarin and TMP-SMZ. There is also a potential for increased hypoglycemic effects of glyburide. The nurse will need to carefully monitor lab work, including BUN and creatinine levels for renal function as well as liver panel (AST, ALT, ALP). The nurse would also need to monitor for life-threatening adverse effects, including electrolyte imbalances (hyperkalemia, hyponatremia, hypoglycemia), seizures, angioedema, anemias, leukopenia, pseudomembranous colitis, and Stevens-Johnson syndrome (erythema multiforme major). Stevens-Johnson syndrome is characterized by fever, malaise, joint pain, and skin lesions. Severe cases can be life threatening and may require intensive care hospitalization and the use of immunoglobulins.

CHAPTER 30: ANTITUBERCULARS, ANTIFUNGALS, AND ANTIVIRALS

1. acid-fast, tuberculosis
2. do not
3. speak, sneeze, cough; inhale
4. latent tuberculosis infection
5. kidney, liver; renal or hepatic disorders, alcoholism, diabetic retinopathy, severe hypersensitivity to pyrazinamide or ethionamide, concurrent MAOI therapy
6. is not (Psychotic behavior is an adverse effect and isoniazid should be discontinued should it occur.)
7. Combination
8. vitamin B_6 (pyridoxine)
9. isoniazid (INH), 6–9 (Other answer: INH with rifampin for 4 months)
10. a
11. a
12. a
13. b
14. a
15. b
16. b
17. b
18. a
19. opportunistic
20. histamine-mediated
21. cold sores, genital herpes

22. shingles, dermatome
23. A, B
24. does not
25. B, C
26. b. Other life-threatening effects include blood dyscrasias (such as agranulocytosis, hemolytic anemia, aplastic anemia, thrombocytopenia, and eosinophilia), encephalopathy, and exfoliative dermatitis (such as Stevens-Johnson syndrome).
27. b. Alcoholism is a contraindication for treating tuberculosis with isoniazid. Alcohol ingestion with this drug can increase the incidence of peripheral neuropathy and hepatotoxicity.
28. c. Rifapentine has a long half-life. To minimize drug toxicity but maintain therapeutic level, the drug must be taken twice per week with a minimum interval between doses of 72 hours.
29. a, b, d. Side effects can occur 1–3 hours after starting amphotericin B infusion. Side effects include chills, flushing, fever, nausea, vomiting, headache, dyspnea, and tachypnea. To alleviate side effects, diphenhydramine, acetaminophen, and hydrocortisone can be administered 30–60 minutes before administering amphotericin B.
30. d. Ribavirin is labeled to treat hepatitis C virus. Acyclovir is given for herpes virus, amphotericin B is an antifungal, and zanamivir is for influenza.
31. b, c, d. It will be important to obtain a history of drugs taken and drug allergies before starting treatment. A history of tuberculosis (TB) exposure and the results and dates of most recent purified protein derivative (PPD) and chest x-rays will also be important information. Blood glucose level is not pertinent in this patient; important baseline laboratory values include monitoring liver and renal functions.
32. b. 400 mg/day. The initial dose is 5 mg/kg per day (5 × 80 = 400) or over 5 days/week. Other regimen includes 15 mg/kg given up to 3 days/week. Maximum dose is 900 mg/day.
33. c. INH can be hepatotoxic; therefore liver functions must be monitored on a regular basis. Hepatic disease is a contraindication for INH. Patients on INH should be taught adverse drug effects, including abdominal pain, yellowing of skin/eyes, and clay-colored stool. INH is metabolized, not excreted, by the liver. INH has not been implicated in causing liver cancer.
34. c. Aluminum hydroxide/magnesium hydroxide is an antacid. Antacids should not be taken at the same time as INH. Antacids decrease the absorption of INH.

35. a, b. Vitamin B_6 supplements or increased intake may be necessary to prevent peripheral neuropathy. Alcohol should be avoided since INH can be hepatotoxic. Rifampin, not INH, may turn body fluids brownish-orange.
36. b. Combination therapy is more effective in eradicating TB infection than any single drug.
37. b. The nurse will administer amphotericin B intravenously since it is not absorbed from the GI tract. Because of its risk of toxicity, close monitoring is needed while administering the drug.
38. b. The standard dose range is 0.25–1.5 mg/kg per day. The drug should be further diluted and infused intravenously slowly via an in-line filter while monitoring for side effects, such as fever, chills, flushing, nausea, and vomiting. The drug must be protected from light.
39. c. Amphotericin B is given only intravenously, and its side effects include flushing, nausea, vomiting, hypotension, and chills. The patient does not need to be NPO before receiving a dose of amphotericin B, and it may in fact be beneficial to have a light, nongreasy meal or even some crackers to help decrease the nausea. Amphotericin B is nephrotoxic, so any changes in urination should be reported immediately to the healthcare provider.
40. a, c, d, e. Patient should be instructed to maintain hydration and it can be taken at mealtime. Acyclovir can cause orthostatic hypotension and patient should be instructed to change or stand up slowly. The patient should report decreased urination, dizziness, or confusion. The patient should abstain from sexual intercourse or use a barrier method, such as condoms, correctly and consistently. Use of spermicide does not prevent spread of infection.
41. a, b, c. Peginterferon can cause mild to serious side effects. Mild side effects such as flu-like symptoms and myalgia can be treated with antiinflammatories. Other side effects are more serious; peginterferon can cause papilledema (which can lead to vision changes), pancytopenia (placing the patient at risk for infection, so fever should be reported), and mood changes (which may indicate depression).
42. b. Each tablet has 100 mg. The dose is 150 mg. Therefore patient should take 1.5 tablets.
43. a, b, c, e. Laboratory values that assess hepatic and renal function should be obtained at baseline and trended. Fluconazole can cause hypokalemia. Prothrombin time (PT) may be altered if the patient is taking warfarin.

Clinical Judgment Standalone Case Study

Answers:

Nursing Actions	Appropriate	Inappropriate
Hold rifampin if body fluids, such as urine, sweat, and saliva, turn red-orange color		X
Administer isoniazid on empty stomach	X	
Obtain initial follow-up appointment with a medical provider prior to patient being discharged	X	
Explain that his partner does not need to be treated		X
Obtain sputum samples to test for acid-fast bacilli	X	
Anticipate in administering pyridoxine with isoniazid	X	
Place patient in reverse isolation		X
Assess for numbness, tingling, or burning sensations	X	
Assist the patient in developing a plan to remain adherent to the drug regimen	X	

Rationale:

It is inappropriate to instruct patients to hold rifampin if body fluids, such as urine, sweat, and saliva, turn red-orange color; rifampin turns body fluids orange, and soft contact lenses may become permanently discolored. It is appropriate to administer isoniazid to be taken on an empty stomach. Absorption is decreased with food. To improve drug adherence the nurse would obtain an initial follow-up appointment with a healthcare provider prior to hospital discharge. Anyone in close contact with the patient, including sexual partners, should be tested and most likely will receive prophylactic drug treatment. It is appropriate to obtain sputum sample to test for acid-fast bacilli. Sputum specimens for acid-fast bacilli should be negative for several weeks or months after taking antitubercular drugs. Pyridoxine prevents peripheral neuropathy, such as numbness, tingling, or burning sensations, to extremities that are caused by isoniazid. Patients with tuberculosis do not need to be in reverse isolation. To increase drug adherence, treatment plan for tuberculosis should be discussed with the patient and significant others. healthcare personnel should assist them in developing a plan to remain adherent to the drug regimen.

Reference

McCuistion, L.E., DiMaggio, K.V., Winton, M.B., & Yeager, J.J. (2025). Pharmacology: A patient-centered nursing process approach, 12th ed. St. Louis, MO: Elsevier. pp. 354–368.

CHAPTER 31: ANTIMALARIALS, ANTHELMINTICS, AND PEPTIDES

1. c
2. e
3. a
4. b
5. d
6. g
7. f
8. b. The most common site for helminths is the intestine. Person can be infected from soil containing helminths. Other sites include the vascular system and the liver, but they are not common sites.
9. c. Malaria is caused by multiple species of protozoan parasites that are carried by mosquitos, and it remains one of the most prevalent protozoan diseases.
10. b. They are all antimicrobials, but chloroquine is a commonly prescribed drug for protozoans causing malaria. If drug resistance to chloroquine occurs, then other treatments can be used. Acyclovir and delavirdine are antivirals. Tobramycin is an antibacterial.
11. c, d, e, f. With the use of chloroquine, red blood cell count, hemoglobin, and hematocrit levels may be lowered. Liver enzymes such as AST may be elevated. Baseline laboratory values should be obtained and monitored.
12. b. Chloroquine is taken for 2 weeks before travel and continued for another 8 weeks while traveling in an endemic area for malaria to prevent growth of the parasites. Abdominal cramping, nausea, and vomiting are among the expected side effects. Ringing in the ears may be an indication of ototoxicity and needs to be reported immediately. Taking either antacids or laxatives may decrease the effectiveness of chloroquine.
13. b. Patient has most likely developed resistance to chloroquine. Artemether/lumefantrine is a combination drug that has a high success rate and may be used if other drugs have failed because of resistance.

Administering more chloroquine will not improve the health of the patient. Thiabendazole is an anthelminthic. Zidovudine is an antiviral to treat HIV.

14. b, d, e. Proper hygiene for a patient who has helminths includes frequent handwashing, especially after using the toilet and before eating. Because helminths may live on a variety of materials, all clothing, towels, and bedding should be changed daily and washed in hot water. The patient should shower instead of sitting in a bathtub and should not swim in pools or use hot tubs while infected. To prevent trichinosis, caused by *Trichinella spiralis*, all pork and pork-containing products must be thoroughly cooked to destroy the larvae.

15. c, d, e. Taeniasis is a parasitic infestation with tapeworms. Praziquantel is prescribed to treat taeniasis. Possible side effects include dizziness, headache, and weakness. Other side effects can include anorexia, malaise, nausea, vomiting, and abdominal pain. Vision and hearing deficits are not side effects.

16. a, c, d. Antibiotics, such as colistimethate, should be taken as prescribed and the full course should be completed, even if the person feels better.

Case Study: Critical Thinking

1. Helminths are parasitic worms that have been transmitted from infected soil to the person. Helminths feed on the person's tissue.
2. Groups of helminths that infest humans include tapeworms, flukes, and roundworms. They enter humans when the person eats contaminated food, the person is bitten by carrier insects, or the helminth directly penetrates the skin.
3. Helminths are treated with anthelmintics taken orally. The type of helminth infestation will determine the type(s) of anthelmintic(s) prescribed.

CHAPTER 32: HIV- AND AIDS-RELATED DRUGS

1. a
2. d
3. c
4. f
5. b
6. b
7. e
8. a
9. e
10. a
11. binding, fusion, replication, assembly
12. should
13. 100
14. CYP450
15. Efavirenz
16. dosing frequency, food requirement, fluid requirement, pill burden, drug interaction potential, side effect profile

17. IRIS (immune reconstitution inflammatory syndrome)

18. a, d. HIV is transmitted via contact with blood and body fluids, such as semen, vaginal fluids, and breast milk; this also includes donated sperm from an HIV-infected person. Increased risk occurs in those who have unprotected sex; those who have sex with multiple partners; and IV drug users who share contaminated personal care items, such as razors.

19. b. CD4+ T-cell count can be used to determine when to initiate drug therapy and to monitor the efficacy of therapy. Other laboratory tests include plasma HIV RNA quantitative assay (or viral load) and HIV resistance testing.

20. c. Two laboratory tests used to determine the efficacy of treatment include CD4+ count and HIV viral load. CD4+ count reflects the immune status and should increase in response to ART. HIV viral load is indicative of the virus circulating in the blood, which should decrease in response to ART.

21. a, c, e. It is recommended that all who are HIV positive be treated. Tools to promote drug adherence should be provided, which include using a pill planner and setting alarms. The drugs are selected based on results of genotypic resistance testing, comorbidities, potential drug-drug interactions, pregnancy status, and patient's willingness and readiness to start therapy. There are many drugs used in various combinations to increase drug adherence. While patient's age and support system are important considerations, they are not a determining factor for initiating ART.

22. b, c. Adherence is improved because newer drug formulations decrease dosing frequency or pill burden. Also, some ARTs have been combined into one pill to further reduce pill burden. Newer ARTs have increased potency and/or have fewer side effects.

23. b. Zidovudine's usual adult dosage is 300 mg every 12 hours. Another dosing schedule is 200 mg every 8 hours.

24. b. The oral dose for neonates at 4 weeks old is 12 mg/kg every 12 hours. 9 mg/kg dosing is for intravenous administration. 120 mg/kg and 300 mg/kg would be overdosing the neonate.

25. a, b, c. Zidovudine can cause hepatotoxicity, lactic acidosis, pancytopenia, and myelosuppression. Therefore CBC with differentials will be monitored for indications of pancytopenia and myelosuppression. A metabolic panel will be checked for signs of hepatotoxicity (elevated ALT/AST) and lactic acidosis (creatinine).

26. a, b, c, d. Seizures would be an adverse reaction, not a side effect.

27. c. Efavirenz is the only NNRTI that crosses the blood-brain barrier (cerebrospinal fluid); neural tube defects to fetuses can occur. Neuropsychiatric symptoms, such as dizziness, sedation, nightmares, euphoria, and loss of concentration, can occur.

28. d. Efavirenz is scheduled daily, usually at night to reduce CNS side effects, such as dizziness. However, efavirenz can cause insomnia and euphoria.

29. d. All NNRTIs can cause hepatotoxicity, including hepatic failure; therefore liver panels should be monitored.

30. a, c, d. Most side effects associated with efavirenz are CNS related such as dizziness, insomnia, agitation, and hallucinations. Gastrointestinal side effects include nausea and diarrhea. Other side effects include rash. Seizures are adverse reactions, not side effects.

31. a, c, d. Efavirenz has effects on the liver and increases the potential for liver failure. Efavirenz crosses the cerebrospinal fluid. Alcohol can increase the risk of hepatotoxicity and neuropsychiatric symptoms and should not be consumed while taking efavirenz. The patient should discuss the use of any herbal preparations with the healthcare provider. St. Johns wort should not be taken with efavirenz. Vomiting is one of the common side effects, not an adverse reaction.

32. b, c, d. Tenofovir is a nucleoside/nucleotide reverse transcriptase inhibitor (NNRTI) used to treat certain viral infections, such as HIV. Monitoring of liver enzymes and lipid panels (cholesterol and triglycerides) is important while taking tenofovir.

33. a, b, d. St. Johns wort should not be taken with any antiretrovirals, as it may change the levels in the blood. A benefit of tenofovir is that it may be taken with or without food. This is important because nausea, vomiting, diarrhea, and flatulence are potential GI side effects.

34. a. Combination therapy is the standard of care for both treatment of maternal HIV infection and prophylaxis to reduce the risk of transmitting HIV to the fetus. During intrapartum, zidovudine IV should be given if the viral load is greater than or equal to 400 copies/mL, regardless of current ART.

35. a, b, c, e. Atazanavir has few side effects. They include rash, cough, diarrhea, vomiting, and nausea.

36. a, b, d, e. Anything that will help the patient keep track of timing of drug and increase adherence will be of benefit. This can be in the form of pill organizers, timers to remind the patient of dosing schedule, and wall calendars or charts where the drug can be crossed off after it has been taken. Also, taking the drug at the same time each day can increase adherence.

Clinical Judgment Standalone Case Study
Answer:

Options for 1	Options for 2	Options for 3	Options for 4
Postexposure prophylaxis (PEP) treatment	4 weeks	CD4+ T cell	HIV RNA

Rationale:

HIV can be transmitted when a person encounters body fluid of a person who is HIV positive. Body fluids include blood, semen, vaginal fluids, and breast milk. Various modes of exposure to body fluids include accidental needle injury with a used needle. When occupational exposure occurs, the area should be thoroughly washed with soap and water, report the incident, and seek medical care. Postexposure prophylaxis (PEP) treatment should be started within 72 hours of exposure and will continue for at least 4 weeks. Periodic laboratory testing is conducted to assess the levels of CD4+ T cell and HIV RNA quantitative assay (viral load).

Preexposure prophylaxis (PrEP) treatment is provided to persons who are HIV negative but are at high risk for encountering others who are HIV positive to reduce the risk of acquiring HIV. Non-HIV antiviral treatment is not used for treating occupational exposure to HIV. 6 months of treatment is longer than the recommendation of 4 weeks. While elevated WBCs can indicate infection, CD4+ T lymphocytes are more determinant of HIV activity. Neutrophils may be elevated, but CD4+ T cells are more indicative. HIV is an RNA retrovirus, not DNA. Currently, there is no treatment for HIV mRNA.

References

McCuistion, L.E., DiMaggio, K.V., Winton, M.B., & Yeager, J.J. (2025). Pharmacology: A patient-centered nursing process approach, 12th ed. St. Louis, MO: Elsevier. pp. 381–394.

O'Byrne, P., et al. (2019). *PrEP-RN: Clinical considerations and protocols for nurse let PrEP.* The Journal of the Association of Nurses in AIDS Care: JANAC, 30(3), 301–311. https://doi.org/10.1097/JNC.0000000000000075

CHAPTER 33: TRANSPLANT DRUGS

1. cadaveric transplantation
2. lymphocytes
3. posttransplant lymphoproliferative disorder, Epstein-Barr virus
4. mTOR inhibitor, T-cell and B-cell (antibodies)
5. hypokalemia
6. skin, sun
7. Induction therapy includes transplant drugs that provide *immunosuppression*, which is a decreased immune response.
8. An example of a living-donor transplantation is when *one kidney* donated by a living person is transplanted into the body with *end-stage kidney* disease. Another example of a living-donor transplantation is when a *portion of a liver* by a living person is transplanted into the body with *severe liver disease*.
9. Transplant recipients receiving immunosuppressive drugs *cannot* receive live vaccines.
10. Sirolimus is primarily excreted in the *feces*.

11. Antithymocyte globulin alters *T-cell* function and prolongs T-cell *deletion*.
12. c
13. e
14. g
15. c
16. f
17. e
18. a
19. d
20. b
21. a, c, e. Cytokine release syndrome is a complex event associated with cytokine release because of an infusion reaction. When cytokines are released into the circulation, systemic symptoms can occur, such as hypotension, tachycardia, dyspnea, and fever (hyperthermia). Other symptoms include chills, nausea, headache, rash, scratchy throat, and asthenia.
22. a. Before receiving immunosuppressive drugs, antipyretics, antihistamines, and/or corticosteroids are administered to reduce the severity of the symptoms associated with cytokine release syndrome.
23. d. Grapefruit and grapefruit juice affect the metabolism of cyclosporine; they increase the blood concentration of cyclosporine.
24. c. Many drugs can interact with cyclosporine, including antibiotics, histamine$_2$-receptor blockers (e.g., cimetidine), antiinflammatories (e.g., ibuprofen), and herbal preparations. Fever can indicate an infection, and the patient should call the healthcare provider.
25. a. The dose ordered is incorrect. The maintenance dose for belatacept is 5 mg/kg starting week 17 post renal transplant. The nurse should not give the drug; instead, the nurse should notify the physician for the correct dose. Giving belatacept without an order is not within the scope of nursing practice.
26. d. Mammalian target rapamycin inhibitor (mTOR) is appropriate for persons who had a kidney transplant. Individuals who had other organ transplants are at risk for lymphoma and other malignances.
27. a, c, d. Mycophenolate mofetil prevents the proliferation of T-lymphocyte cells and formation of antibodies by the B lymphocytes. It is recommended for recipients of kidney, heart, or liver transplant.
28. c. The adrenal cortex produces and secretes natural glucocorticoids that are necessary for the immune system. High doses of corticosteroids, such as prednisone, suppress adrenal function, more specifically the adrenal cortex. If corticosteroids are discontinued abruptly, the adrenal cortex does not have time to adjust and is not able to produce and secrete its hormones.
29. d. To decrease the incidence and severity of adverse reactions while receiving antithymocyte globulin, a corticosteroid and an antihistamine should be administered. A prophylactic antibiotic is not necessary.
30. a. Infection is a major risk factor for patients on immunosuppressive therapy. Patients and their families and/or caregivers should be taught to wash hands frequently, especially after toileting, and to avoid sick people or crowds. Taking daily blood pressure and temperature is not necessary. Exercise and proper nutrition are encouraged, but cooking all fruits and vegetables is not necessary.

Case Study: Critical Thinking

1. Cyclosporine modified is a calcineurin inhibitor that inhibits T-lymphocyte proliferation and reduces the synthesis of cytokines. Methylprednisolone sodium succinate is a corticosteroid that decreases the inflammatory response; suppresses neutrophils, the immune system, and adrenal function; and alters vascular permeability.
2. Common side effects for cyclosporine and methylprednisolone sodium succinate include hypertension, edema, acne, hirsutism, nausea and vomiting, headache, and insomnia, among others. Adverse effects include diabetes mellitus, malignancy, infections, and seizures.
3. Immunosuppressive drugs such as cyclosporine and methylprednisolone sodium succinate suppress the immune response and place the patient at risk for disseminated infection resulting from the live virus.

CHAPTER 34: VACCINES

1. d
2. f
3. e
4. c
5. b
6. a
7. g
8. 20
9. vaccinations, ages, dosage, and route
10. mosquitoes
11. VAERS (Vaccine Adverse Events Reporting System)
12. Herpes, varicella
13. d. Toxoids are inactivated toxins that stimulate the formation of antitoxins but can no longer produce harmful disease. Examples of toxoids are diphtheria and tetanus.
14. b, c, e. Acquired passive immunity is provided through administration of antibodies pooled from another source. Receiving preformed immunoglobulins (Ig) is necessary when exposed persons are at high risk for complications of the disease, when time does not permit active vaccinations, or when persons suffer from an immune deficiency and do not have effective immune response. Fetuses are automatically protected by the maternal immune system. Pregnant females should not receive immunizations, including preformed Ig, with a few exceptions such as the seasonal flu vaccine.

15. c. Passive immunity involves receiving antibodies that are preformed and have short duration of action. On the other hand, active immunity is when the body's own immune response recognizes a pathogen and produces antibodies. Active immunity provides long-term protection.

16. d. Seroconversion occurs when a person acquires detectable antibodies after receiving vaccines.

17. d. Vaccines involve the administration of a small amount of antigens, which stimulate an immune response. Not all persons will develop antibodies, thereby immunity. Vaccines are perceived by the body as foreign particles or antigens. Vaccines rarely cause an allergic reaction, and they do not produce a mild form of the disease. Mild reactions, such as swelling and pain at the injection site and low-grade fever, can occur. Persons can develop a hypersensitivity reaction due to vaccine's components.

18. a. A patient actively infected stimulates their own immune response and acquires natural immunity.

19. a. First vaccine is usually administered at birth. Hepatitis B is the only vaccine that is recommended at birth.

20. a. Rubella is also known as German measles. Herpes zoster is also known as shingles.

21. a. Adolescents should receive the two doses of varicella zoster vaccine (VZV) 4–8 weeks apart.

22. c. Healthcare providers must report any vaccine-related adverse reactions to the Vaccine Adverse Events Reporting System (VAERS). VAERS is a surveillance system that receives and acts on any reports of adverse events.

23. a. Td is a vaccine that contains inactivated tetanus and diphtheria toxins that stimulate the formation of antitoxins to produce active immunity.

24. c. Attenuated vaccines are composed of live, weakened microbes. Vaccines against MMR and varicella zoster are composed of live, attenuated viruses. Vaccine against hepatitis B is a recombinant subunit vaccine that contains some of the genetic material. Td (tetanus) is a toxoid vaccine.

25. c. Fever, myalgia, and cough are typical signs and symptoms of influenza. Other manifestations include headaches, malaise, and nasal congestion. Gastrointestinal distress, such as abdominal pain, vomiting, and diarrhea, is usually not associated with influenza.

26. d. When MMR is not administered on the same day as varicella, then the administration of the two vaccines should be separated by at least 4 weeks.

27. a. The nurse would explain that redness and tenderness are common side effects and prepare to administer the DTaP as scheduled. DTaP should be given intramuscularly, not subcutaneously. Of the routine childhood immunizations, MMR, varicella, and meningococcal are administered subcutaneously.

28. a, b, c, e. Parents should be given a copy of the immunization record as well as an appointment card with a contact phone number for the clinic at the time of discharge. A Vaccine Information Statement (VIS) should be given to any patient, not just children, before receiving any immunizations.

29. a. Those traveling abroad should have their immunizations updated based on their age, immunization history, and destination of travel. Current vaccine recommendations for international travel can be obtained from the Centers for Disease Control and Prevention (CDC).

30. c. Although diphenhydramine is used for mild allergic reactions, in the case of an anaphylactic reaction, epinephrine should be readily available.

Case Study: Clinical Judgment Standalone

Answers:

_____ A. Influenza, live attenuated

_____ B. Varicella

__X__ C. Zoster recombinant

__X__ D. Tetanus, diphtheria, and pertussis

_____ E. Meningococcal B

__X__ F. Pneumococcal

Rationale:

A puncture wound with gardening tools places the person at risk for tetanus. Since the patient has not received immunizations in the last 20 years, the immunizations appropriate for this patient include tetanus, diphtheria, and pertussis (Tdap); zoster recombinant (herpes zoster); and pneumococcal. Tdap booster should be received every 10 years to prevent tetanus. Zoster prevents shingles. Since the patient has had chicken pox, they are at risk for shingles. The zoster recombinant is given in two doses. Pneumococcal 13-valent conjugate vaccine is recommended in all persons older than 65 years to prevent against 13 serotypes of *S. pneumoniae* pneumococcal pneumonia.

Reference

https://www.cdc.gov/vaccines/schedules/

McCuistion, L.E., DiMaggio, K.V., Winton, M.B., & Yeager, J.J. (2025). Pharmacology: A patient-centered nursing process approach, 12th ed. St. Louis, MO: Elsevier. pp. 407–420.

CHAPTER 35: ANTICANCER DRUGS

1. h
2. j
3. a
4. d
5. i

6. c
7. g
8. b
9. f
10. e
11. Acute myelogenous leukemia
12. Skin cancer
13. Non-Hodgkin lymphoma or Hodgkin disease, or nasopharyngeal cancers
14. Cancer of the colon, rectum, breast, uterus, prostate, and ovary
15. Cancer of mouth, throat, esophagus, liver, and breast
16. a. Combination chemotherapy is used as a treatment across all (or most) phases of cell life; therefore it tends to be more effective and has better response rate than single-drug treatment. Also, combination therapy decreases drug resistance. However, combination therapy results in increased side and adverse drug effects.
17. d. Viruses, such as human papillomavirus (HPV) and Epstein-Barr virus (EBV), have been implicated in cancer. HPV is associated with cervical cancer and EBV with Burkitt lymphoma and nasopharyngeal cancer. Benzene can cause acute myelogenous leukemia. Hepatocellular cancer is caused by aflatoxin.
18. c. General side effects and adverse drug reactions are due to the actions on rapidly growing normal cells, such as skin and hair. Anticancer drugs affect all phases of the cell cycle and are not cell specific. Many of the side effects of anticancer drugs are temporary.
19. a. The goal of palliative chemotherapy is not to cure but to help improve the patient's quality of life by treating symptoms such as pain or shortness of breath that may be associated with advanced disease.
20. a. White blood cells are used to fight infection. If the white blood cell count is decreased (leukopenia), the patient is at higher risk for an infection. Temperature changes, even if slight, may be an indication of a developing illness.
21. a. Chemotherapy causes myelosuppression, involving red cells, white cells, and platelets. Platelets are involved with clotting and healing injured tissue. If the platelet count is low (thrombocytopenia), the patient is more prone to occult bleeding (from the GI tract, for example) and may be unable to effectively develop clots to prevent bleeding.
22. d. Caffeine may have a laxative effect, so it should be limited in patients with diarrhea. Fresh fruits and vegetables and high-fiber foods will increase the number of stools. Foods with extreme temperature are not a concern.
23. b. When digoxin and cyclophosphamide are given orally, cyclophosphamide decreases digoxin levels by impairing GI absorption. This can decrease serum digoxin level and have a subtherapeutic effect, thereby increasing the risk of atrial fibrillation. Digoxin dose may need to be altered.
24. d. Metronidazole may increase the toxicity of 5-FU by inhibiting elimination. The dose of 5-FU may need to be decreased. An increase in toxicity will increase the risk of adverse drug effects.
25. c. Doxorubicin may cause cardiac toxicity, including congestive heart failure. Shortness of breath and crackles could be an indication of early heart failure. Methotrexate can cause hematologic and GI toxicities. Although cyclophosphamide can cause hematologic, pulmonary, and cardiac toxicity, CHF is more prevalent in patients taking doxorubicin.
26. c. Antiemetics decrease the severity of nausea and vomiting and should be administered 30–60 minutes prior to administering 5-FU.
27. c. Hemorrhagic cystitis is a result of severe bladder inflammation, which may occur with cyclophosphamide. Adequate hydration before and while giving this drug is important to potentially prevent this complication.
28. a. Hemorrhagic cystitis can occur with cyclophosphamide. Signs of cystitis include hematuria, urinary frequency, or dysuria. Patient needs to remain hydrated. Hydration should be started before treatment and maintained throughout. Antiemetics should be given 30–60 minutes before beginning treatment prophylactically.
29. a. Doxorubicin is a vesicant, and tissue necrosis can occur 2–4 days after administration. Dexrazoxane is a parenteral chemoprotectant drug used to treat anthracycline extravasation.
30. d. Two pairs of disposable gloves, preferably powder-free gloves (nitrile, polyurethane), should be worn when preparing chemotherapy and changed every 30 minutes or if they become punctured or contaminated.
31. b. The patient and his family will need to be alert for signs of infection attributable to the effects of chemotherapy. Assessing the temperature will need to become a part of his routine.
32. a. Aromatases are enzymes that convert other hormones into estrogens that can increase the risk of breast cancer. Aromatase inhibitors block the conversion of androgens to estrogens and slow tumor growth.
33. d. Vincristine lowers the effects of phenytoin, so the patient must be carefully observed for an increase in seizure activity.
34. c. An alcohol-based mouthwash will be very uncomfortable for a patient with stomatitis. Also, if the skin barrier is broken, using an alcohol-based mouthwash will potentially cause further irritation.

Case Study: Critical Thinking

1. Cyclophosphamide is an alkylating drug. It works by causing the DNA strand to cross-link, strands to break, and abnormal base pairing to occur. This prevents the cancer cells from dividing.

Cyclophosphamide is also a CCNS (cell cycle–nonspecific) drug that kills cells across the lifespan.

2. Some major side effects of cyclophosphamide include nausea and vomiting, anemia, risk for infection, and bleeding. Some side effects specific to this medication include the potential for hemorrhagic cystitis, discoloration of the nails, cardiomyopathy, and syndrome of inappropriate antidiuretic hormone (SIADH) secretion.

3. A thorough nursing history and physical assessment are crucial for this patient throughout the course of therapy. A baseline assessment of laboratory values, x-rays, and vital signs is very important. A psychosocial assessment should also be completed. Careful monitoring of the patient's temperature daily is crucial to watch for early signs of infection.

4. The patient should be taught that adequate fluid intake (both oral and IV) will be very important to prevent hemorrhagic cystitis. Even if the patient is nauseated, small sips of water at frequent intervals may be beneficial. The goal for fluid intake is 2–3 L/day. The patient should be advised not to become pregnant while undergoing treatment. Also, before using any OTC drugs or herbal preparations, the patient should confer with her healthcare provider since there are several herbs (ginseng, garlic, kava kava, echinacea, ginkgo, St. Johns wort) that may have interactions with chemotherapy. If the patient has a desire for complementary therapy, it should be respected as much as possible.

CHAPTER 36: TARGETED THERAPIES TO TREAT CANCER

1. Growth factors
2. Proteasomes
3. growth, spread
4. EGFR (epidermal growth factor receptor)
5. Kinases
6. d
7. b
8. a
9. e
10. c
11. d. Shortness of breath could be an indication of an anaphylactic reaction. The infusion must be stopped immediately and the reaction treated.
12. c. Bevacizumab blocks the VEGF which inhibits tumor angiogenesis. This prevents the tumor from receiving blood and nutrients, thereby inhibiting tumor's microvascular growth.
13. b. Diarrhea is a common side effect for gefitinib. Other side effects include skin reactions, anorexia, vomiting, and elevated liver enzymes.
14. a, b, e. mAbs are antibodies that are specific to tumor cells that express the target antigen. The class mAbs include fully human antibodies, murine antibodies, chimeric antibodies, and humanized antibodies.

15. a. Gefitinib is extensively metabolized by the liver, and it can increase the levels of other drugs, such as warfarin, which can increase the international normalized ratio (INR).
16. b. Other drugs, such as ketoconazole, that are CYP3A4 enzyme inhibitors can increase the plasma concentration of sunitinib, leading to toxicity.
17. c. Erlotinib can cause interstitial lung disease. Assessing lung sounds for adventitious sounds is the most important action by the nurse in a patient beginning to receive erlotinib. Patients who have preexisting respiratory problems are cautioned in receiving erlotinib because pulmonary fibrosis may occur.
18. a. Imatinib may cause thrombocytopenia and increase the risk for bleeding. This may be initially apparent with bleeding gums, bruising, and petechiae.
19. c. Ziv-aflibercept is an angiogenesis inhibitor. Its primary action is to prevent the development of new blood vessels.
20. b. Notify the healthcare provider. Rituximab can worsen hypotension when given with antihypertensive drugs. The dose may need to be decreased or the nurse may need to give a bolus of IV fluids, but the nurse must first notify the provider for the order.

Case Study: Critical Thinking

1. For metastatic ovarian cancer, bevacizumab 10 mg/kg is administered intravenously every 2 weeks in combination with paclitaxel.
2. Bevacizumab binds to vascular endothelial growth factor (VEGF) and prevents the binding of VEGF with its receptors. It blocks angiogenesis, and the goal is to slow the disease progression.
3. Side effects include hypertension, headache, rhinitis, asthenia, dry skin, and back pain. Adverse effects of bevacizumab are GI perforations, encephalopathy, renal toxicity, thromboembolic events, and congestive heart failure. Although there are many side effects and/or adverse effects, bevacizumab is used for those patients with metastatic disease where the benefits outweigh the risks.
4. Because of the many potential side and adverse effects, the patient should be informed of when to notify the healthcare provider. The patient should notify her provider if she develops any GI symptoms, such as nausea, vomiting, or diarrhea, because of the risk for GI perforation or formation of fistulas. Chest pain, abdominal pain, or swelling with redness or pain in the legs should be reported immediately. She should also report any blood in the stools. The patient should not take NSAIDs because of the risk for bleeding. The patient should avoid dehydration and should wear loose clothing to prevent thrombosis.

CHAPTER 37: BIOLOGIC RESPONSE MODIFIERS

1. biologic response modifiers; restore
2. recombinant DNA; hybridoma technology
3. immunomodulation; metastasizing
4. monocytes
5. red blood cells
6. endothelium; neutrophils
7. capillary leak syndrome
8. b
9. c
10. a
11. d
12. a, b, d. The main function of BRMs is to assist the immune system by the following: enhance the immune system, have cancer cells behave like healthy cells, inhibit normal cells from changing into cancer cells, enhance the body to repair or replace damaged cells, and prevent from metastasizing.
13. d. Granulocytes may become sequestered in the pulmonary system and cause dyspnea. This will cause an additional stress on the already compromised patient. Special attention should be paid to complaints of difficulty breathing.
14. b. It is important to assess the hemoglobin level. Risk for complications is higher when EPO is administered to patients with a hemoglobin level >11 g/dL.
15. a, b, c. Interferons should be stopped if patients develop severe depression, hematologic toxicity (severe neutropenia and thrombocytopenia), and hepatic decompensation. Dosages are adjusted for hematologic toxicity other than neutropenia or thrombocytopenia.
16. a. Common side effects of interferons are flu-like symptoms, such as fever, chills, malaise, and myalgia. Other common side effects include neurological symptoms, such as paresthesia; alopecia, xerostomia, and dizziness. These and other side effects will subside after the drug is stopped.
17. a, c, d. Dermatologic effects include alopecia, xerostomia, and rash. Ecchymosis is not a common dermatologic effect from interferons.
18. a, b, d. The patient should be educated regarding side effects, adverse effects, and how to administer interferon alpha. The side effects from BRM administration usually disappear 72–96 hours after discontinuation of therapy.
19. b, c. GM-CSF should be administered to both allogeneic and autologous BMT recipients. It is not recommended for Kaposi sarcoma. GM-CSF is used for an ANC <1500/mm³, and it should not be used within 24 hours of chemotherapy.
20. a, c, e. Conventional high-dose aldesleukin is associated with significant adverse effects that can affect essentially every organ. Many of the adverse effects are due to capillary leak syndrome, which results from extravasation of plasma proteins into the extravascular space. The dose should be interrupted or discontinued when the nurse observes new arrhythmia, blood in stool, hypoglycemia, any changes to mentation, new skin eruption, myocardial infarction/myocarditis, sepsis, and hepatic failure, among others.

Case Study: Critical Thinking

1. G-CSF is not a chemotherapeutic drug but is used in conjunction with myelosuppressive chemotherapy to increase production of neutrophils and enhance phagocytosis to help fight infection. It is an adjunct to chemotherapy.
2. Side effects of G-CSF are like those of other BRMs (nausea, vomiting, fatigue, etc.); however, bone pain is consistently reported with G-CSF because of the action on the bone marrow. Bone pain occurs more frequently in patients receiving higher doses.
3. Priority teaching instructions include the use of nonopioids to help relieve bone pain. Should the patient want to become pregnant, the healthcare provider should be notified immediately, as caution should be used in administering this G-CSF to pregnant patients. The patient should also report any abdominal pain, including pain referred to the left shoulder, as well as chest pain or unusual bleeding, such as hematuria or bloody stool.

CHAPTER 38: UPPER RESPIRATORY DISORDERS

1. c
2. a
3. d
4. b
5. H₁, smooth
6. first-generation; dry mouth; drowsiness
7. nonsedating; anticholinergic
8. tolerance; rebound nasal congestion; 3 days
9. alpha-adrenergic; vasoconstriction; hypertension
10. a
11. b
12. b
13. a
14. b
15. a
16. b. Antihistamines block H₁ receptors found in the extravascular smooth muscles resulting in an anticholinergic effect. This antagonist effect can cause dryness of the mouth and decreased secretions. Antihistamines can also decrease nasal itching. Antihistamines do not have an analgesic (pain relief) property. Antitussives suppress cough rather than decrease secretions. Antihistamines have an anticholinergic, not cholinergic, effect.
17. a. Second-generation antihistamines have fewer anticholinergic effects than first-generation antihistamines. Drowsiness is less with second-generation antihistamines.

18. d. Phenylpropanolamine was discontinued in all over-the-counter cold remedies and weight-loss aids because of an increased risk of stroke, hypertension, renal failure, and cardiac dysrhythmias.

19. a. The recommended dose to treat allergies with diphenhydramine is 25–50 mg every 4–6 hours, with a maximum dose of 300 mg/day.

20. d. Diphenhydramine is an H_1 antagonist and is one of the most frequently used over-the-counter antihistamines. Diphenhydramine has antitussive effects, in addition to treating allergic rhinitis, sneezing, pruritus, urticaria, and motion sickness.

21. c. Breastfeeding patients need to be instructed that small amounts of diphenhydramine can pass into breast milk. Since children are more susceptible to the antihistamine effects, use of diphenhydramine while breastfeeding is contraindicated.

22. d. Both nasal and systemic decongestants have different mechanisms of action. Nasal decongestants have sympathomimetic actions which stimulate the alpha-adrenergic receptors that cause vasoconstriction. Frequent use of nasal decongestants can have a rebound effect. Systemic decongestants are alpha-adrenergic agonists primarily used for allergic rhinitis. The advantage of systemic over nasal decongestants is that they last longer. But, nasal decongestants have quicker action.

23. c. Expectorant reduces the viscosity of secretions so that they can be eliminated by coughing. The most common ingredient in cold remedies is guaifenesin. However, the best way to help loosen mucus is by maintaining hydration.

24. a, b, c, d. The class of drugs used to treat cold symptoms include antihistamines (H_1 blockers for vasoconstriction), decongestants (vasoconstriction), antitussives (control cough), and expectorants (to thin secretions).

25. a, b, c, d. Decongestants are not contraindicated in obesity unless the patient also has any of the other diagnoses.

26. c, d. Antihistamines may cause drowsiness. Diphenhydramine is a common ingredient in OTC sleeping preparations. Should the patient choose to take any OTC drugs, the patient should be instructed to read the label carefully to check for interactions. The best option, however, is to check with the healthcare provider or pharmacist. Decongestants taken at bedtime may cause insomnia or jitteriness. Antibiotics are ineffective against a virus.

Case Study: Critical Thinking

1. Oxymetazoline is a decongestant nasal spray that is used to help constrict the vessels within the nasal cavity. The nasal mucous membranes shrink, and it is easier for the patient to exchange air through the nose.

2. The correct dose for this patient would be two or three sprays in each nostril, morning and night. It should not be used for longer than 3–5 days because of the potential for rebound congestion.

3. Rebound congestion occurs because of irritation of the nasal mucosa leading to vasodilation instead of vasoconstriction.

4. Use of nasal decongestants can also lead to nasal dryness and, if overused, epistaxis. Some brands of oxymetazoline are listed as moisturizing.

5. Another option is to use saline nasal drops, although this will only moisturize and not serve as a decongestant. Oral decongestants such as phenylephrine or pseudoephedrine may also be used. Also important with this patient is to determine the cause of the nasal congestion. Allergies may be treated with intranasal glucocorticoids and first- or second-generation antihistamines. A common cold will not be treated with glucocorticoids.

CHAPTER 39: LOWER RESPIRATORY DISORDERS

1. d
2. e
3. b
4. f
5. c
6. a, b
7. b
8. f
9. cyclic adenosine monophosphate (cAMP)
10. epinephrine
11. beta$_2$-adrenergic agonists
12. cAMP
13. increases
14. synergistic
15. shorter
16. methylxanthine (xanthine); asthma
17. glucocorticoids
18. prophylactic; histamine
19. rebound bronchospasm
20. beta$_2$
21. is
22. evening
23. 10 mg/day
24. mucolytics
25. antibiotic
26. c. The inhaler should be shaken well before each use. Inhalers do not require refrigeration. By testing the inhaler each time to see if the spray works, the patient is losing a dose of the medication.
27. a, b, d, e. Inhaled doses of drugs for asthma have a more rapid onset and fewer side effects than oral preparations. Inhalers are shorter acting than oral drugs. Some inhaled and oral drugs can be taken together.
28. a. The bronchodilator helps open the airway which increases the effectiveness of the inhaled steroid. Beta agonist can cause tachycardia, but it is not the reason to take the beta agonist before the inhaled steroid.
29. a, c. Long-term use of glucocorticoids can cause impaired immune response, hyperglycemia, fluid

retention, electrolyte imbalance, hypertension, thinning of the skin, abnormal subcutaneous fat distribution, and purpura. Insomnia, vomiting, and weight loss can be seen with short-term use.

30. b. Ipratropium is an anticholinergic drug that is administered via meter dose inhaler (MDI). It can also be administered via aerosol nebulizer treatment. Unlike albuterol, ipratropium has few side effects which include headache, blurred vision, tachycardia, urinary retention, and constipation.

31. d. Taking theophylline and ephedra together may increase the risk of theophylline toxicity. Hyperglycemia is a sign of theophylline toxicity.

32. a, b, c, d. It is not necessary to wait 5 minutes between inhalations.

33. a, b, c, e. Beta-blockers increase the half-life of theophylline. Theophylline increases the risk of digitalis toxicity and decreases the effects of lithium. Phenytoin decreases theophylline levels.

34. b. Cromolyn sodium is used as a prophylactic medication to prevent asthma attacks by preventing the release of histamine and suppressing inflammation in the bronchioles. It will not stop an attack once it has started and is not a bronchodilator.

35. c. The therapeutic range for theophylline is 10–20 mcg/mL.

Case Study: Critical Thinking

1. Albuterol is a selective beta$_2$ agonist. It is considered a "rescue inhaler" and can be used on an as-needed basis during an acute asthma attack. Montelukast sodium is a leukotriene modifier. Fluticasone propionate/salmeterol 100/50 is a glucocorticoid combination drug that contains fluticasone propionate 100 mcg and salmeterol 50 mcg.

2. Albuterol is a fast-acting selective beta$_2$ agonist and provides bronchodilation. It has fewer side effects than nonselective beta agonists. Leukotrienes are chemical mediators that cause airway edema and increase mucous production. Leukotriene modifiers, such as montelukast sodium, decrease inflammation. They must be taken daily and are not effective to treat an acute asthma attack. Glucocorticoids, such as fluticasone propionate/salmeterol, have antiinflammatory properties, and they work synergistically with beta$_2$ agonists.

3. Patients should be encouraged to keep all appointments as scheduled and to contact the healthcare provider before taking any over-the-counter drugs. If the patient smokes, information on smoking cessation programs should be given. Female patients should be advised to notify the healthcare provider if contemplating pregnancy. Patients with asthma should be encouraged to stay hydrated and report any increased use of "rescue inhalers" like albuterol. A patient with asthma should also be encouraged to wear a medical identification bracelet or necklace to indicate the drugs being taken.

CHAPTER 40: CARDIAC GLYCOSIDES, ANTIANGINALS, AND ANTIDYSRHYTHMICS

1. b
2. e
3. c
4. d
5. a
6. weakens; enlarges
7. increase
8. digitalis glycosides; inhibit
9. increase; decrease
10. positive inotropic action (increases heart contraction); negative chronotropic action (decreases heart rate); negative dromotropic action (decreases conduction of the heart cells); and increased stroke volume
11. decrease
12. warfarin (or other anticoagulants)
13. hypokalemia, hypomagnesemia, hypercalcemia
14. dilating; arterioles; renal; decreases
15. extensive first-pass metabolism by the liver
16. smooth muscle of blood vessels
17. 1–3; 3
18. headache
19. beta-blockers and calcium channel blockers
20. verapamil; diltiazem
21. reflex tachycardia; pain
22. stressed (or exerted)
23. frequently, unpredictable, and progressive
24. is at rest
25. spasm
26. reduction of venous tone or coronary vasodilation
27. hypoxia; hypercapnia
28. fast sodium channel blockers; beta-blockers; calcium channel blockers; also drugs that prolong repolarization
29. alcohol; cigarettes
30. b
31. a
32. a
33. c
34. d
35. c. Phosphodiesterase inhibitors, such as milrinone, promote positive inotropic response and vasodilation, not vasoconstriction. Phosphodiesterase inhibitors do not increase serum sodium and potassium levels. Increasing serum sodium can promote water retention, which will worsen heart failure.
36. Quinidine is a fast sodium channel blocker that decreases sodium influx into cardiac cells. The response is slowed conduction speed, suppressed automaticity, and increased repolarization time.
37. Amiodarone prolongs repolarization and is given intravenously in emergency treatment for ventricular dysrhythmias when other antidysrhythmics are not effective. Atropine is for symptomatic bradycardia; acebutolol is for premature ventricular contractions and is given orally.

38. Lidocaine is used to treat ventricular dysrhythmias. Atrial fibrillation, bradycardia, and complete heart block are atrial dysrhythmias.

39. a, c. Constipation is a side effect of verapamil, which is taken three times per day. Verapamil may cause hypotension, not hypertension.

40. Calcium channel blockers can affect kidney and liver function, so baseline liver enzymes and renal function should be obtained and trended.

41. ANP and BNP are elevated in persons with HF. Both are secreted from the atrial cells of the heart.

42. Normal values are less than 100 pg/mL. Greater than 100 pg/mL is considered elevated. Older females tend to have higher normal BNP levels than older males; however, a level of 630 pg/mL is markedly elevated and is of concern for heart failure.

43. Digitalis drugs, such as digoxin, can be used for heart failure or atrial fibrillation. Atrial fibrillation is a cardiac dysrhythmia of the atria.

44. The usual maintenance dose of digoxin is 0.125–0.5 mg/d. Answers b and c are too low and answer d is too high of a dose. The therapeutic serum level for digoxin is 0.8–2 ng/mL.

45. b. Digoxin has a long half-life of 30–40 hours and has low protein-binding power of 20%–30%. Because of the long half-life, drug accumulation can occur causing digoxin toxicity. Serum digoxin levels are drawn to assess for possible toxicity. The therapeutic serum level when taken for dysrhythmias is 0.8–2 ng/mL. When digoxin is taken for heart failure, the therapeutic level is 0.5–1 ng/mL.

46. Digoxin-immune Fab can be given to treat severe digitalis toxicity. This drug binds with digoxin so that it can be excreted in the urine.

47. a, b, c. Cortisone, furosemide, and hydrochlorothiazide all promote loss of potassium, which increases the effect of digitalis and can lead to digitalis toxicity. A person taking a potassium-wasting diuretic or cortisol should avoid hypokalemia by eating potassium-rich foods or taking potassium supplements.

48. There are no specific drug-food contraindications for digoxin. The patient should be encouraged to eat foods high in potassium such as fruits and vegetables (including potatoes). A patient with heart failure should avoid hot dogs because of their high sodium content.

49. a, b. Nitroglycerin tablets should not be chewed but should be placed under the tongue. There are no dietary restrictions when taking nitroglycerin. Tablets must be stored in their original amber glass container and away from light to prevent decomposition. A very dry mouth will hinder absorption, so sips of water may be taken. If chest pain persists or worsens after three tablets, the patient should seek emergency assistance by calling 911 rather than notifying their healthcare provider.

50. The duration of action for NTG patch is 18–24 hours. However, patients should be instructed to remove the patch nightly to allow for 8–12 hours of nitrate-free interval to avoid building tolerance.

51. Acebutolol is a beta-blocker and should not be abruptly stopped because abrupt discontinuation can lead to reflex tachycardia or dysrhythmias.

52. a, d, e. Aloe, ma-huang, and ginseng should be avoided while taking digoxin. Aloe and ma-huang can increase the risk of digoxin toxicity; ginseng can falsely elevate digoxin levels.

53. a, b, e. Electrolyte imbalances, especially potassium, calcium, and magnesium, can lead to cardiac dysrhythmias. Excessive catecholamines may lead to rapid atrial or ventricular rates as well as ectopy. Hypoxia and hypercapnia may also cause dysrhythmias.

Case Study: Critical Thinking

1. The three different types of angina are classic, unstable, and variant. Classic angina is fairly predictable and occurs with stress or exertion. Unstable angina is also known as *preinfarction angina*. It is unpredictable and increases in frequency and severity. Unstable angina may or may not be related to stress. Variant angina is also known as *vasospastic* or *Prinzmetal angina*. It occurs at rest. Patients frequently have a combination of both classic and variant angina. Classic angina is caused by an actual narrowing of the coronary arteries, whereas variant angina is caused by vessel spasms. Unstable angina often indicates an impending myocardial infarction (MI).

2. Vasospastic angina or variant angina occurs at rest. But since stress plays a part in anginal attacks, avoiding strenuous activities, heavy meals, and emotional upset may be beneficial nonpharmacologic methods to treat vasospastic angina. Smoking cessation is very important to overall cardiac health. Preventive measures include adequate rest and relaxation techniques.

   Pharmacologic treatments for angina include nitrates, beta-blockers, and calcium channel blockers. Antianginal drugs either increase oxygen supply or decrease oxygen demand by the myocardium. Nitrates reduce venous tone, promote vasodilation, and decrease cardiac workload. Beta and calcium channel blockers decrease oxygen demand by decreasing the workload of the heart. Nitrates and calcium channel blockers are effective for treating vasospastic angina.

3. Beta-blockers and calcium channel blockers can be used to treat angina. Beta-blockers include atenolol, metoprolol, and nadolol. Calcium channel blockers include amlodipine, diltiazem, and verapamil hydrochloride. Beta-blockers should be used in persons with stable angina. Nitrates and calcium channel blockers can be used for variant angina. Nitrates are also used for unstable angina.

4. Nitrates cause relaxation and dilation of blood vessels, including coronary vasculature, which

decreases resistance; hence, blood pressure drops. Nitrates also decrease preload and afterload, reducing myocardial oxygen demand.

CHAPTER 41: DIURETICS

a. Tubules: *Proximal tubule*
   Class of diuretic: *Osmotic and carbonic anhydrase inhibitors*
   Electrolytes: *Na⁺*

b. Tubules: *Loop of Henle*
   Class of diuretic: *Loop diuretics*
   Electrolytes: *Na⁺ and K⁺*

c. Tubules: *Distal tubule or distal convoluted tubule*
   Class of diuretic: *Thiazides*
   Electrolytes: Na⁺ and K⁺

d. Tubules: *Collecting tubule*
   Class of diuretic: *Potassium sparing*
   Electrolytes: *K⁺*

Laboratory Test	Normal Levels	Abnormal Results
1. Potassium	3.5–5 mEq/L	Hypokalemia
2. Magnesium	1.5–2.5 mg/dL	Hypomagnesemia
3. Calcium	8.6–10.2 mEq/L	Hypercalcemia
4. Chloride	96–106 mEq/L	Hypochloremia
5. Bicarbonate	24–28 mEq/L	Minimal bicarbonate loss
6. Uric acid	2.8–8 mg/dL	Hyperuricemia
7. Blood sugar	70–99 mg/dL	Hyperglycemia
8. Blood lipids	Total chol: <200 mg/dL LDL: <100 mg/dL Trig: <150 mg/dL	Hyperlipidemia

9. The two main purposes of diuretics are to decrease fluid and decrease hypertension (lower blood pressure).

10. Most diuretics promote sodium and water loss by blocking sodium and chloride reabsorption from the renal tubules. This causes a decrease in fluid volume in the tissues and circulation, which lowers blood pressure.

11. b, d, e. Diuretics are classified according to their mechanisms of action. Loop diuretics promote the loss of potassium and sodium, potassium-sparing diuretics promote the loss of sodium while retaining potassium, and thiazide diuretics promote the loss of sodium and some potassium. All diuretics promote the loss of water. While osmotic diuretics promote the loss of water and sodium, they are not used to treat hypertension and congestive heart failure; instead, they are used to decrease edema,

especially cerebral edema. Carbonic anhydrase inhibitors also promote water and bicarbonate loss with minimal influence on electrolytes. Their use is to decrease intraocular pressure, not hypertension and heart failure.

12. b. Spironolactone is a potassium-sparing diuretic. It promotes potassium retention in the renal tubules.

13. a. Furosemide is a loop diuretic, which promotes excretion of water, sodium, and potassium, primarily in the loop of Henle and some in the distal renal tubules. Other electrolytes that are excreted include magnesium, ammonium, phosphate, and calcium.

14. c. Spironolactone blocks the action of aldosterone and inhibits the sodium-potassium pump, so potassium is retained. This is important in maintaining a regular cardiac rhythm. It is frequently prescribed and is not contraindicated in patients who have had a myocardial infarction. Sodium is excreted with this drug. Patients should be advised not to overindulge in foods rich in potassium such as bananas, because this could cause above-normal levels of potassium (hyperkalemia).

15. d. To prevent hearing loss, furosemide must be administered by slow IV push over at least 1–2 minutes. It does not need to be diluted and does not require a central line for administration. Cardiac monitoring is not essential, because furosemide does not generally cause arrhythmias.

16. a, b, d. Hypokalemia, or low serum potassium level, is a risk for patients taking thiazides. This could be a life-threatening condition. Sodium is also lost, causing hyponatremia. Calcium level is elevated because thiazides block calcium excretion. There is minimal effect on bicarbonate levels. Cautious use in patients with hepatic failure is recommended, but trending of AST/ALT levels is not always indicated. Baseline values may be beneficial.

17. a. The normal range for serum potassium level is 3.5–5 mEq/L. A level of 5.8 mEq/L is considered hyperkalemic. The dose of spironolactone may need to be held or decreased, and the patient should decrease their intake of potassium-rich foods such as bananas, apricots, leafy greens, and salmon.

18. a. Acetazolamide is a carbonic anhydrase inhibitor. It blocks the action of carbonic anhydrase, which is an enzyme that affects hydrogen ion balance. If the action is blocked, more bicarbonate will be excreted, leading to metabolic acidosis.

19. d. Because the onset of action HCTZ is 2 hours, it may be best to take the drug when the patient will be awake for several hours so sleep is not disturbed. Hydrochlorothiazide can be taken with food to prevent GI upset. The drug needs to be taken consistently, even if the patient is not having symptoms of heart failure.

20. a. Furosemide will cause an increased loss of potassium (hypokalemia) when given with amiodarone, which may predispose the patient to ventricular arrhythmias.

21. c. Muscle weakness, abdominal distention, severe leg cramping, and cardiac arrhythmias are indications of hypokalemia (low potassium levels). Low potassium levels may occur with the use of loop diuretics.

22. a. Loop diuretics are contraindicated in patients with anuria (no urine). Giving diuretics to a patient without any urine output will not force urine production. Patients allergic to sulfa drugs should not take furosemide or bumetanide; these are derivatives of sulfonamides.

23. d. Daily weights and vital signs need to be trended at home on a daily basis. The patient and family should be educated on how to take these measurements or arrangements should be made for assessment by home health services, at least initially. The onset of action for hydrochlorothiazide is 2 hours. Hyperglycemia is a side effect of hydrochlorothiazide, so blood sugar level should be monitored. This medication can be taken with food to prevent nausea.

Case Study: Critical Thinking

1. Mannitol is an osmotic diuretic that is used for patients with increased intracranial pressure and increased intraocular pressure. Osmotic diuretics increase osmolality and sodium reabsorption which will allow fluid to shift from the brain tissue to the vasculature. Sodium, chloride, potassium, and water are then excreted. This shift in fluid will cause, at least temporarily, a decrease in intracranial pressure.

2. The standard dosage range in adults for increased intracranial pressure (ICP) for mannitol is 0.25–1 g/kg, followed by 0.25 mg/kg to 1 g/kg infused over 30–60 minutes. The drug can be repeated every 6–8 hours. While there is no true maximum dose, the nurse must closely monitor patient's renal function. Mannitol crystallizes easily, so it must be warmed before administration. It is given through an IV administration set with a filter.

3. For this patient the correct initial dose and maintenance dose would be 20–80 g over 30–60 minutes.

CHAPTER 42: ANTIHYPERTENSIVES

1. beta-adrenergic blockers; centrally acting alpha$_2$ agonists; alpha-adrenergic blockers; also adrenergic neuron blockers, alpha$_1$- and beta$_1$-adrenergic blockers

2. diuretics, direct-acting arteriolar vasodilators; also ACE inhibitors, angiotensin II–receptor blockers, and calcium channel blockers

3. beta-blockers; ACE inhibitors; also angiotensin II–receptor blockers, potassium-sparing diuretics, centrally acting alpha$_2$ agonist

4. diuretics

5. diminished; lowered

6. cardioselective

7. decreased; increased

8. c

9. d

10. b

11. a

12. e

13. f

14. g

15. h

16. b. Nonselective alpha-adrenergic blockers are used for severe hypertension associated with pheochromocytomas (catecholamine-secreting tumors of the adrenal medulla).

17. d. Direct-acting vasodilators relax the smooth muscles of the blood vessels, mainly the arteries, resulting in vasodilation. This promotes blood flow to the brain, kidneys, and other vital organs. Vasodilation causes the blood pressure to decrease.

18. d. Diuretics are frequently given with a variety of antihypertensive to decrease fluid retention and peripheral edema.

19. a, b, c. Angiotensin II binds to cell receptors to increase blood pressure. Angiotensin II also causes vasoconstriction and increases vascular resistance. ARBs inhibit the binding of angiotensin II at receptor sites, thereby decreasing blood pressure. Without the binding, vasoconstriction does not occur and the peripheral resistance is not increased. ARBs do not increase sodium retention or decrease heart rate.

20. b. ARBs inhibit the binding of angiotensin II to receptor sites; thereby, blood pressure does not increase. Diuretics, such as thiazides, assist in lowering blood pressure by promoting water and sodium loss.

21. a. The primary side effect of captopril (ACE inhibitors) is a constant, irritated cough (which could be an early sign of angioedema) which may be relieved upon discontinuation of the drug. Valsartan (ARBs) have less incidences of coughing. However, patients still need to be monitored for angioedema with ARBs. Patients may become dizzy due to either captopril or valsartan due to hypotension. Constipation could occur with either drug, but they are not the most limiting reason for the use of either drug. Sneezing does not occur with either drug.

22. d. Lisinopril is an ACE inhibitor. African Americans are not as responsive to ACE inhibitors as a monotherapy but may respond better if they are combined with a diuretic.

23. c. Calcium channel blockers and alpha$_1$ blockers may be more effective in African American patients for treating hypertension. They do not respond well to direct renin inhibitors, beta-blockers, and ACE inhibitors. ARBs have similar mechanism of action as ACE inhibitors, affecting the RAAS.

24. a. Ma-huang decreases or counteracts the effects of antihypertensives and can even increase the hypertensive state.

25. b. ACE inhibitors, such as captopril, when taken with nitrates, diuretics, or adrenergic blockers can increase the risk of hypotension. Nitrates cause vasodilation, diuretics cause sodium and water loss, and adrenergic blockers decrease sympathetic tone.

26. b. Aldosterone, a hormone secreted by the adrenal cortex, promotes sodium retention and potassium excretion. Captopril is an ACE inhibitor that inhibits the release of aldosterone. This action can increase serum potassium level, and if captopril is taken with a potassium-sparing diuretic, such as spironolactone, hyperkalemia is more likely.

27. b. Adherence to the medication regimen can be very frustrating to a patient who "feels better." Stopping an antihypertensive abruptly can lead to rebound hypertension.

28. a. Amlodipine, a calcium channel blocker, is highly protein bound (93%).

29. a, b, d. Metoprolol is a cardioselective beta-blocker that lowers blood pressure, which can cause dizziness, nausea, vomiting, and headache.

30. b. Ankle edema may occur with calcium channel blockers such as amlodipine because of its vasodilatory effect. There are other options that may be utilized to treat the patient's hypertension.

31. d, e. Cardioselective beta-blockers will help maintain renal blood flow and have fewer hypoglycemic effects than those associated with noncardioselective beta-blockers. Rebound symptoms are a possibility if the medication is stopped abruptly. Cardioselectivity does not confer absolute protection from bronchoconstriction.

32. b. Aliskiren can be used for mild to moderate hypertension, either as a monotherapy or with combination of other antihypertensives or diuretics. Aliskiren is not effective in reducing blood pressure among African American patients. Because aldosterone concentration is decreased, aliskiren can cause hyperkalemia, not hypokalemia.

Clinical Judgment Unfolding Case Study
Question 1

Assessment findings:
Reports dizziness
Reports "feels like a band around my head"
Serum sodium 149 mEq/L
Reports occasional epistaxis
Blood pressure 232/136 mm Hg
Blood urea nitrogen (BUN) 23 mg/dL
Creatinine 1.9 mg/dL

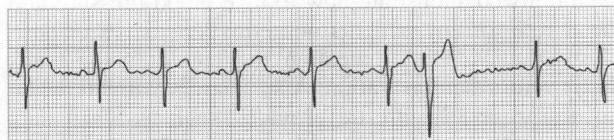

Rationale:

A nurse would follow up immediately for complaints of dizziness, reports of "feels like a band around my head," epistaxis, and hypertension with a blood pressure of 232/136 mm Hg. Hypertensive crisis is when the systolic blood pressure is over 180 or diastolic is over 120. Clonidine is a centrally acting alpha$_2$ agonist that decreases the sympathetic response from the brainstem to the peripheral vessels. This causes decreased peripheral vascular resistance and increased vasodilation, thereby reducing blood pressure. Because clonidine can cause fluid retention, a diuretic, such as chlorthalidone, is frequently prescribed. Rebound hypertensive crisis can occur if a centrally acting alpha$_2$ agonist, such as clonidine, is abruptly stopped. The patient reported that doses are missed here and there. Signs and symptoms of hypertensive crisis include hypertension, headache, and dizziness. If not treated, then it will progress to hypertensive emergencies, which are episodes of uncontrolled blood pressure that can cause acute impairment of one or more systems. If the hypertensive emergency is left untreated, permanent damage can occur. The renal function (BUN/creatinine) indicates mild elevation. The nurse would further assess the patient's renal function. This patient's blood pressure needs to be lowered but in a controlled setting. All other assessment findings are either normal or do not warrant immediate attention. The ECG shows normal sinus rhythm with occasional premature ventricular contractions.

Reference

McCuistion, L.E., DiMaggio, K.V., Winton, M.B., & Yeager, J.J. (2025). Pharmacology: A patient-centered nursing process approach, 12th ed. St. Louis, MO: Elsevier. pp. 536–550.

Question 2

Potential Issues	Risk to the Patient
	Orthostatic hypotension
	Fluid retention
	Renal insufficiency
	Rebound hypertension
	Hypernatremia

Rationale:

Clonidine is a centrally acting alpha$_2$ agonist that decreases the sympathetic response from the brainstem to the peripheral vessels. This causes decreased peripheral vascular resistance and increased vasodilation, thereby reducing blood pressure. One of the most troubling side effects of antihypertensives among older adults is orthostatic hypotension. The episode of sudden low blood pressure presents as dizziness due to blood pooling in the lower extremities. Older adults' sympathetic nervous system does not respond quickly to correct their hemodynamics. Additionally, rebound hypertensive crisis can occur if a centrally acting alpha$_2$ agonist, such as clonidine, is abruptly stopped. The patient reported that doses are missed here and there. Signs and symptoms of hypertensive crisis include hypertension, headache, and dizziness. If not treated, then it will progress to hypertensive emergencies, which are episodes of uncontrolled blood pressure that can cause acute impairment of one or more systems. If the hypertensive emergency is left untreated, permanent damage can occur. The renal function (BUN/creatinine) indicates mild elevation. The nurse would be concerned for possible end organ damage to the kidneys (renal insufficiency). Because clonidine can cause sodium and fluid retention, a diuretic, such as chlorthalidone, is frequently prescribed. Hypokalemia, not hyperkalemia, is a risk for the patient.

Reference

McCuistion, L.E., DiMaggio, K.V., Winton, M.B., & Yeager, J.J. (2025). Pharmacology: A patient-centered nursing process approach, 12th ed. St. Louis, MO: Elsevier. pp. 536–550.

PHASE 2:
Question 3

Options for 1	Options for 2	Options for 3	Options for 4
8739	Metabolic acidosis	Hypotension	Tachycardia

Rationale:
The patient received a total of 8739 mcg [$0.6 \times (178/2.2) \times 60$ min $\times 3$ h]. Nitroprusside is a very potent vasodilator that rapidly decreases blood pressure but retains water and sodium. Its actions are on both arterial and venous vessels. Its major metabolite or by-product is thiocyanide (cyanide). The nurse would assess the patient for signs and symptoms of cyanide toxicity, such as metabolic acidosis, profound hypotension, dyspnea, dizziness, and vomiting. Nitroprusside can also cause reflex tachycardia and palpitations. Other side effects/adverse drug reactions of nitroprusside are agitation, nausea, and confusion.

Reference

McCuistion, L.E., DiMaggio, K.V., Winton, M.B., & Yeager, J.J. (2025). Pharmacology: A patient-centered nursing process approach, 12th ed. St. Louis, MO: Elsevier. pp. 536–550.

Question 4

Nurse's Responses	Patient Questions	Appropriate Nurse's Response for Each Patient Question
	"Why do I need to take two pills when I used to take only one?"	"The metoprolol and hydrochlorothiazide come as a single pill."
	"Couldn't I just continue with my other blood pressure medicine?"	"The other pill caused a significant rebound high blood pressure. People generally tolerate the metoprolol better than clonidine."
	"How do I know if the medicine is working?"	"Let me show you how to take your blood pressure and heart rate. If your blood pressure is really low or you feel dizzy or your heart rate is less than 60, call your doctor."
	"Hopefully this medicine will not cause my blood pressure to skyrocket."	"Metoprolol has less tendency to cause rebound high blood pressure."

Rationale:
To increase medication adherence, diuretics, such as hydrochlorothiazide (HCTZ), are often combined with other antihypertensive drugs, such as beta-blockers or angiotensin-converting enzyme (ACE) inhibitors. Instead of needing to take two pills a day, the patient will be taking a single pill. Centrally acting alpha$_2$ agonist, such as clonidine, has the propensity to cause rebound hypertension when abruptly discontinued. Even though beta-blockers, such as metoprolol, can cause rebound hypertension in select individuals, it is generally well tolerated. A nurse would also demonstrate how to take blood pressure and heart rate for any patients on antihypertensives or antidysrhythmics. Best indication the patient understands is by return demonstration. Also instruct patients when to notify their healthcare provider, such as when they are dizzy or their heart rate is less than 60. Telling the patient "As long as you do not stop taking the medicine,

you will not have problems with high blood pressure" is accusatory.

Reference

McCuistion, L.E., DiMaggio, K.V., Winton, M.B., & Yeager, J.J. (2025). Pharmacology: A patient-centered nursing process approach, 12th ed. St. Louis, MO: Elsevier. pp. 536–550.

PHASE 3:
Question 5:

Nursing Actions	Indicated	Contraindicated
Administer with heart rate 54		X
Hold for blood pressure 90/68	X	
Administer when patient complains of fatigue		X
Hold for urine output of 90 mL in 4 hours	X	
Check blood pressure in sitting and standing	X	

Rationale:

Beta-blockers are sympatholytics that decrease basal sympathetic tone and reduce cardiac output. Vascular resistance is reduced, thereby lowering blood pressure. Beta-blockers also reduce heart rate, contractility, and renin release. The nurse would hold the antihypertensive for hypotension, such as a blood pressure of 90/68. Since beta-blockers influence renal function, the antihypertensive would be held for decreased urine output. Appropriate urine output would be 30 mL or greater per hour. In 4 hours the patient should have 120 mL, not 90 mL. Renal function can also be determined by blood urea nitrogen (BUN) and serum creatinine. The nurse would hold, not administer, metoprolol/hydrochlorothiazide for a heart rate less than 60. One of the side effects of beta-blockers is fatigue possibly due to hypotension and bradycardia. The cause of the fatigue should be explored prior to administering metoprolol/hydrochlorothiazide. Since antihypertensives can cause orthostatic hypotension, it would behoove the nurse to assess the patient's blood pressure and heart rate in sitting and standing positions.

Reference

McCuistion, L.E., DiMaggio, K.V., Winton, M.B., & Yeager, J.J. (2025). Pharmacology: A patient-centered nursing process approach, 12th ed. St. Louis, MO: Elsevier. pp. 536–550.

Question 6
Progress Notes:

- Blood pressure 98/64, apical pulse 86 and radial pulse 72 beats/min.
- Lung sounds with few crackles to bases bilaterally.
- Mild tenderness to lower quadrants. Reports no bowel movements for 3 days. Trace edema to ankles bilaterally.
- Sodium 132 mEq/L, potassium 3.4 mEq/L, calcium 11.3 mg/dL.
- First-degree atrioventricular (AV) block.

Rationale:

Beta-blockers are sympatholytics that decrease basal sympathetic tone and reduce cardiac output. Vascular resistance is reduced, thereby lowering blood pressure. Beta-blockers also reduce heart rate, contractility, and renin release. The nurse would hold the antihypertensive for hypotension, such as a blood pressure of 98/64. Beta-blockers, such as metoprolol, can cause bradycardia and dysrhythmias, such as first AV block. The dysrhythmias can progress into more lethal rhythm. Lungs with crackles can indicate an onset of pulmonary edema, which is an adverse reaction to metoprolol and hydrochlorothiazide. Abdominal pain can be related to constipation. The patient had not had a bowel movement for 3 days, which may indicate the patient is constipated. Hydrochlorothiazide can cause constipation because of fluid loss. Trace ankle edema could be an early sign of heart failure, which is an adverse reaction to metoprolol. Electrolyte imbalance (hyponatremia, hypokalemia, and hypercalcemia) can be due to hydrochlorothiazide and can become life threatening.

Reference

McCuistion, L.E., DiMaggio, K.V., Winton, M.B., & Yeager, J.J. (2025). Pharmacology: A patient-centered nursing process approach, 12th ed. St. Louis, MO: Elsevier. pp. 536–550.

CHAPTER 43: ANTICOAGULANTS, ANTIPLATELETS, AND THROMBOLYTICS

1. artery; vein
2. clot formation; do not
3. do not have
4. venous thrombus; pulmonary embolus
5. subcutaneously; intravenously
6. standard; bleeding
7. warfarin
8. decrease
9. 3–4
10. plasminogen; plasmin
11. bleeding/hemorrhage
12. fondaparinux
13. Order of heparin activity: d, b, a, c

14. c
15. d
16. a
17. a
18. e
19. d
20. f
21. b
22. f
23. c. Warfarin is an oral anticoagulant used to prevent blood clots. Fibrinolytics, not anticoagulants, dissolve existing clots.
24. a, b, c. Most patients on warfarin therapy are maintained at an international normalized ratio (INR) between 2 and 3 seconds. Patients with mechanical heart valves or recurrent systemic embolism should have an INR of 2.5–4.5 seconds.
25. b, d. Clopidogrel is an antiplatelet, and apixaban is a selective factor Xa inhibitor.
26. a. Abciximab is an antiplatelet drug in the glycoprotein (GP) IIb/IIIa receptor antagonist family. It is used primarily for acute coronary syndromes and for preventing reocclusion of coronary arteries following PTCA. Aminocaproic acid is an antagonist to thrombolytics (antithrombolytic) to stop bleeding by inhibiting thrombolysis. Protamine sulfate is an antidote to stop bleeding attributable to heparin or LMWH. Warfarin is an oral anticoagulant.
27. a. The correct dose for continuous infusion is 0.125 mcg/kg per minute. This patient weighs 76 kg (168 pounds ÷ 2.2 = 76 kg). 76 kg × 0.125 mcg/kg/min = 9.5 mcg/min.
28. d. Clopidogrel is an antiplatelet drug used frequently after a myocardial infarction. When used together with aspirin, the therapeutic effect is more effective than when used alone.
29. a. Various laboratory values will be monitored while a patient is taking warfarin. The most important levels to trend will be PT and INR. The INR and PT are closely related.
30. d. Vitamin K is the antidote for warfarin poisoning or overdose. Protamine sulfate is the antidote for heparin overdose. Anagrelide and ticagrelor are antiplatelets.
31. b. Warfarin is highly protein bound (over 90%). In drugs that are highly protein bound, such as fluoxetine, there is the potential for drug displacement of warfarin, leading to higher free drug levels in the blood. This can result in bleeding.
32. a. Fondaparinux is a synthetically manufactured antithrombotic that selectively inhibits factor Xa. The structure is closely related to heparin and LMWH. Uncontrolled bleeding, such as GI bleed, is considered an adverse reaction to fondaparinux. The drug should be discontinued.
33. b. Aminocaproic acid is an antithrombolytic drug that inhibits plasminogen activation, which inhibits thrombolysis. Reteplase is a thrombolytic. Calcium gluconate treats calcium deficiency. Protamine sulfate is the antidote for heparin overdose.
34. a, c, e. Vital signs should be continually assessed while a patient is receiving thrombolytics. Cardiac monitoring should be performed to observe for reperfusion arrhythmias. The nurse should also monitor for signs and symptoms of bleeding. Hemorrhage is a serious complication of thrombolytic therapy. Aminocaproic acid can be given as an antidote. Tenecteplase is given as an IV bolus. Liver enzymes are not usually affected. Typing and crossmatching blood products is not necessary unless there is significant blood loss requiring blood transfusions.
35. a, b, d, e. Anticoagulants would be beneficial for patients with a history of deep vein thrombosis, cerebrovascular accident (embolic stroke), and for those who have received an artificial heart valve. They are also beneficial in patients who have had major orthopedic surgeries, such as hip or knee replacements, to prevent pulmonary emboli.

Clinical Judgment Standalone Study

Answers:

Option 1	Option 2	Option 3	Option 4
Anticoagulants	Warfarin	Enoxaparin	2–3 seconds

Rationale:

The patient with a pulmonary embolus may become restless and complain of dyspnea and sharp chest pain. The patient will most likely be started on oral and/or parenteral anticoagulants, such as oral warfarin and parenteral enoxaparin. In addition to monitoring the patient's hemoglobin, hematocrit, and any evidence of active bleeding, the international normalized ratio would be maintained at 2–3 seconds if the patient is receiving oral warfarin.

Reference

McCuistion, L.E., DiMaggio, K.V., Winton, M.B., & Yeager, J.J. (2025). Pharmacology: A patient-centered nursing process approach, 12th ed. St. Louis, MO: Elsevier. pp. 551–562.

CHAPTER 44: ANTIHYPERLIPIDEMICS AND DRUGS TO IMPROVE PERIPHERAL BLOOD FLOW

1. Low-density lipoproteins (LDL), very-low-density lipoproteins (VLDL), high-density lipoprotein (HDL), chylomicrons
2. protein; fat
3. atherosclerotic plaques; heart disease
4. apolipoprotein
5. HMG-CoA reductase; HMG-CoA reductase inhibitors
6. homocysteine

7. arteriosclerosis; hyperlipidemia
8. b
9. c
10. a
11. a
12. b
13. e
14. d
15. c. There are two forms of apolipoproteins, apoB-48 and apoB-100. Of the two, apoB-100 is a better indicator for CAD.
16. d. Atorvastatin is a statin drug that inhibits HMG-CoA reductase in synthesizing cholesterol in the liver. Rhabdomyolysis is a severe side effect associated with statin drugs, such as atorvastatin. This occurs when muscle tissue breaks down. Rhabdomyolysis can be fatal. Also, serum liver enzymes should be monitored.
17. b. High levels of homocysteine have been linked to loss of flexibility (elasticity) to the vessel walls. Other effects associated with homocysteine include cardiovascular disease, stroke, blood clotting, damage to the vascular endothelial lining, and thickening of the vasculature.
18. c. Intermittent vascular claudications cause vasospasms, and vasodilators improve blood flow to the extremities. Gingko has been taken to treat intermittent claudication.
19. d. LDL contains 50%–60% of cholesterol in circulation and, with an elevated level, increases the risk for atherosclerotic plaques and heart disease.
20. a. An HDL level of 22 mg/dL is low. The normal value should be greater than 60 mg/dL. Low levels of HDL put the patient in the high-risk category for cardiovascular disease. A value less than 35 mg/dL is considered high risk.
21. b. Lifestyle changes, such as eating a low-fat, low-cholesterol diet, generally lower the cholesterol level by only 10%–30%. Other activities should be instituted, such as implementation of routine exercises to increase HDL level and cessation of smoking.
22. c. Diet, exercise, weight loss, and medication all play a vital role in decreasing cholesterol level. Diet continues to play a vital role, despite the antihyperlipidemic drug that is taken.
23. b, d, e. Cilostazol should be taken 30 minutes before or 2 hours after meals. Grapefruit juice will increase the levels of cilostazol, so it should be avoided. There is no contraindication for the use of acetaminophen. Headache and abdominal pain are both side effects of cilostazol. Blood pressure should be monitored frequently, and the patient should be encouraged to change positions slowly to prevent a precipitous drop in blood pressure.

Case Study: Critical Thinking

1. Atorvastatin is an HMG-CoA reductase inhibitor, or a "statin" drug. By inhibiting cholesterol synthesis in the liver, atorvastatin decreases LDL ("bad") cholesterol, slightly increases HDL ("good") cholesterol, and decreases triglycerides.

2. Atorvastatin is contraindicated to be used during pregnancy, including labor and delivery, and breastfeeding (lactation). The patient should use a reliable birth control to prevent pregnancy while on atorvastatin. Another form of treatment, other than statin drugs, may be needed to lower LDL.

3. Monitoring the patient for the desired effect is an obvious priority, although it is important for the nurse to advise the patient that changes in lipid profiles may take several weeks for lipid levels to decline. Liver enzymes should also be drawn at baseline and monitored throughout therapy. Many statin drugs are contraindicated in acute hepatic disease. Vision should be tested at least yearly, because there have been some studies that indicate an increased risk of cataracts in patients taking statins. This risk is higher in those with diabetes.

4. The nurse would emphasize that treatment of hyperlipidemia is a lifelong commitment. Making dietary changes, exercising, and using pharmacologic therapy will help decrease LDL levels and therefore potentially decrease the risk of heart disease. Other important points in the health teaching plan for the patient include the importance of keeping follow-up appointments with healthcare providers, taking the medication as scheduled even if she does not feel she is making any progress, and reporting any muscle pain or tenderness immediately. These symptoms can be an indication of the life-threatening adverse effect of rhabdomyolysis. She would report any vision changes. The nurse would also emphasize to not abruptly stop taking atorvastatin because of a serious rebound effect that could lead to a heart attack.

CHAPTER 45: GASTROINTESTINAL TRACT DISORDERS

1. f
2. d
3. e
4. b
5. g
6. c
7. a
8. chemoreceptor trigger zone (CTZ); medulla
9. antihistamines, bismuth subsalicylate, phosphorated carbohydrate
10. anticholinergics
11. glaucoma
12. antiemetics; chemoreceptor
13. nausea, vomiting; serotonin or $5HT_3$
14. cannabinoid
15. Laxatives; cathartics
16. sodium; magnesium
17. deficit; electrolyte

18. antihistamines, anticholinergics, dopamine antagonists, benzodiazepines, serotonin antagonists, glucocorticoids, cannabinoids, miscellaneous

19. fecal impaction, chronic laxative use, neurologic disorders, bowel obstruction, immobility, delayed defecation, insufficient fluid intake, poor dietary habits, certain drugs such as opioids and anticholinergics

20. Mix psyllium in 8–10oz of water, stir, and drink immediately, followed by another glass of water.

21. False. Prescription or nonprescription antiemetics *are not safe* for pregnant females to take. Antiemetics are not recommended for pregnant females to consume because of the risk to the fetus. Instead, nonpharmacologic treatment should be tried, such as flat soda or weak tea and crackers.

22. False. A person *can have one or more* per day to be "normal." A "normal" bowel movement varies from one person to another. A "normal" number of bowel movements can range from one per day to three per week.

23. True. Chronic use of laxatives can cause a person to become dependent on the laxative for a bowel movement, especially in older adults.

24. False. Even though castor oil is a natural substance, it is *still not safe* for females in early pregnancy to use for occasional constipation because it can stimulate uterine contractions.

25. a, b, c, e. All but the opioids can be used as antiemetics. Opioids can cause constipation that can decrease intestinal motility, thereby decreasing peristalsis; opioids can be used as antidiarrheals.

26. b. Promethazine is a phenothiazine that blocks H_1-receptor sites on effector cells, impedes histamine-mediated responses, and inhibits the CTZ.

27. a, b, c, d. Drinking weak tea and sodas that have gone flat may help with nausea. Open a can or bottle of soda and let it sit for several hours to remove its carbonation. Unsweetened gelatin may also be helpful. Crackers and dry toast may provide substance in the stomach. Dry toast (without butter) can be beneficial.

28. a. When poison is ingested, vomiting should not be induced because regurgitating these substances can cause esophageal injury. Instead, activated charcoal is administered to absorb the poison.

29. a, b, e. Diphenoxylate with atropine is an antidiarrheal. Usual side effects are caused by atropine, an anticholinergic; these include headache, drowsiness, and urinary retention. It also causes hypotension (not hypertension), nausea, and vomiting. It does not cause hypoglycemia.

30. b, d, e. Laxatives and/or cathartics include bulk forming, emollients, and stimulants. Adsorbents are considered antidiarrheal, and emetics are used to induce vomiting.

31. a. Bisacodyl is a stimulant laxative used for bowel preparation and for prevention and short-term treatment of constipation. Its action increases peristalsis

by directly affecting the smooth muscle of the intestine.

32. b. Mineral oil absorbs the fat-soluble vitamins so the body cannot absorb them. This can lead to vitamin deficiency.

33. d. Patients with any kind of bowel obstruction or severe abdominal pain should not take laxatives.

34. a, c, d, e. Promethazine is an antihistamine given for nausea and/or vomiting. Antihistamines inhibit histamine-mediated responses and have anticholinergic side effects, which include blurred vision, drowsiness, dry mouth, and hypotension.

35. c, d. A patient with diarrhea should avoid "heavy" fried foods and milk products. Promoting fluid intake and replacing electrolytes are priority interventions when the patient is experiencing diarrhea.

Case Study: Critical Thinking

1. Constipation has a variety of causes, including decreased fluid intake, poor diet, lack of exercise, and current drugs. Lack of appetite is a frequent complaint among the older adult. Poor dentition may lead to inability to eat raw fruits and vegetables. The opioid the patient is taking for postoperative hip pain, as well as the potential for decreased mobility and lack of exercise, may also lead to constipation.

2. Bisacodyl is a stimulant laxative that promotes defecation by irritating the smooth muscle of the intestine.

3. Omeprazole and other proton pump inhibitors will decrease the effect of bisacodyl, so dosage adjustments may need to be made. Calcium supplements can decrease the dissolving of bisacodyl. There are no serious interactions with either digoxin or hydrocodone.

4. It will be important for the nurse to encourage the patient to eat well and exercise as much as possible. Including bran and whole grain in the diet may be beneficial. Bulk-forming laxatives can provide the fiber that the patient may not be getting in a regular diet. When possible, the patient should discontinue use of the opioid pain reliever. The nurse would also advise the patient that the drug should be taken whole, with a glass of water. Milk should be avoided around the time of administration, because milk also reduces the effectiveness of the laxative. The patient should be instructed on the side effects of bisacodyl, such as abdominal cramps.

CHAPTER 46: ANTIULCER DRUGS

1. g
2. a, h
3. e
4. b
5. f
6. c

7. i
8. a
9. e
10. d
11. c
12. d
13. a
14. d
15. c
16. e
17. b
18. d
19. b
20. b. Antacids neutralize hydrochloric acid and should be taken 1–3 hours after meals and at bedtime. Chewable and liquid antacids should be followed by 2–4 oz of water to ensure the drugs reach the stomach. They should not be taken with meals because of the delayed gastric emptying time, which can increase acid production. Some antacids can cause acid rebound (increased acid production). Antacids should not be taken with other oral drugs concomitantly due to multiple drug-drug interactions.
21. b, c, d, f. Antiulcer drugs include anticholinergics, antacids, H_2 blockers/antagonists, and PPIs. Other antiulcer drugs include tranquilizers, pepsin inhibitors, and prostaglandin E_1 analogs.
22. c, e. Commonly used drugs to treat GERD include H_2 blockers/antagonists and PPIs. Anticholinergics and pepsin inhibitors are commonly used to treat ulcers. Antacids are used to decrease acid production, which can prevent ulcers.
23. d. Propantheline is an anticholinergic that inhibits gastric secretions and is used to treat peptic ulcers. Anticholinergics should be taken before meals to decrease acid secretion and at bedtime. It should not be used as a monotherapy.
24. a, b, c. Nizatidine should not be taken with meals, because it will delay absorption. The abdominal pain should have improved within 1–2 weeks, depending on the cause. Healing of the ulcer may take 4–8 weeks.
25. a, b, d, e. Side effects of famotidine and other H_2 blockers/antagonists include dizziness, headache, erectile dysfunction, and nausea. Other side effects include agitation, constipation, abdominal pain, diarrhea, vomiting, blurred vision, malaise, and weakness.
26. a, b, c. There are no documented interactions between esomeprazole and either lisinopril or propranolol. Esomeprazole interferes with the absorption of ampicillin, digoxin, and ketoconazole.
27. c. Hyperglycemia is an adverse reaction to sucralfate. Although the normal range for blood glucose may vary, a blood glucose level of 185 mg/dL is considered elevated. Another adverse reaction includes hypophosphatemia. Hgb, serum potassium, and INR are all normal.

Clinical Judgment Standalone Case Study

Answers:

- side
- hypercalcemia
- 40–60 mL

Rationale:

Antacids promote ulcer healing by neutralizing acid and reducing pepsin activity. Antacids containing aluminum hydroxide have a nonsystemic effect. Constipation (difficulty in "passing stool") is a common side effect of aluminum hydroxide. Continued use of the antacid can promote hypercalcemia, hypophosphatemia, and hypomagnesemia. Calcium is resorbed from the bones which promotes osteoporosis and nephrolithiasis. The usual dosage for aluminum hydroxide is 40–60 mL every 3–6 hours or 1–3 hours after meals and at bedtime. Patients should be encouraged to not "drink" from the bottle but instead use a medication dispensing system for proper dosage to minimize side effects.

Reference

McCuistion, L.E., DiMaggio, K.V., Winton, M.B., & Yeager, J.J. (2025). Pharmacology: A patient-centered nursing process approach, 12th ed. St. Louis, MO: Elsevier. pp. 590–602.

CHAPTER 47: EYE AND EAR DISORDERS

1. locally
2. artificial eyes
3. NSAIDs; corticosteroids
4. tear
5. intraocular; trabecular
6. angle-closure glaucoma (closed-angle glaucoma)
7. diuretics; glaucoma
8. cycloplegics
9. increase
10. conjunctivitis
11. carbonic anhydrase inhibitors
12. parasympathomimetic
13. h
14. f
15. i
16. a
17. b
18. d
19. c
20. j
21. g
22. e
23. c. Mydriatics dilate pupils for better visualization during a diagnostic procedure. Carbonic anhydrase inhibitors decrease intraocular pressure by decreasing the production of aqueous humor. Cerumenolytics soften and break up the cerumen in the external ear canal.

24. c. Acetazolamide is a systemic carbonic anhydrase inhibitor used to decrease IOP. Acetazolamide is also a diuretic and can cause fluid and electrolyte imbalances.

25. b. Carbamide peroxide is an OTC cerumenolytic that softens the cerumen to help break up cerumen so it can be washed away. Bimatoprost is a prostaglandin inhibitor to treat open-angle glaucoma to decrease IOP. Echothiophate is a cholinergic agonist used to treat open-angle glaucoma. Proparacaine is a topical anesthetic instilled in the eyes to conduct a comprehensive examination.

26. a, c, d, e. Pilocarpine is a cholinergic agonist with minimal systemic effects, but they can occur. The side effects are similar to that of cholinesterase inhibitors, which include blurred vision, eye pain, and headache. Cardiac dysrhythmias and respiratory depression are adverse reactions and are deemed an emergency.

27. e. There are two types of age-related macular degeneration, wet and dry. Dry AMD is more common, with vision being gradually lost. There is no known treatment or drug for dry AMD. Treatment for wet AMD targets vascular endothelial growth factor (VEGF).

28. a, b, c, d. Tetracaine is a topical anesthetic. The other medications listed are decongestants to help with the eye irritation attributable to allergies. Ophthalmic allergy drugs contain antihistamines and/or mast cell stabilizers.

29. b. A cotton wick is placed inside the external auditory canal (EAC) for medication to reach the length of the EAC. When the swelling subsides, the wick will fall out or it can be manually removed.

Case Study: Critical Thinking

1. Open-angle glaucoma occurs when there is too much aqueous humor that causes pressure and damages the optic nerve, which leads to decreased vision. As aqueous humor is formed, excess fluid drains through the trabecular meshwork structure of the eye. In open-angle glaucoma the trabecular network is clogged, and the excess fluid cannot drain. Open-angle glaucoma occurs gradually, and the cause is unknown.

2. There are several different classes of medications that are used to treat glaucoma. Timolol is a nonselective beta-adrenergic blocker. Beta-blockers are usually the first-line drugs in glaucoma treatment. Beta-blockers work by decreasing the production of aqueous humor.

3. The patient should wash hands before administration of the drug and be very careful not to touch the tip of the bottle to the eye. The head should be tipped back, and one drop instilled in the conjunctival sac of the lower lid. The patient should not rub the eyes after the drug is instilled. A tissue can be used to dab at the extra drug. Eyedrops should be instilled before any eye ointment.

4. No. This dose is too high. The standard dose is 1 gtt of 0.25%–0.5% solution bid initially; then it can be decreased to 1 gtt/day as the condition stabilizes. The patient must be carefully observed for bradycardia, bronchospasm, and indications of developing or worsening heart failure, since this drug may cause systemic effects.

CHAPTER 48: DERMATOLOGIC DISORDERS

1. c
2. d
3. b
4. a
5. f, h
6. h
7. b, c, d, e
8. a
9. b, c, d
10. athlete's foot, ringworm
11. Comedones; whiteheads; blackheads
12. teratogen; iPLEDGE
13. multisystem; skin; joints
14. rebound
15. T-cell
16. desquamation
17. thinning; atrophy
18. a, c, d. Acne vulgaris is a common skin disorder treated nonpharmacologically or with pharmacotherapy. Drugs used to treat acne include antibiotics, corticosteroids, and keratolytics. Antifungals can be used for skin disorders caused by tineas. Nonsteroidal antiinflammatories are not effective for skin inflammation. A T-cell antagonist, such as methotrexate, is a folate antimetabolite for systemic treatment of psoriasis.

19. a. Calcipotriene is a synthetic vitamin D analog that enhances keratinocyte differentiation while inhibiting their proliferation. There is no cure for psoriasis, but there are periods of remissions and exacerbations.

20. b. Infliximab is a biologic response modifier; specifically, it inhibits tumor necrosis factor and is given in a controlled environment via IV injection at prescribed intervals.

21. b, c, e. Contact dermatitis, a common form of eczema, can cause local manifestations, such as rash, swelling, and stinging at the affected skin site. Common skin irritants include cosmetics, dyes, and plants. Anesthetics and peanuts can also cause an allergic response, but usually the manifestations are systemic, such as anaphylaxis.

22. a. The standard initial dose for tetracycline is 500 mg q12h for 1–2 weeks; then the dose can be decreased to 125–500 mg daily or every other day.

23. a, b, d. The patient should be encouraged to report to the healthcare provider if she is pregnant or plans on becoming pregnant because tetracycline has

possible teratogenic effects. Harsh cleansers may be irritating to skin that may already be sensitive. Tetracycline taken in combination with isotretinoin will increase the potential for adverse effects. Sunscreens with SPF 30 and higher are recommended for all adults. Also, tetracycline can cause tooth discoloration to developing teeth.

24. c. Hair loss or alopecia can be treated with minoxidil solution to stimulate hair growth. Acitretin and methotrexate are for psoriasis. Tretinoin can be used for acne and warts.

25. a, b, c. Contact dermatitis attributable to skin irritants can be treated with antiinflammatories or topical corticosteroids, such as triamcinolone and dexamethasone, and/or antihistamines, such as diphenhydramine. Fluconazole is an antifungal. Salicylic acid is used to treat acne, psoriasis, or verruca vulgaris.

Case Study: Critical Thinking

1. Full-thickness burns extend down and include the epidermis, the dermis, and the subcutaneous tissue. They have also been referred to as *third-degree burns*. Full-thickness burns may appear red, black, or white and are not painful because the nerve endings have been destroyed. Partial-thickness burns do not extend as deep; there may be blistering. Partial-thickness burns are very painful. Frequently partial-thickness (second-degree) burns surround a full-thickness burn.

2. Mafenide acetate is a broad-spectrum antibiotic that is applied topically (1.6 mm thick once or twice daily) to the burned area. Mafenide is a sulfonamide derivative, and it interferes with bacterial cell-wall synthesis and metabolism.

3. Another treatment option is silver sulfadiazine. It is also applied topically to the burned surface. Silver sulfadiazine acts on the cell membrane and cell wall. It is less likely to cause metabolic acidosis than mafenide.

4. Priority nursing interventions for this patient are adequate fluid resuscitation, pain control, and prevention of infection by providing sterile dressing changes. It will be easier for this patient to receive skin grafting when appropriate with minimal to no infections.

CHAPTER 49: PITUITARY, THYROID, PARATHYROID, AND ADRENAL DISORDERS

1. f
2. h
3. i
4. a
5. m
6. b
7. l
8. n
9. c
10. g
11. d
12. j
13. k
14. e
15. **Addison Disease**: Adrenal hyposecretion (hypocortisolism): anemia, hyponatremia, hyperkalemia, hypoglycemia, weight loss, fatigue, hypotension, tachycardia, diarrhea, hyperpigmentation.

    Cushing Syndrome: Adrenal hypersecretion (hypercortisolism): weight gain, hyperglycemia, buffalo hump, edema, delayed wound healing, hyperlipidemia, peptic ulcers, hirsutism, hypertension, hypernatremia, hypokalemia.
16. a
17. d
18. e
19. g
20. c
21. b
22. f
23. c. The normal dose is 25–50 mcg/day initially, with a maintenance dose of 50–200 mcg/day.
24. d. Manifestations from hypothyroidism are usually alleviated within 2–4 weeks without having symptoms of adverse reactions. Activity level is usually improved within 4 weeks of thyroid treatment.
25. a, c, d. Symptoms of hyperthyroidism include palpitations, excessive perspiration, and tachycardia. Constipation is a symptom of hypothyroidism, not hyperthyroidism.
26. a. Levothyroxine should be taken on an empty stomach at least 30–60 minutes before breakfast.
27. a, e. Over-the-counter drugs are generally contraindicated in patients with hypothyroidism. Patients with thyroid disorders should be encouraged to wear a medical alert identification. Drugs for hypothyroidism should be taken on an empty stomach. Numbness and tingling of the hands occur with hypoparathyroidism, not hypothyroidism. Hypothyroidism causes weight gain; it is not a priority to teach patients to increase food and fluid intake.
28. d. Prednisone is a glucocorticoid steroid. Long-term use can cause sodium and fluid retention.
29. b. Prednisone is a corticosteroid and should be taken with food to prevent irritation of gastric mucosa.
30. b, c, d, e. Concurrent use with NSAIDs including aspirin can increase the risk of GI bleed; phenytoin can decrease the effect of glucocorticoids; digitalis toxicity can occur and may cause dysrhythmias; and diuretics can increase potassium loss, increasing the risk of hypokalemia.
31. c, d, e. Obtaining a drug history is important before starting a patient on prednisone, because there are many drug interactions possible with glucocorticoids. Vital signs and daily weights should be monitored. Hypernatremia, not hyponatremia, can

occur with prednisone. Weight gain is a side effect of prednisone.

32. b. Glucocorticoids can lead to fluid retention. Adequate fluid intake should be ensured but not forced.

33. b. Corticosteroids can decrease serum potassium and cause hypokalemia. Herbal laxatives or diuretics taken concurrently with corticosteroids can worsen hypokalemia.

34. b. Corticosteroids increase metabolism and can cause insomnia; these effects can worsen when taken with herbal stimulants, such as ginseng.

35. a, b, e. Levothyroxine has many drug-drug interactions. Levothyroxine can increase the effects of an anticoagulant, such as warfarin. Levothyroxine can decrease the effects of digoxin and oral antidiabetic drugs. There are no strong interactions with diuretics and NSAIDs.

Clinical Judgment Standalone Case Study
Answers:

- adrenal
- Addison
- cosyntropin
- glucocorticoids
- fludrocortisone

Rationale:

The nurse recognizes that the patient's clinical manifestations of irregular menses, nervousness, muscle weakness, lethargy, electrolyte imbalance, and hypoglycemia could be a complication from adrenal insufficiency, also known as Addison disease. To determine primary deficiency, cosyntropin is used to assess if the problem is related to the pituitary gland or the adrenal glands. Persons with Addison disease lack glucocorticoids and mineralocorticoids. Treatment for this patient's insufficiency would include glucocorticoids, such as cortisone acetate, and mineralocorticoids, such as fludrocortisone.

Reference

McCuistion, L.E., DiMaggio, K.V., Winton, M.B., & Yeager, J.J. (2025). Pharmacology: A patient-centered nursing process approach, 12th ed. St. Louis, MO: Elsevier. pp. 633–648.

CHAPTER 50: ANTIDIABETICS

1. d
2. f
3. h
4. c
5. g
6. e
7. a
8. b
9. 3
10. obesity, stress, insulin resistance
11. abdomen
12. gastrointestinal secretions
13. lipodystrophy; rotating
14. insulin resistance; allergy
15. c
16. a
17. f
18. b
19. e
20. d
21. regular
22. Somogyi effect
23. Hyperglycemia; dawn
24. hypoglycemia
25. biguanide; glucose; absorption; receptor; peripheral
26. 48 hours; lactic acidosis
27. type 2
28. a, b, e. Three major symptoms of diabetes are characterized by the three Ps that include polydipsia (increased thirst), polyphagia (increased hunger), and polyuria (increased urination).
29. a, b, d. Certain drugs increase serum glucose level (hyperglycemia), including cortisone, hydrochlorothiazide, and epinephrine. Doxepin is a tricyclic antidepressant that can lower blood glucose level. Thiazolidinediones are a class of oral antidiabetic drugs that lower blood glucose level.
30. b, c, d, e. The patient experiencing hypoglycemia can have headache, sweating, nervousness, and tremor. Abdominal pain and vomiting can occur because of a reaction to oral antidiabetic drugs.
31. b, c, d, e, f. Signs and symptoms of ketoacidosis include dry mucous membrane, fruity breath odor, Kussmaul respirations, polyuria, and thirst. The patient can also develop tachycardia, not bradycardia.
32. d. Tolazamide is a first-generation intermediate-acting oral antidiabetic drug. Oral drugs in this class should not be used by patients with type 1 diabetes; instead, insulin is used.
33. a, b, c, d. Oral antidiabetic medications should be taken on a regular, prescribed basis and not adjusted by glucose testing results.
34. a. Unopened insulin vials should be kept in the refrigerator, and an opened vial can be kept in the refrigerator or kept at room temperature. They should not be stored in the freezer, exposed to direct sunlight, or left in a high-temperature area.
35. c. Cloudy insulin is mixed by rolling the vial. Shaking the vial can cause bubbles, which can lead to an inaccurate dose.
36. a, c, e. The patient needs to develop a rotation pattern to prevent lipodystrophy and promote insulin absorption. Insulin is not administered IM. The ADA's suggested actions do not include injection into a different area of the body every day.
37. a. Regular insulin is short acting, with an onset of 30 minutes to 1 hour. If the patient administers

regular insulin at 0700, the patient may start experiencing hypoglycemic reaction around 0800–0900.

38. b, d, e. Insulin glargine is a long-acting insulin that is evenly distributed over a 24-hour duration of action and is usually administered in the evening (bedtime). It is available in a prefilled cartridge, and some patients have complained of pain at the injection site. Hypoglycemia can still occur, but it is not as common as with other insulins. Some patients may need coverage with rapid-acting or short-acting insulins.

39. c. Insulin pumps are used for type 1 diabetics, and they reduce the number of hypoglycemic reactions. An insulin pump is not used with intermediate insulin, such as NPH, because of unpredictable glucose control. Insulin pumps use a needle to insert a cannula under the skin; the needle does not stay inserted.

40. a. Depending on the class of oral antidiabetic drugs, they can increase the insulin cell receptor sensitivity, increase insulin release from the pancreas, decrease hepatic production of glucose, decrease glucose absorption from the small intestine, and/or increase peripheral glucose uptake at the cellular level. They do not increase the number of insulin-producing cells, nor do they replace receptor sites or insulin.

41. b. Metformin, which is a biguanide, decreases glucose production by the liver. They can cause hypoglycemic reactions. Metformin does not decrease hepatic production of glucose from stored glycogen. Metformin decreases, not increases, the absorption of glucose from the small intestine. Metformin is an oral antidiabetic drug that lowers serum glucose level, not increase it.

42. b. Ginseng and garlic can lower blood glucose; garlic may increase insulin level which assists in lowering the blood glucose. Concomitant use of these complementary and alternative drugs may necessitate a change in the insulin or oral antidiabetic drug dose.

43. b, c, d, e. Aspirin, oral anticoagulants, and cimetidine can increase the action of sulfonylureas, especially with the first generations, by binding to plasma proteins and displacing sulfonylureas. The action of sulfonylureas may be decreased by taking several different types of medications, including anticonvulsants such as phenytoin.

Clinical Judgment Standalone Case Study
Answers:

- hypoglycemia
- glucagon
- glucose
- increase

Rationale:

Persons with type 1 diabetes will be prescribed insulin since their pancreas is unable to produce insulin. If the person does not consume adequate carbohydrates, hypoglycemic reaction can occur. The person may exhibit nervousness, trembling, lack of coordination; cool and clammy skin; and may complain of a headache. They can also exhibit combativeness and be incoherent. As hypoglycemia continues, the person can become unresponsive which is a medical emergency. Since the patient is unresponsive, the nurse would anticipate administering glucagon intravenously to treat insulin-induced hypoglycemia; intramuscularly and subcutaneously are other routes of administration. Glucagon is a hyperglycemic hormone that stimulates glucose production by the liver (glycogenolysis), which increases blood sugar. Oral sugar-containing products, such as hard candy or drinks, are contraindicated in an unresponsive patient because of an increase in aspiration.

Reference

McCuistion, L.E., DiMaggio, K.V., Winton, M.B., & Yeager, J.J. (2025). Pharmacology: A patient-centered nursing process approach, 12th ed. St. Louis, MO: Elsevier. pp. 649–664.

CHAPTER 51: URINARY DISORDERS

1. b
2. e
3. d
4. f
5. e
6. d
7. c
8. a
9. e
10.

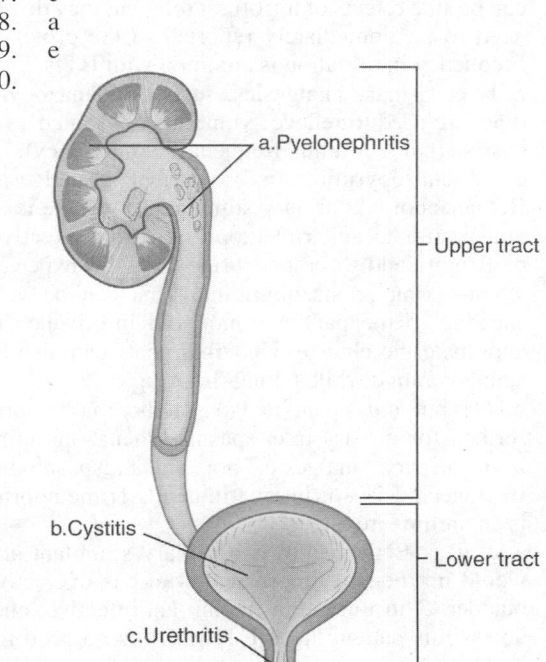

11. c. When methenamine is given with sulfonamide, crystals in the urine can form. Methenamine can cause hematuria, even when used alone. Chest pain and intestinal distention are not known to occur when given with sulfonamide.

12. b. Cranberry juice can help lower the pH and make the urine more acidic. Whole milk may make urine more alkaline and increase the pH. Although increased fluid intake is important when a patient has a urinary tract infection (UTI), simply increasing the amount of water alone will not decrease the urine pH. Prune juice will make the urine acidic, not alkalotic.

13. b. Flavoxate is an antispasmodic that has a direct action on the smooth muscles and is contraindicated in patients with glaucoma. Antispasmodic has the same effects as anticholinergics.

14. c, d, e. Ertapenem, an antiseptic, has side effects that include diarrhea, headache, and nausea. Other side effects include drowsiness, confusion, agitation, and elevated hepatic enzymes.

15. a, c, d. Urinary antiseptics can inhibit and/or prevent bacterial growth in the kidneys and bladder but are not effective for systemic infections. Antacids decrease absorption of other oral drugs when taken together.

16. d. Dyspnea could indicate an adverse drug reaction to nitrofurantoin. Other signs and symptoms to report immediately include chest pain, cough, fever, and chills. Also, tingling or numbness of extremities could be a sign of neuropathy, which can be irreversible and needs to be evaluated immediately. Brown- or rust-colored urine and diarrhea can be side effects of nitrofurantoin, but they do not need to be immediately reported to the provider. Frequency in urination is common with UTIs.

17. a, b, e. Urinary analgesics, such as phenazopyridine, are used to relieve symptoms associated with cystitis (pain, burning, frequency, and urgency).

18. c. Phenazopyridine is a urinary analgesic. Bethanechol is a urinary stimulant, flavoxate is an antispasmodic, and trimethoprim is an antiinfective.

19. d. Bright reddish-orange urine is to be expected when taking phenazopyridine. This can be very startling to the patient if not told in advance to anticipate the change. Undergarments can also be stained orange while taking this drug.

20. b. Oxybutynin is an antispasmodic that is prescribed for urinary tract spasms. Phenazopyridine is a urinary analgesic, not an antispasmodic. Bethanechol is a urinary stimulant. Trimethoprim is an antiinfective.

21. a, c, d, e. Bethanechol is a urinary stimulant and would not benefit this patient who has overactive bladder. Nitrofurantoin is an antiinfective and, unless this patient has a UTI, there is no need for it. Oxybutynin and tolterodine tartrate, although beneficial to patients with overactive bladder, are contraindicated in patients with glaucoma. Dimethyl sulfoxide (DMSO) is a urinary analgesic that is used to treat urinary frequency and urgency.

22. b. Bethanechol chloride is a urinary stimulant that increases bladder tone. It is prescribed when bladder function is lost because of spinal cord injuries, such as with paralysis.

Case Study: Critical Thinking

1. Oxybutynin chloride is a urinary antispasmodic that has direct action on the smooth muscles of the urinary tract. By relaxing these muscles the spasms are decreased.

2. Patients who have urinary or GI obstruction as well as those with narrow-angle glaucoma should not take oxybutynin. Oxybutynin blocks acetylcholine receptors that mediate parasympathetic function. Should the patient experience severe abdominal pain, constipation, or urinary retention, the healthcare provider should be contacted immediately.

3. Common side effects include dry mouth, drowsiness, blurred vision, headache, insomnia, tachycardia, GI distress, and constipation. The patient should be encouraged not to participate in any activities where dizziness could be an issue (climbing, skateboarding, etc.). The patient should be warned not to drive or operate heavy machinery until it is known how the drug will affect the body. If any of these symptoms are severe, the healthcare provider should be contacted.

4. No dosage adjustment needs to be made unless the current dosage of 5 mg bid is not adequate, then the dose may be increased. The dosage range is 5 mg bid/qid, with a maximum of 20 mg/day.

CHAPTER 52: PREGNANCY AND PRETERM LABOR

1. g
2. f
3. j
4. i
5. a
6. b
7. d
8. e
9. h
10. c
11. c, d, e. Maternal physiologic changes seen during pregnancy affecting drug actions include increased maternal circulating volume, resulting in dilution of drugs; increased glomerular filtration rate and rapid elimination of drugs; and increased liver metabolism. Other changes are reduced GI motility and increased gastric pH, making the environment more alkaline; and the clearance of drugs is altered during late pregnancy, resulting in decreased serum concentration.

12. a. Drugs crossing the placenta are analogous to drugs infiltrating breast tissue. Lactation causes increased blood flow to the breast and drugs accumulate in the adipose tissue through simple diffusion.

13. a, b, d. Timing, dose, and duration of drug exposure are crucial in determining the drug's teratogenicity. The teratogenic period begins 2 weeks after conception, and exposure to teratogens can result in birth defects and/or death of the fetus.

14. b. Corticosteroids, such as betamethasone, accelerate lung maturity and surfactant development in the fetus in utero, thereby decreasing the incidence and severity of respiratory distress.

15. b, d, e. Gestational hypertension can have devastating maternal and fetal effects. Gestational hypertension can progress to preeclampsia and/or eclampsia, increasing the risk of HELLP syndrome and seizures. The goals for patients who develop gestational hypertension include prevention of HELLP syndrome, delivery of an uncompromised fetus, reduction of vasospasms, and prevention of seizures.

16. a, c, d. GI complaints, such as heartburn, nausea, and vomiting, are the most common during pregnancy, possibly resulting from elevated levels of progesterone, which causes decreased gut motility and relaxation of the cardiac sphincter.

17. c. In maternal iron deficiency anemia, iron supplements will show a modest reticulocyte count increase in 5–10 days; a rise in the hemoglobin level will be seen in 2–4 weeks.

18. a, c, d, e. Nausea and vomiting or "morning sickness" are frequent complaints during early pregnancy. To decrease nausea and vomiting, patients should avoid fatty or spicy foods; eat high-protein snack. Also, eating crackers, dry toast, or other carbohydrates before rising can also decrease frequency and severity of nausea. Fluids taken between meals rather than during meal can also help. Fluids should not necessarily be avoided before arising. Sometimes small sips of flat soda or apple juice may be beneficial.

19. b, c, e. Iron supplements should be taken 2 hours before or 4 hours after antacids so the medication can be absorbed. Although best taken on an empty stomach, iron can be taken with food if necessary. Jaundice should be reported immediately to the healthcare provider. Vitamin C found in orange juice can enhance iron absorption.

20. a. Foods that are rich in iron include broccoli, red meat, nuts, spinach, and iron-fortified cereal.

21. b. The recommended dosage of folic acid is 400–800 mcg. If planning pregnancy, folic acid should be started 1 month before and for the first 2–3 months after conception. The American Congress of Obstetricians and Gynecologists recommends that all females of childbearing age take 400 mcg of folic acid and 600 mcg during pregnancy.

22. a. Acetaminophen is the most commonly OTC drug for pain relief during pregnancy. It is safe to use during all trimesters of pregnancy. Aspirin and ibuprofen use during pregnancy is contraindicated. Diphenhydramine is an antihistamine.

23. a. Beta-sympathomimetic drugs, such as terbutaline, stimulate beta-2 receptors on uterine smooth muscle to decrease the frequency and severity of uterine contractions. Terbutaline has significant adverse effects. Pulmonary edema and cardiac arrhythmias can occur. Breath sounds should be auscultated at least every 4 hours and assessed for the presence of wheezes, crackles, or coughing.

24. b, d, e. The loading dose of magnesium sulfate 4–6 g is given over 20–30 minutes as an IVPB. It is administered via a pump. Too rapid administration of magnesium sulfate can lead to cardiac arrest. Patients receiving magnesium sulfate are on bed rest while receiving therapy and should be monitored continuously. Calcium gluconate is the antidote for magnesium sulfate toxicity and should be at the bedside for emergency. Decreased or loss of DTRs is an adverse reaction to magnesium sulfate.

25. a, b, c. NSAIDs, such as aspirin and ibuprofen, can cause maternal anemia and greater blood loss at delivery, and the overall homeostasis of the fetus can be compromised. Additionally, ibuprofen, when taken late in pregnancy, can prematurely close the ductus arteriosus.

26. a, b, d. Side effects and adverse reactions are generally dose related and include flushing, nausea, and slurred speech. Other side effects include feelings of increased warmth, perspiration, nasal congestion, lethargy, decreased gut motility, tachycardia, and hypotension.

Case Study: Critical Thinking

1. Some priority questions to ask include if the patient has been receiving regular prenatal care and the date of her last visit. The nurse should inquire if there are any known complications with this pregnancy such as gestational diabetes, gestational hypertension, or hyperemesis gravidarum. The patient should also be questioned regarding membrane rupture and for any bleeding or changes in fetal movement. Other questions should include substance use, including herbals, caffeine, and tobacco use.

2. The patient is at high risk because of her age, history of miscarriage, and previous PTL.

3. Nonpharmacologic measures that the nurse can suggest while the patient is waiting to hear back from the healthcare provider include lying down on her left side or, if that is not possible, at recline and put her feet up. Dehydration may lead to PTL, so the patient should maintain hydration. Having an empty bladder may also help, so the patient should be advised to void. If nonpharmacologic measures are not effective, the patient may require tocolytics.

There are no FDA-approved drugs for PTL. But, beta sympathomimetics (terbutaline), magnesium sulfate, or prostaglandin inhibitors are used "off label" to halt or delay labor. One of the major goals in tocolytic therapy is to interrupt or inhibit uterine contractions to create additional time for fetal maturation in utero.

4. Although the survival rate of a fetus at 33 weeks is fairly high, the baby is preterm and will require close observation. The mother may be given corticosteroids, such as betamethasone or dexamethasone, to accelerate fetal lung maturity and development of surfactant to decrease the incidence of respiratory distress syndrome in preterm infants.

CHAPTER 53: LABOR, DELIVERY, AND POSTPARTUM

1. a. spinal block; b. epidural block
2. b
3. d
4. e
5. a
6. c
7. b
8. d
9. a
10. c
11. latent; active; transition
12. neonatal
13. mu; kappa
14. should not
15. saddle block
16. oxytocin; other uterotropic drugs include ergot alkaloids, prostaglandins
17. decreases
18. $Rh_0(D)$ immune globulin
19. d. Postdural headaches are caused by leakage of cerebrospinal fluid through a puncture site. The decrease in pressure exerted by the CSF causes the headache.
20. a, b, c, d. Postdural headaches can occur with regional anesthesia, such as epidural or spinal anesthesia. Patient should be advised that bed rest, oral analgesics, and/or caffeine can help relieve the headache. At times, an autologous blood patch may be needed.
21. d. Opioids can cause maternal or neonate respiratory depression. A reversal agent, naloxone, is given.
22. a. Before administering general anesthesia, antacids or other drugs that decrease gastric secretions are given to decrease gastric acidity. They may also prevent nausea and vomiting, but these are not the primary reasons for their administration just before general anesthesia.
23. d. Patients with hypotension are positioned on their left side to facilitate placental perfusion. Isotonic fluids will need to be rapidly infused, and ephedrine or phenylephrine may need to be administered. Oxygen may be needed but it is not the first thing the nurse would do.
24. c. Bishop score is an objective measurement to determine the readiness for labor induction. The elements assessed by the Bishop score are dilation, effacement, station, cervical consistency, and cervical position. Scores of 8 or greater are associated with a successful labor induction.
25. d. Ergot alkaloids should not be used during labor. Instead, they are used after delivery to sustain uterine contractions, to prevent or control postpartum hemorrhage, and to promote uterine involution. The fourth stage of labor is the "early postpartum" that consists of the first 4 hours after the delivery of the placenta.
26. a. Patients with hypertension should not receive methylergonovine. When this drug is given IV, dramatic increases in blood pressure can occur.
27. a, c. During assistance in all types of regional/local anesthesia the nurse would continuously monitor the patient. If the anesthetic is injected into a vessel, the patient may experience dizziness and metallic taste in the mouth. Other indications of vascular access are ringing in the ears or numbness. Hypotension, not hypertension, can occur with local anesthesia. If hypotension, the patient should be placed on her left side to increase placental blood flow.
28. b, c, d, e. Deep tendon reflexes are usually assessed on a patient receiving magnesium sulfate, not oxytocin. A type and crossmatch should be obtained in the event that the patient will need an emergent cesarean section. The fetus may become hypoxic, and there is an increased risk for uterine rupture. If uterine rupture is suspected, assess for FHR deceleration, sudden increased pain, loss of uterine contractions, and hemorrhage.
29. c, d. Somatic pain occurs during the transition phase and the second stage of labor. Pain is caused by the stretching of the perineum and vagina.
30. b, c, e. Anesthesia for cesarean delivery may be general, spinal, or epidural. General anesthesia allows for rapid anesthesia induction and control of the airway.
31. a, d. Topical agents used for pain relief for perineal wounds include benzocaine and witch hazel.
32. b. Use of heat lamp after applying benzocaine topical spray to relieve perineal pain is not recommended. Heat lamp can cause tissue burn.
33. b. $Rh_0(D)$ immune globulin is given when there is a maternal/fetal blood mixing of incompatible blood. The Ig should be given at 28 weeks' gestation and within 72 hours of giving birth. It is not given at 38 weeks' gestation or before amniocentesis. It can be given after amniocentesis.
34. a, b, d, f. Zuranolone is a drug that was approved in 2023 to treat postpartum depression. Since it can

cause somnolence and confusion, patients should not drive until they know how the drug affects them. Also, the drug is passed through the breast milk; therefore it is recommended that breastfeeding is stopped until 1 week after the last dose. The drug should be taken with a high fatty food, not on an empty stomach, for better absorption. The medication is taken for 14 days, not 1 year.

Clinical Judgment Standalone Case Study

Answers:

Nursing Action	Potential Complication	Appropriate Nursing Action for the Complication
	Uterine rupture	Monitor fetal heart rate for any decelerations
	Maternal hypoxia	Have oxygen readily available
	Uterine hyperstimulation	Ensure terbutaline is readily available
	Seizures	Review labs for any electrolyte imbalance

Rationale:

Oxytocin is used to augment or induce labor and stimulate uterine contractions. Before administering oxytocin, gestational age and the fetus' position must be ascertained. At 38 weeks the patient is considered full term. The position of the fetus should include its head down and deep in the pelvis. The cervix must be soft and ripened, progressing in effacement and partial dilation. Prior to administering oxytocin, the drug must be diluted in 1000 mL of intravenous (IV) fluid (usually lactated ringers) at a concentration of 10 milliunits/mL and connected to the primary IV line using a separate IV pump. The patient would be closely monitored for complications. The nurse would continuously monitor fetal heart rate to determine any decelerations, which could indicate uterine rupture. The nurse would also have oxygen readily available for maternal hypoxia. Another nursing action would include ensuring terbutaline is readily available to reverse uterine hyperstimulation. Uterine hyperstimulation is defined as uterine contractions lasting at least 2 minutes or five or more contractions in a 10-minute window or six or more uterine contractions in a 20-minute window. Uterine hyperstimulation can cause fetal distress and markedly increase maternal pain. Yet another nursing action would include reviewing labs for any electrolyte imbalance (such as hyponatremia and hypokalemia), which could induce seizures. Increasing the rate of oxytocin infusion would worsen the complications. While the patient would be receiving hydration intravenously, administering 1 L of 0.9% sodium chloride is not the most appropriate answer for any of the listed complications. Since this patient is not complaining of pain or desiring analgesia,

preparing the patient for regional anesthesia would be an incorrect response.

Reference

McCuistion, L.E., DiMaggio, K.V., Winton, M.B., & Yeager, J.J. (2025). Pharmacology: A patient-centered nursing process approach, 12th ed. St. Louis, MO: Elsevier. pp. 689–707.

CHAPTER 54: NEONATAL AND NEWBORN

1. Respiratory distress syndrome; surfactant
2. endotracheal
3. Hyperoxia; hypocarbia
4. newborn
5. ophthalmia neonatorum
6. d. Surfactant replacement, such as beractant, is given to premature newborns with immature lung development.
7. c. Exogenous surfactant must be warmed before administration by warming it in the hands for 8 minutes or at room temperature for 20 minutes. The vial should not be shaken.
8. b, d, e. Exogenous surfactants are administered to newborn to treat respiratory distress syndrome due to premature lung development. Drugs of this class include beractant, poractant alfa, and calfactant.
9. a, b, d. Complications during and following administration of surfactant can cause bradycardia and hyperoxia. Desaturation can also occur because transient esophageal reflux can obstruct the ET tube. Cyanosis, not pallor, is another complication.
10. b. Generally, complications such as cyanosis and hypoxia after surfactant administration do not lead to severe complications when properly managed. The nurse should assist in repositioning the neonate to disperse the drug throughout the lung. Suctioning is appropriate if an obvious sign of airway obstruction is noted.
11. d. HBIG should be given to the newborn if the mother is hepatitis B positive. The first of three series doses of recombinant hepatitis B should be given as a separate injection at a separate site. The HBIG provides passive protection while the newborn's body develops acquired immunity to the recombinant hepatitis B vaccine.
12. b. Erythromycin is an antiinfective administered to a newborn's eyes within the first hours of birth to prevent blindness. Blindness in newborns can occur because of vaginal infections, such as chlamydia and gonorrhea.

Case Study: Critical Thinking

1. Hepatitis B virus transmission occurs vertically, also known as perinatal transmission, at the time of delivery when the neonate is exposed to the mother's blood and body fluids.

2. The nurse should acknowledge the patient's concerns and inform her that her baby will receive medications to decrease the risk of developing hepatitis B.

3. The nurse would anticipate administering hepatitis B immune globulin (HBIG) and the first dose of recombinant hepatitis B. HBIG should be administered within 12 hours of birth. HBIG provides immediate passive protection against liver damage. Recombinant hepatitis B stimulates the body to produce antibodies against hepatitis B viruses.

4. Recombinant hepatitis B vaccine is given in three series. The first one is given within 24 hours after birth. Subsequent doses are given at 1 month and again at 6 months of age.

CHAPTER 55: WOMEN'S REPRODUCTIVE HEALTH

1. b
2. e
3. d
4. c
5. a
6. menarche; menopause
7. estrogen
8. spironolactone; diuretic
9. 48
10. anovulation; amenorrhea
11. hypoestrogenic
12. b
13. d
14. c
15. a
16. e
17. c. A female with breast cancer should not take oral contraceptives because the hormones could accelerate tumor growth. Other contraindications include history of endometrial cancer, history of thromboembolic disorders, liver disease, coronary artery disease, undiagnosed vaginal bleeding, and endometriosis. A person who is not sexually active may not need oral contraceptives; however, it is not contraindicated.

18. a, b, c. There are no contraindications for using combined hormone contraceptives (CHCs) in epilepsy, but other medications that the patient takes must be evaluated. There is no contraindication for a patient with depression taking CHCs. The 45-year-old patient is, in all likelihood, perimenopausal, so there may not be a need for CHCs, but they are not absolutely contraindicated. A person who smokes or has diabetes requires extra caution because of the risk for thromboembolism.

19. c. If only one dose has been missed, the patient should take the dose as soon as possible and then resume the regular schedule with the next dose.

20. a, b, c, d, e. Common side effects with conjugated estrogen include acne, breast tenderness, leg cramps, fluid retention, and nausea. Other common side effects are vomiting, breakthrough bleeding, and chloasma.

21. a, d, e. Aspirin toxicity can occur, increasing the anticoagulant effects. Barbiturates such as phenobarbital and topiramate, which can be used either for seizures or for migraines, are contraindicated in patients taking oral contraceptives. All females of childbearing age should take supplemental folic acid.

22. c. Potassium levels should be monitored closely. Drospirenone causes the body to retain potassium. Hyperkalemia is possible, especially in patients with undiagnosed kidney disease.

23. c. Ethinyl estradiol and etonogestrel transvaginal rings are inserted vaginally and left in place for 3 consecutive weeks. After 3 weeks the ring should be removed. The patient should wait at least 1 week before inserting a new one. If the ring has been out for less than 3 hours, it can be rinsed with lukewarm water and reinserted. If the ring has been out for more than 3 hours, it should be reinserted, and use an alternative form of contraception until the ring has been in place for 7 days.

24. b. As part of the ACHES mnemonic (Abdominal pain [severe], Chest pain or shortness of breath, Headache [severe], Eye disorders, Severe leg pain), severe headaches could be indicative of cardiovascular side effects and should be reported to the healthcare provider immediately.

25. c. Progestin hormone therapy decreases the risk of ovarian and cervical cancers but progestin does increase a person's risk for breast cancer and cardiovascular events, such as blood clots and hypertension.

26. b. Vitamin D enhances the absorption of dietary calcium.

Case Study: Critical Thinking

1. With these presenting symptoms and at her age the patient is likely menopausal. Dyspareunia, frequency, urgency, thinning vaginal epithelium, and decreased elasticity on speculum examination are due to estrogen deficit. Frequency and urgency can also be associated with a urinary tract infection (UTI), so a urinalysis should be obtained; however, a UTI would not account for the findings on speculum examination. By definition, a lack of menstruation for 1 year is defined as menopause. Other symptoms associated with menopause may include hot flashes and night sweats.

2. Treatment may be symptomatic and include taking cool baths, using a fan, and sleeping in light clothing. Another option is hormone therapy (HT). HT should be administered at the lowest doses and for the shortest amount of time possible. HT improves vasomotor symptoms such as hot flashes, and it also improves vaginal dryness and irritation. It does,

however, come with increased risks of cardiovascular events, such as DVT, stroke, and MI, and certain cancers (breast, ovarian, and lung). The healthcare provider should discuss the risk-to-benefit ratio with the patient to help her decide the best option.

3. HT also decreases the risk of osteoporosis. The patient is thin and White, which are two risk factors for osteoporosis. Using HT, increasing vitamin D and calcium intake, and exercising (such as walking) may help prevent bone loss. The medications used for osteoporosis include bisphosphonates and SERMs. These medications help prevent the breakdown of bone.

CHAPTER 56: MEN'S REPRODUCTIVE HEALTH

1. g
2. h
3. j
4. f
5. e
6. i
7. b
8. c
9. a
10. d
11. d. Sildenafil is indicated for erectile dysfunction. Its action is enhancing blood flow to the penis to facilitate an erection. Sildenafil is contraindicated in patients with significant cardiac disease or persons with anatomic deformities or conditions that predispose them to priapism. Sildenafil is also contraindicated in persons who are on nitrates. Age is not a contraindication.
12. d. Androgens (i.e., testosterone) are male sex hormones to control the development and maintenance of sexual processes, accessory sexual organs (i.e., hypogonadism), cellular metabolism, and bone/muscle growth.
13. c. The use of hormones to "bulk up" or improve performance occurs at all levels of sports competition. Side/adverse effects from the use of excessive intake of anabolic steroids include increased low-density lipoprotein cholesterol, decreased high-density lipoprotein cholesterol, acne, high blood pressure, liver damage, and dangerous changes in the left ventricle of the heart. Adverse effects may not be recognized until years later.
14. a. Blood glucose levels may be decreased in patients with diabetes when taking androgens. The patient should be instructed to carefully monitor blood glucose levels for changes so the insulin dose can be adjusted.
15. a, c. Androgens can be used to treat advanced breast cancer and endometriosis in females. Other uses include management of severe menopausal symptoms in females, refractory anemia in both sexes, and tissue wasting associated with severe illness.

16. a, b, d. Males on androgens can experience frequent, and often time painful, continuous erection called priapism. They can also experience gynecomastia, and sperm counts can decrease or even stop. Other side and/or adverse effects include abdominal pain, nausea, insomnia, diarrhea, or constipation. Androgens can cause hypercalcemia which can cause frequent urination.
17. a, c, e. Androgen antagonist blocks the synthesis or action of androgens and is indicated for benign prostatic hypertrophy (BPH), advanced prostate cancer, and endometriosis. Androgen antagonists are also used to treat male-pattern baldness, acne, hirsutism, virilization syndrome in females, and precocious puberty in boys.

Case Study: Critical Thinking

1. Erectile dysfunction can occur in males at any stage of life. It occurs due to lack of sufficient blood flow to the penis. It may be seen in males with diabetes. Some of the drugs used to treat hypertension, such as diuretics and beta-blockers, may also cause erectile dysfunction.
2. One class of drugs that the patient may be referring to is the phosphodiesterase (PDE-5) inhibitors, which include sildenafil, tadalafil, and vardenafil. They work by increasing blood flow to the penis so the patient can maintain an erection.
3. Side effects may include upset stomach, blurred vision, flushing, and headache. The most serious side effect is a sustained erection (priapism) that lasts longer than 4 hours. Priapism is an emergency because a thrombosis may form in the corpora cavernosa, which can lead to permanent loss of function.
4. The nurse would teach the patient not to use any herbal preparations without discussing their side effects with his healthcare provider. The patient would also be advised to not use any nitroglycerin or nitrate-containing drugs while taking PDE-5 inhibitors because the combination can cause marked hypotension. PDE-5 inhibitors should also not be taken with grapefruit or grapefruit juice because it increases the amount of PDE-5 available. Side effects, such as headache and vision changes, should be taught to the patient.

CHAPTER 57: SEXUALLY TRANSMITTED INFECTIONS

1. c
2. e
3. b
4. f
5. a
6. d
7. b
8. d

9. e
10. c
11. a
12. d
13. True
14. False. Washing bed linens of a patient diagnosed with scabies *is* necessary. All bedding and clothing should be decontaminated and anyone in close contact with an infected person should also be examined and treated if necessary.
15. False. Nitroimidazoles and alcohol *are* contraindicated. Like metronidazole, drinking alcohol concomitantly can cause a disulfiram-like reaction.
16. False. Pediculosis pubis is treated with topical *permethrin 1% cream rinse*. Alternatively, malathion lotion can be applied. Both will need to be rinsed off after certain period of time has lapsed. An oral drug, ivermectin, can be taken to treat pediculosis pubis.
17. c. Patients with gonorrhea should also be tested for HIV, *Chlamydia*, and syphilis.
18. a. Abstaining from sexual activity is the safest practice to prevent any further transmission; however, if that is not an option, all partners should wear a condom during sex. Partners do not need to take antibiotics; however, all partners should be tested.
19. d. If the patient wants to participate in sexual activity, using a condom is the safest, even if gonorrhea was treated. However, if abstaining or using a condom is not possible, then the patient should wait at least 7 days after treatment to resume sexual activities.
20. a. Gonorrhea and syphilis are two different types of sexually transmitted infections. If a patient is diagnosed with one sexually transmitted infection, then they should be tested for the other, including HIV and *Chlamydia*.
21. a, b, c, d. HIV is a virus that is spread through sexual contact and blood and body fluids. Blood and body fluids include breast milk, blood, and vaginal secretions. There are no indications that HIV is transmitted through mosquitoes.

Case Study: Critical Thinking

1. The presumptive diagnosis is gonorrhea involving both her genitourinary and oral mucous membranes caused by *Neisseria gonorrhea*. Oral infections caused by *N. gonorrhea* cause pharyngitis and dysphagia. She may also have a fever, and if left untreated, her infection can cause tubal scarring.
2. Single-drug therapy is recommended with ceftriaxone 500 mg IM as a single dose. Dual therapy is no longer recommended due to the increased cases of resistance to azithromycin. The patient should be encouraged to abstain from sexual encounters for a minimum of 7 days after treatment.
3. The patient should be informed that she is at risk for other infections, such as chlamydia, HPV, and HIV, and that she should be further tested. She should abstain from sexual activities until therapy is completed and her partners should be treated. If she cannot abstain from intercourse, then instruct her to use condoms. Review with the patient how STIs are transmitted and how they could be avoided.

CHAPTER 58: ADULT AND PEDIATRIC EMERGENCY DRUGS

1. h
2. g
3. k
4. e
5. i
6. a
7. f
8. b
9. d
10. c
11. j
12. f
13. d
14. a
15. d
16. b
17. c
18. e
19. g
20. a. Nitroglycerin is a vasodilator and can cause a rapid drop in blood pressure, especially in first-time users. Tachycardia or bradycardia can also occur, but it is not as common as hypotension.
21. a. Morphine can cause respiratory depression so the patient's respiratory status must be monitored closely. Naloxone can be used to reverse respiratory depression if needed.
22. d. Myocardial ischemia can occur when a patient is receiving dobutamine. The nurse must monitor carefully for signs of myocardial ischemia, including chest pain and dysrhythmias. Dobutamine can cause tachycardia, not bradycardia.
23. b. Procainamide is an antiarrhythmic for ventricular dysrhythmias that are unresponsive to adenosine. Procainamide is discontinued if hypotension develops. Other end points to procainamide include ECG changes (i.e., widening of the QRS complex by 50% or more), when the maximum dose has been given (17 mg/kg), or when the dysrhythmia is successfully treated.
24. b, e. Amiodarone is appropriate to treat ventricular tachyarrhythmia, such as ventricular fibrillation and atrial fibrillation that is not controlled by other measures. The dose to administer is dependent on the presence or absence of a pulse. Amiodarone is not given in patients with bradycardia or

atrioventricular blocks, such as second-degree block.

25. a. Sodium bicarbonate is indicated to treat severe metabolic acidosis as well as hyperkalemia related to specific drug overdose situations. It is not a first-line drug to treat cardiac arrest.

26. c. Intracranial pressure can increase following head trauma or malignancy. Mannitol is an osmotic diuretic used to treat increased intracranial pressure by causing fluid to shift from the brain tissue back into the vasculature. Strict fluid intake and output must closely be monitored due to possible significant fluid loss.

27. c. Swelling of the tongue and lips is the indication of an allergic reaction and is considered an emergency. Diphenhydramine should be administered intravenously. Diphenhydramine reduces histamine-induced swelling and itching that occur in allergic reactions.

28. c. Naloxone is an opiate antagonist and naloxone 0.4 mg IVP is within the dose range to be administered. If this is an opioid overdose, the drug should reverse fairly rapidly, and typically, a patient with ventricular dysrhythmias is given a 1–1.5 mg/kg bolus of lidocaine, followed by 0.5–0.75 mg/kg every 5–10 minutes until the dysrhythmia is controlled or a total dose of 3 mg/kg will become responsive. If this is not an opioid overdose, there will be no response. Benzodiazepines, such as diazepam, are also used for back spasms, but they do not produce pinpoint pupils. Flumazenil is the reversal agent for benzodiazepines.

29. a, d, e. Dopamine is a vasopressor and may be used to treat hypotension in cardiogenic, neurogenic, and septic shock after adequate fluid and/or blood product resuscitation. However, norepinephrine may be preferred in neurogenic shock. Hypovolemic shock should be treated with fluids, either crystalloids or blood. *Insulin shock* is actually misnamed and refers to a hypoglycemic reaction. It should be treated with glucose, not vasopressors.

30. a. Dobutamine is a sympathomimetic drug with beta-adrenergic activities. It is used in shock states. Blood pressure is elevated only through the increase in cardiac output.

31. b. Norepinephrine is a catecholamine that acts on the alpha-adrenergic receptors and has potent vasoconstrictor actions, and as with other adrenergic agonists, abrupt discontinuation can cause a profound drop in the blood pressure.

32. d. D_{50} is used to treat severe hypoglycemia, most commonly attributable to insulin shock. Increased urine output and hyperglycemia can occur because of D_{50}. D_{50} is highly irritating to the vein and should be administered through a large peripheral or central vein.

33. c. Adenosine is a first-line drug for supraventricular tachycardia. It has a very short half-life of less than 5 seconds. Adenosine 6 mg is given IV push over 1–3 seconds followed by 20 mL of saline. If a second dose is needed, a 12-mg bolus is given 1–2 minutes after the initial dose.

34. a. Once the dysrhythmia has been suppressed, if a total of 3 mg/kg has not been exceeded, the patient should be monitored for signs and symptoms of lidocaine toxicity which include confusion, drowsiness, hearing impairment, cardiac conduction defects, myocardial depression, muscle twitching, and seizures. Typically, a patient with ventricular dysrhythmias is given a 1–1.5 mg/kg bolus of lidocaine, followed by 0.5–0.75 mg/kg every 5–10 minutes until the dysrhythmia is controlled or a total dose of 3 mg/kg.

35. b. The correct solution to utilize for IM injection is 1:1000 solution.

36. a. The standard concentration of 1:10,000 epinephrine is used in cardiac arrest.

37. a. Usual dosage for atropine in adults is 1 mg and may be repeated q3–5 min. Anything less than 0.5 mg can produce a paradoxical bradycardia.

38. b. Diazepam is a benzodiazepine. Flumazenil is a reversal drug for benzodiazepines. Naloxone is a reversal drug for opioids.

39. c, e. Magnesium sulfate is an essential element needed by the body for multiple functions. The primary indications for emergent magnesium are cardiac arrest and torsades de pointes. It is not indicated for atrial dysrhythmias or hypokalemia.

40. d. Furosemide is a loop diuretic that inhibits reabsorption and promotes renal excretion of water, sodium, potassium, magnesium, calcium, and hydrogen. It also promotes vasodilation and diuresis, which can lower blood pressure.

41. b, d, e. Nitroprusside sodium is a drug used to reduce arterial blood pressure in hypertensive emergencies. Blue or brown color indicates the solution has degraded and should not be used. The bottle should be protected from light. Because this drug is a potent antihypertensive, the patient will need to be monitored continuously in the critical care unit. As nitroprusside breaks down, the by-products include thiocyanate or cyanide; therefore levels must be monitored closely, and the drug should be used for the shortest amount of time necessary. Nitroprusside should be tapered, not discontinued abruptly.

42. a, c, d. Atropine is an anticholinergic and can cause dry mouth, mydriasis (not miosis), and urinary retention. It can also cause myocardial ischemia, restlessness, anxiety, and thirst.

Case Study: Critical Thinking

1. The patient self-administered three nitroglycerin (NTG) tablets before calling EMS. NTG dilates the coronary arteries to improve blood flow and oxygenation to the ischemic myocardium. IV NTG infusion is reserved for chest pain related to unstable angina or acute myocardial infarction. BP and HR must be continuously monitored because hypotension is a common adverse effect.

2. An aspirin is given to patients having chest pain to decrease platelet aggregation in acute coronary syndrome and for acute myocardial infarction. Oxygen is given to provide adequate supply to the myocardium. It can be administered either by nasal cannula, nonrebreather mask, simple mask, or endotracheal intubation to maintain the oxygen saturation within a defined clinical parameter. Morphine is used to relieve pain, dilate venous vessels, and reduce the workload of the heart. IV nitroglycerin is reserved for patients with unstable angina or an AMI. A nitroglycerin drip is usually initiated at a rate of 5 mcg/min and increased by 5 mcg/min every 3–5 minutes, based on chest pain and blood pressure response.

3. The nurse would prepare to administer epinephrine 1 mg IV q3–5 minutes while continuing CPR and shocking any shockable rhythm. If the patient continues in ventricular tachycardia, then amiodarone 300 mg IV can be given and may be repeated once at a dose of 150 mg. The vagal activity is considered completely blocked and should be evaluated periodically for a pulse and/or change in rhythm.